Heparin

Heparin

New Biochemical and Medical Aspects

Proceedings of the Symposium of the
Deutsche Gesellschaft für Klinische Chemie
Titisee, Breisgau, Germany
June 29th – July 1st, 1981

Editor Irene Witt

W DE G

Walter de Gruyter · Berlin · New York 1983

Editor
Prof. Dr. Irene Witt
Klinisch-Chemisches Labor
Biochemisches Labor
Universitäts-Kinderklinik Freiburg
Mathildenstraße 1
D-7800 Freiburg

CIP-Kurztitelaufnahme der Deutschen Bibliothek

Heparin: new biochem. and med. aspects;
proceedings of the symposium of the
Dt. Ges. für Klin. Chemie, Titisee, Breisgau, Germany,
Jun 29th – July 1st, 1981 / ed. Irene Witt. –
Berlin; New York : de Gruyter, 1983.
ISBN 3-11-008637-9.
NE: Witt, Irene [Hrsg.]; Deutsche Gesellschaft
für Klinische Chemie

Library of Congress Cataloging in Publication Data

Main entry under title:

Heparin: new biochemical and medical aspects.
Includes bibliographical references and index.
1. Heparin – Congresses.
2. Thrombosis – Chemotherapie – Congresses. I. Witt, Irene.
II. Deutsche Gesellschaft für Klinische Chemie.
[DNLM: 1. Heparin – Congresses. QV 193 D486h]
RC694.3.H46 1983 616.1'57061 82-22164
ISBN 3-11-008637-9

 Printing: Druckerei Gerike GmbH, Berlin. – Binding: Dieter Mikolai, Berlin. – Printed in Germany.

Preface

The aim of the symposium was to assess the current status of monitoring heparin therapy.

This assessment was feasible only with the aid of reviews on new aspects of heparin structure, its biosynthesis and mechanism of action as well as the medical usage of heparin.

In the light of this background information, the first clinical experiences related to monitoring the heparin activity in blood by means of photometric methods were presented. Although heparin has been used for nearly 50 years in the therapy and prevention of venous thrombosis and thromboembolism, this conference has illustrated that our ever increasing knowledge about this heterogeneous molecule is far from complete.

Multifarious open questions were outlined in the lectures themselves and raised during the subsequent discussions.

For the sake of shortening publication time, the discussions following each lecture have been condensed to include only the most important aspects and have been edited in the interest of readability. It is hoped that the opinions of the participants have been faithfully represented.

I wish to express special thanks to Dr. Helmut Lill for his thorough and critical help with the editing of the discussions and also Mr. David James for his valuable assistance with the English language of the manuscripts and discussions.

Sincere gratitude is extended to Mrs. Evelyne Glowka, Mrs. Ingeborg Klak and Dr. Rudolf Weber of Walter de Gruyter Publishers, whose helpful co-operation has made the task of editing this book a pleasant one.

Freiburg i. Br., November 1982 Irene Witt

Introductory Welcome

Ladies and Gentlemen,
I cordially welcome you to the symposium of the German Society of Clinical Chemistry entitled "Monitoring of Heparin Therapy".

Special appreciation is due those participants who have travelled a great distance to participate in this heparin meeting in the small village of Titisee tucked away in the Black Forest.

For a number of colleagues, it is the second meeting here in Titisee concerned with problems of blood coagulation. It was exactly five years ago that we held the first meeting in Germany on "New Methods for the Analysis of Coagulation Using Chromogenic Substrates".

While that first meeting concerned itself primarily with methodological questions, the purpose of this meeting is to emphasize the clinical relevance of photometric tests for the determination of heparin.

It is not my intention to imply that in the meantime all methodological problems have been solved. Although a method for the photometric determination of heparin was already reported by Teien at the meeting in 1976, difficulties continue to increase rather than decrease. The difficulties for the monitoring of heparin arise from several sources.

In the last years, we have learned a great deal about the heterogenous composition of the various preparations. The different heparins in a preparation presumably follow different mechanisms of anticoagulatory and antithrombotic action. This is most likely one of the basic problems in the monitoring of the anticoagulatory action of heparin.

Although something is known about the fate of the administered heparin in vivo, this seems to be only the tip of the iceberg. The same holds true for the variations in the individual response of patients to heparin.

This illustrates only some of the reasons why the evaluation of heparin analyses is very difficult. Therefore, most of the numerous heparin determinations with chromogenic or fluorogenic substrates are performed only for scientific purposes and not for the control of patients treated with heparin.

Now, what is the aim of this symposium?

I hope we can clarify what we know about the structure of heparin, the mechanisms of its action, its synthesis and catabolism and its fate in the organism.

On the basis of our present knowledge, we should discuss what the most effective method of monitoring heparin activity in the patients seems to be.

The primary aim of our efforts should be to improve heparin therapy and prophylaxis and to minimize the side effects.

In view of these intentions, we shall first hear plenary lectures on the structure of heparin, on its mechanism of action and on its synthesis and catabolism.

After the presentation of the currently available methods for the determination of heparin, we shall have lectures and discussions relative to the clinical use of heparin and the present experience with monitoring heparin therapy with photometric tests.

We should conclude by evaluating what we have learned during this symposium and what we must do when we return to our laboratories and hospitals.

Irene Witt

List of Participants

Prof. Dr. M. Aronson	Tel-Aviv University Sackler School of Medicine Dept. of Histology and Cell Biology Ramat-Aviv 69978
Dr. A. S. Bhargava	Dept. Exp. Toxikologie Schering AG Postfach 65 03 11 D-1000 Berlin 65
Dr. Dr. N. Bender	Zentrum der Inneren Medizin Abteilung für Angiologie Klinikum der Johann Wolfgang Goethe Universität Theodor-Stern-Kai 7 D-8000 Frankfurt
Dr. Joan Dawes	Medical Research Council Immunoassay Team 2 Forrest Road GB-Edinburgh
Prof. Dr. F. Duckert	Zentrallaboratorium Universitätskliniken Kantonsspital Basel CH-4004 Basel
Dr. F. Fabris	Istituto Di Semeiotica Medica Dell Universita Di Padova Via Ospedale Civile 105 I-Padova
Dr. P. Friberger	AB KABI Peptide Research S-43122 Mölndal
Dr. J. Harenberg	Medizinische Universitätsklinik Abteilung KLinische Pharmakologie Bergheimer Straße 58 D-6900 Heidelberg
Prof. Dr. D. L. Heene	1. Medizinische Klinik Klinikum der Stadt Mannheim Theodorf-Kutzer-Ufer D-6800 Mannheim
Dr. H. A. Holm	Medical Department A Aker University Hospital N-Oslo 5

Prof. Dr. V. V. Kakkar
King's College Hospital Medical School
University of London
Thrombosis Research Unit
Department of Surgery
Denmark Hill
GB-London SES 8RX

Dr. H. Lill
Boehringer Mannheim GmbH.
Biochemica Werk Tutzing
Bahnhofstraße 5
D-8132 Tutzing/Obb.

Dr. G. A. Marbet
Gerinnungslaboratorium
Universitätskliniken
Kantonsspital Basel
CH-4004 Basel

Dr. K. H. Müller
Klinisch-chemisches Zentrallaboratorium
der Med. Fakultät
Technische Hochschule
Goethestraße 27-29
D-5100 Aachen

Prof. Dr. A. Oberdorfer
Institut für Klinische Chemie und
Pathobiochemie der
Technischen Universität München
Ismaningerstraße 22
D-8000 München 80

Dr. J. Riesenfeld
Swedish University of Agricultural
Sciences
College of Veterinary Medicine
Dept. of Medical and Physiological
Chemistry
Biomedicum Box 575
S-75123 Uppsala

Prof. Dr. L. Róka
Institut für Klinische Chemie und
Pathobiochemie am Klinikum der
Justus-Liebig-Universität
Klinikstraße 32 b
D-6300 Gießen

Prof. Dr. R. D. Rosenberg
Sidney Farber Cancer Institute
Harvard Medical School
44 Binney Street
Boston, Mass. 0215
USA

Dr. U. Schmitz-Huebner
Medizinische Klinik und Poliklinik der
Westfälischen Wilhelms-Universität
Abteilung Innere Medizin A
Westring 3
D-4400 Münster

Doz. Dr. T. H. Schöndorf	Zentrum für Innere Medizin am Klinikum der Justus-Liebig-Universität Klinikstraße 32 b D-6300 Gießen
Dr. R. Spaethe	Merz & Dade Lerchenstraße 5 D-8000 München 50
Doz. Dr. E. Thaler	1. Medizinische Universitätsklinik Lazarettgasse 14 A-1090 Wien
Prof. Dr. M. Verstraete	Department of Medical Research Katholieke Universität Leuven Herestraat 49 B-3000 Leuven
Prof. Dr. Ellen Weber	Medizinische Universitätsklinik Abteilung Klinische Pharmakologie Bergheimer Straße 58 D-6900 Heidelberg
Prof. Dr. E. Wenzel	Abteilung für Klinische Haemostaseologie und Transfusionsmedizin Universitätskliniken Homburg (Saar) D-6650 Homburg (Saar)
Prof. Dr. Irene Witt	Biochemisches Labor Universitäts-Kinderklinik Mathildenstraße 1 D-7800 Freiburg i. Br.
Dr. E. Zimmer	Boehringer Mannheim GmbH Sandhoferstraße 116 D-6800 Mannheim

Contents

I. Heparin: Structure, Mechanism of Action, Biosynthesis and Catabolism

The Function and Structure of the Heparin Molecule
Robert D. Rosenberg 3

Biosynthesis of Heparin
Johan Riesenfeld 35

Physiological Heparin - its Function and Fate
Joan Dawes 45

Mechanism of Heparin Rebound and Heparin-Protamine Interactions
Moshe Aronson, Ina Fabian, Ilan Bleiberg 69

II. Methods for the Determination of Heparin

Overview on Methods for the Determination of Heparin
Irene Witt 89

Control of Heparin Therapy by Measurement of the Antithrombin III-Heparin-Complex
Helmut Lill 95

Determination of Heparin by a Fluorogenic Synthetic Substrate
Reiner Spaethe, Margot Naumann, Joan Strauß 103

Properties of the Coatest® Heparin Assay
Petter Friberger 117

A Sensitive Competitive Binding Assay for Heparin
Joan Dawes 129

Determination of Low Dose Heparin Activities in Plasma
Ladislaus Róka 139

Characterization of Heparin Preparations in Vivo by
Different Test Systems
Job Harenberg, Fernando Fussi, Werner Junker, Kurt Mattes,
Ellen Weber, Rainer Zimmermann 149

Determination of Heparin and Fractionated Heparin
with Different Molecular Weights
Ulrich Schmitz-Huebner 161

III. Clinical Usage of Heparin

Low Molecular Weight Heparin and the Prevention
of Postoperative Deep Vein Thrombosis
V. V. Kakkar, B. Djazaeri, J. Fok, M. Scully, J. Westwick . . . 175

The Effect of Heparins on Platelet Release Reaction
F. Fabris, G. Cella, M. Randi, A. Casonato, F. Fussi, A. Girolami 207

Characterization of a New Potent Heparin
Akhil S. Bhargava, Peter Günzel 227

Side Effects of Heparin
Ellen Weber, Erhard Walter, Job Harenberg 239

Role of Heparin-Like Molecules in Atherogenesis
Robert D. Rosenberg, John J. Castellot, Jr., Morris J. Karnovsky 261

Unresolved Problems in the Use of Heparin
Marc Verstraete 275

IV. Experience with "Monitoring of Heparin Therapy"

Heparin Treatment of Deep Venous Thrombosis:
Correlation Between Clinical Effects and Heparin Assays
Hans Asbjørn Holm, Ulrich Abildgaard 289

Heparin-, Heparin Cofactor- and Platelet Factor 4 Plasma Levels
Under Heparin Treatment
Norbert Bender, Jürgen Schlegel, Viola Hach,
Carl Maximilian Kirchmaier, Hans Klaus Breddin 301

Determination of Heparin, Partial Thromboplastin Time and
Antithrombin III after Subcutaneous Heparin Administration
Theodor H. Schöndorf, Helena Paplham, Klaus Franz 315

Monitoring of Heparin During Extracorporal Circulation
in Open Heart Surgery
Reiner Spaethe, Margot Naumann 329

Chromogenic and Fluorogenic Assays - a Challenge for
Conventional Monitoring of Heparin Therapy?
German A. Marbet, François Duckert 343

V. Concluding Discussion 365

Subject Index 369

I. Heparin: Structure, Mechanism of Action, Biosynthesis and Catabolism

The Function and Structure of the Heparin Molecule*

Robert D. Rosenberg
Department of Biology,
Massachusetts Institute of Technology,
Cambridge, Massachusetts, U.S.A. 02139 and

Department of Medicine,
Harvard Medical School,
Boston, Massachusetts, U.S.A. 02115

Heparin functions as an anticoagulant by dramatically accelerating the velocity at which antithrombin neutralizes serine proteases of the hemostatic mechanism (Rosenberg, 1977). We have provided evidence that the mucopolysaccharide acts by binding to antithrombin and thereby allosterically increasing the rate of formation of enzyme-inhibitor complexes (1). Gitel (2) and Holmer et al. (3) have postulated that heparin is initially bound by antithrombin but is subsequently able to approximate hemostatic system serine proteases with respect to the protease inhibitor. Machovich (4), Smith and Craft (5), Griffith (6), and Griffith et al. (7) have proposed that the mucopolysaccharide binds preferentially to hemostatic system serine proteases and that the resultant complexes are rapidly inactivated by free antithrombin via allosteric or approximation phenomena. These various potential mechanisms of heparin action are summarized in Fig. 1.

In the present communication, we examine functional and structural aspects of the mucopolysaccharide. The resultant analyses permit us to estimate the relative importance of the four postulated model of heparin action.

*Supported by Grants from the National Institutes of Health HL-2862501 and HL-25066 and the National Foundation for Cancer Research, Bethesda, Maryland, U.S.A.

Heparin · New Biochemical and Medical Aspects

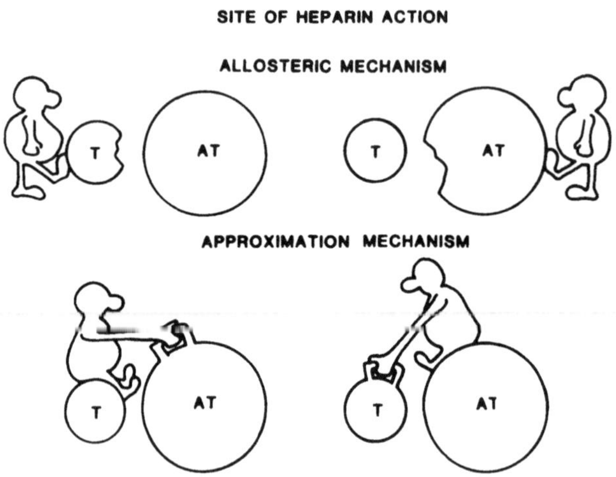

Fig. 1. Mechanisms of Heparin Action.

Functional Aspects of Heparin Species

We initially studied the binding of highly active as well as relatively inactive low molecular weight heparin species to antithrombin (8). Chromatographic isolation of the radiolabeled highly active heparin-antithrombin interaction product permitted us to show that the protease inhibitor possesses only one binding site for the low molecular weight species and therefore can complex with only one molecule of this mucopolysaccharide. The formation of the highly active heparin-antithrombin complex is accompanied by an increase in the intrinsic fluorescence of the protease inhibitor at 330 nm (9). Einarsson and Andersson (10) and Björk and Nordenman (11) have made similar observations with poorly characterized active heparin products of unknown binding stoichiometry. We have demonstrated that the progressive enhancement in the intrinsic fluorescence of antithrombin at increasing concentrations of highly active heparin can be fitted to a mass action equation with a K_{DISS}^{HA} of 5.7×10^{-8} M and a binding stoichiometry of 1 : 1 (9) (Fig. 2 A). The excellent agreement between our experimental observations and this simple, single site model indicates that the mucopolysaccharide behaves as a nearly ideal ligand despite its extraordinary charge density. Data obtained for relatively inactive heparin could also be fitted to the same single site binding model except that K_{DISS} averaged 1.0×10^{-4} M (9) (Fig. 2 B).

As expected variations in protein concentration from 5×10^{-8} M to 4×10^{-7} M did not alter the binding isotherm for the highly active heparin-antithrombin interaction. However, changes in the level of inhibitor from 2×10^{-8} M to 5×10^{-6} M markedly displaced the binding isotherm for the relatively inactive heparin-antithrombin interaction (Fig. 2 B). These results point to the unexpected conclusion that highly active heparin is quite homogeneous, whereas only a small subpopulation within the relatively inactive mucopolysaccharide is able to bind tightly to antithrombin. A computer fit of the experimental data indicates that this anomalous shift in the binding isotherm of relatively inactive heparin is best explained by the contamination of this material with 1 - 2 % of the active mucopolysaccharide (9).

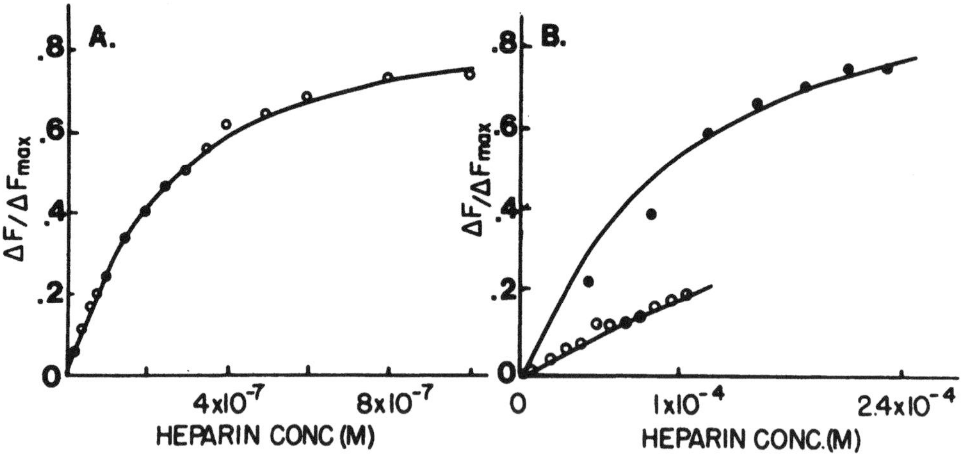

Fig. 2. The binding of heparin species to antithrombin as monitored by fluorescence spectroscopy.

A. Highly active heparin. Antithrombin was admixed with highly active heparin at varying concentrations of mucopolysaccharide and constant concentrations of inhibitor (2×10^{-7} M). The extent of fluorescence enhancement of antithrombin, at 330 nm, ΔF, was determined by quantitating the fluorescence of inhibitor in the presence and absence of highly active heparin. This parameter normalized to its projected maximal increase ($\Delta F/\Delta F_{max}$) is plotted *versus* the total concentration of mucopolysaccharide added.

B. Relatively inactive heparin. The experimental conditions were the same as in A except that the concentration of antithrombin was 2×10^{-7} M in the *upper curve* and 5×10^{-6} M in the *lower curve.* The change in fluorescence of the protease inhibitor at 330 nm was normalized to the projected maximal increase in this parameter observed with highly active heparin under similar conditions. The *solid lines* represent a computer fit of our data to a single site binding model.

We subsequently analyzed the binding of highly active as well as relatively inactive, low molecular weight heparin species to thrombin. For this purpose, we labeled the mucopolysaccharide with a fluorescent tag that did not significantly alter the functional characteristics of this complex sugar (12). This fluorescamine-heparin conjugate could then be utilized in conjunction with fluorescence polarization spectroscopy to monitor interactions between the mucopolysaccharide and thrombin.

The binding of highly active heparin to thrombin was studied with respect to the stoichiometry and avidity of this process. The stoichiometry of this interaction was determined by adding varying concentrations of thrombin that ranged between 5×10^{-7} M and 3×10^{-5} M to a constant level of fluorescamine-heparin maintained at 8.57×10^{-6} M and measuring the ΔP (change in fluorescence polarization) of each of these reaction mixtures. The ΔP_{max} (maximal change in fluorescence polarization) of this process was experimentally defined by observing that ΔP reached a constant level when thrombin concentrations of 1.0×10^{-5} M or greater were employed. This value represents an augmentation in fluorescence polarization of approximately 150 %. In Fig. 3A, we have plotted $\Delta P/\Delta P_{max}$ of the various mixtures *versus* the molar ratio of thrombin to fluorescamine-heparin utilized. As noted, a line drawn through the initial linear portion of the binding isotherm intersects the horizontal asymptote at a molar ratio of thrombin to fluorescamine-heparin of approximately 2.0. This suggests that a single molecule of enzyme is capable of binding two molecules of mucopolysaccharide (12).

We next sought to determine the avidity of highly active heparin to thrombin. To this end, we quantitated the ΔP of fluorescamine-heparin at varying levels of added enzyme as outlined above. However, the concentration of labeled mucopolysaccharide was reduced to 8.58×10^{-7} M wich is optimal for evaluating the dissociation constants of this interaction. Fig. 3B shows the average results of several experiments in which the projected ΔP_{max} of this process are plotted *versus* the molar concentrations of thrombin employed. Our polarization data is most compatibel with a two binding site model (12). The best statistical fit was achieved by utilizing $K^{H_1T}_{DISS} = K^{H_2T}_{DISS} = 8.0 \times 10^{-7}$ M. When the interaction of relatively inactive heparin with thrombin was examined, binding parameters virtually identical to those outlined were obtained.

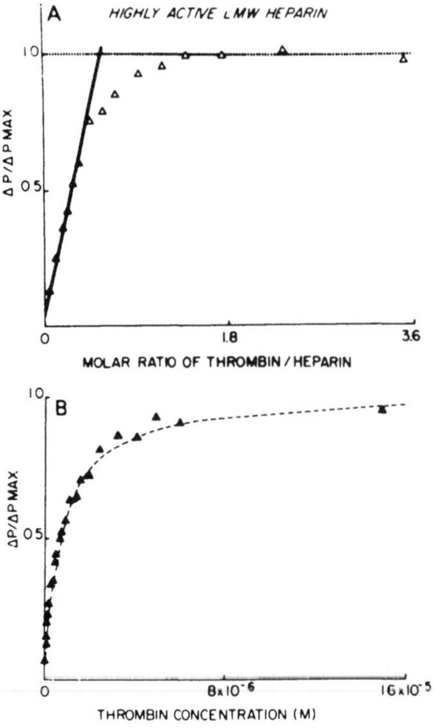

Fig. 3. The binding of fluorescamine-heparin to thrombin as monitored by fluoresecence polarization spectroscopy.

A. Estimate of reaction stoichiometry. The solid line (▬▬) represents a linear least squares fit of binding data contained within the ascending limb of the isotherm (r = 0.99).

B. Determination of $K_{DISS}^{H_1T}$ and $K_{DISS}^{H_2T}$. The dashed line (-----) represents theoretical values calculated from the two binding site model that best fits our experimental data. These estimates were obtained by numerical evaluation of experimental observations with $K_{DISS}^{H_1T} = K_{DISS}^{H_2T} = 8 \times 10^{-7}$ M.

We have also studied the ability of the two heparin species to accelerate thrombin-antithrombin interactions (9). Prior to examining these properties in a quantitative manner it was necessary to probe the kinetic relationships between mucopolysaccharide and protease inhibitor. Various investigators have suspected that heparin might function as a catalyst during the neutralization of thrombin by antithrombin (2, 13, 14).

To examine this possibility, we have utilized levels of reactants sufficiently reduced to permit monitoring of enzyme inactivation by manual assay techniques. The initial concentrations of enzyme and inhibitor were set at 10^{-7} M. When highly active heparin was admixed at final levels of 2.5×10^{-9} M, 5×10^{-9} M, and 1×10^{-8} M, respectively, complete neutralization of thrombin took place over 150 seconds. Minimal amounts of this enzyme are inhibited at the same point in time when mucopolysaccharide is absent. Given the 1 : 1 molar binding stoichiometry of highly active heparin and antithrombin, we calculate that the mucopolysaccharide must be reutilized ten to twenty times during the course of this reaction (Fig. 4).

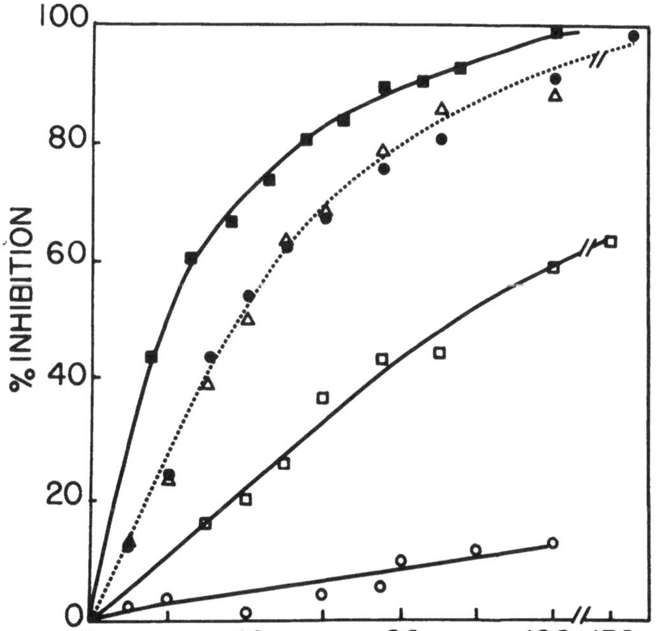

Fig. 4. The acceleration of thrombin-antithrombin interactions with limiting concentrations of highly active heparin.

Curve a (———) depicts the inhibition of enzyme without added heparin when the levels of thrombin and antithrombin were set at 1×10^{-7} M.

Curves b (□ ——— □), *c* (o———o), and *d* (■ ——— ■) show the effect of highly active heparin when present at concentrations of 2.5×10^{-9} M, 5×10^{-9} M, and 1×10^{-8} M, respectively.

The *triangles* (Δ·····Δ) represent a reaction mixture identical with that of *Curve c*, except that purified thrombin-antithrombin complex was added at a level of 2×10^{-6} M.

It is apparent that highly active heparin might function as a catalyst if the mucopolysaccharide were released from antithrombin during formation of the enzyme-inhibitor complex and were able to bind anew to free protease inhibitor. We have validated this hypothesis by demonstrating that three critical aspects of the mechanism are correct. Firstly, we have demonstrated that the binding of thrombin to the highly active heparin-antithrombin complex results in the discharge of mucopolysaccharide from the protease inhibitor on a 1 : 1 molar basis (9). Secondly, we have provided evidence that release of mucopolysaccharide is linked to its ability to bind tightly to the thrombin-antithrombin complex as compared to free inhibitor. Thirdly, we have shown that highly active heparin discharged from the protease inhibitor during enzyme inactivation retains its ability to bind to antithrombin (9).

In most instances, the rate of enzyme is limited by the recycling of mucopolysaccharide. The inactivation of thrombin is exceedingly rapid once the heparin-antithrombin complex has formed. Thus, the amount of highly active heparin-antithrombin complex formed at time zero should determine the initial rate of the thrombin-antithrombin interaction. In Fig. 5, we provide a plot of the initial velocity of this reaction *versus* the concentration of highly active heparin present in the incubation mixture. It is apparent that this profile exhibits an ascending limb, pseudoplateau, descending limb, and final plateau. Also depicted are the levels of heparin-antithrombin complex and the various types of heparin-thrombin interaction products *versus* the concentrations of mucopolysaccharide. These latter components include binary complexes of enzymes and mucopolysaccharide (TH_1), tertiary complexes of these species (TH_2), and a summation of both products ($TH_1 + TH_2$). The concentrations of the various species have been calculated from the binding parameters obtained earlier. It is evident that the ascending limb of the kinetic profile exhibits a higher degree of correspondence to the level of heparin-antithrombin complex than to the concentration of any heparin-thrombin interaction product (Fig. 5A). Thus, our data indicate that the former species must be responsible for the mucopolysaccharide dependent acceleration of this inhibitory process.

In Fig. 5B, we compare the descending limb of the initial velocity plot with the concentration of ($To\text{-}TH_1$), ($To\text{-}TH_2$), and ($To\text{-}TH_1\text{-}TH_2$). It would appear that this region of the kinetic profile coincides best with the level of ($To\text{-}TH_2$). Thus, our data suggest that the TH_2 complex rather than the TH_1 interaction product is neutralized at a significantly slower rate than free enzyme.

A small discrepancy is noted between the concentration of the heparin-antithrombin complex and the uppermost portion of the ascending limb of the initial velocity plot (Fig. 5A). Furthermore, a more significant lack of concordance is observed between the level of ($To\text{-}TH_2$) and the descending limb of the kinetic profile (Fig. 5B). We suspected that these discrepancies were due to two independent phenomena. On the one hand, competition exists between thrombin and antithrombin for limiting quantities of mucopolysaccharide. On the other hand, the heparin-antithrombin complex interacts with the heparin-thrombin complex at a different rate than with free enzyme.

The following equation provides the theoretical relationship between the initial velocity of enzyme neutralization, the concentration of mucopolysaccharide added, and the level of enzyme employed. This algebraic expression takes into account the competition between enzyme and inhibitor for limiting quantities of mucopolysaccharide and the differing rates of interaction of heparin-antithrombin complex with heparin-thrombin complex or free thrombin. This model is valid when equimolar levels of enzyme and inhibitor are utilized and when the concentrations of these reactants are low ($< 10^{-7}$ M). These conditions have been satisfied in the experiment cited above.

$$\text{initial velocity} = b(1-c)k_1 [Eo]^2 + bc\,k_2\,[Eo]^2$$

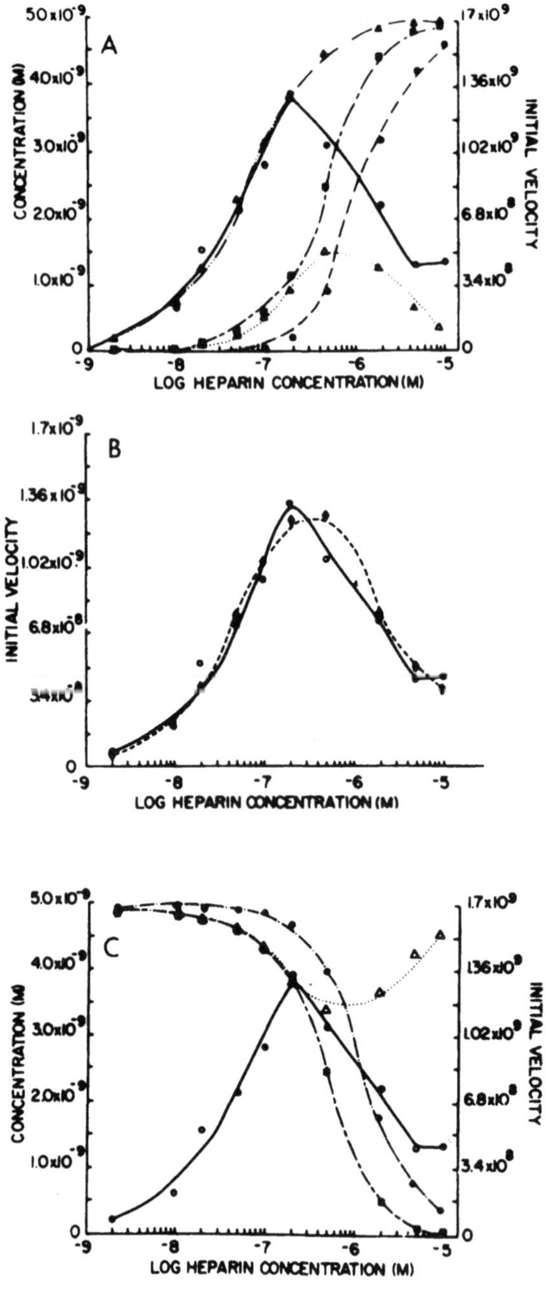
A
B
C
CONCENTRATION (M)
INITIAL VELOCITY
LOG HEPARIN CONCENTRATION (M)

Fig. 5.

Fig. 5. Correlation between the binding of heparin to thrombin as well as antithrombin and the ability of the mucopolysaccharide to accelerate thrombin-antithrombin interactions.

A. Comparisons of the levels of heparin-protein complexes with the kinetics of the thrombin-antithrombin interactions. (0——0), initial velocity, (▲-•-▲), concentrations of heparin-antithrombin complex (■——■), concentration of heparin-thrombin complexes (TH_1 + TH_2) (●- • -●), concentration of tertiary complex of heparin and thrombin (TH_2), and (Δ····Δ), concentration of binary complex between heparin and thrombin (TH_1).

B. Comparison of various combinations of free thrombin and heparin-thrombin complexes with the kinetics of the thrombin-antithrombin interactions. (0——0), initial velocity, (■—■), concentration of free thrombin ($T-TH_1-TH_2$), (●- • -●), concentration of free thrombin and TH_1 ($T-TH_2$, and (Δ····Δ), concentration of free thrombin and TH_2 ($T-TH_1$).

C. Comparison of the observed (0---0) and theoretically predicted (♦ --- ♦) kinetics of the thrombin-antithrombin interaction.

Where Eo is the initial concentration of enzyme, k_1 is the bimolecular rate constant for the interaction of a given enzyme with the heparin-inhibitor complex, k_2 is the bimolecular rate constant for the interaction of a given heparin-enzyme complex with the heparin-inhibitor complex, b is the fractional saturation of antithrombin with mucopolysaccharide and c is the fractional saturation of enzyme with mucopolysaccharide. The latter two parameters are functions of heparin and protein concentration and can be directly calculated from the dissociation constants K_{DISS}^{HA} and K_{DISS}^{HE}, respectfully (15).

The above equation was employed to construct a theoretical plot of the initial velocity of the thrombin-antithrombin interaction as a function of heparin concentration. The experimentally determined values of the various dissociation constants were utilized to generate the theorectical estimate. We also assumed that TH_2 rather than TH_1 exhibited a reduced rate of interaction with the heparin-antithrombin complex. As shown in Fig. 5C, this resulted in a theoretical kinetic plot that is virtually indistinguishable from the experimental profile when $k_1 = 1.7 \times 10^9\ M^{-1}min^{-1}$ (rate of interaction between heparin-thrombin complex and heparin-antithrombin complex). We have previously demonstrated that the bimolecular rate constant (k_1^*) of this interaction in the absence of mucopolysaccharide is $4.25 \times 10^5 M^{-1} min^{-1}$ (15). Therefore, the normalized values of the two parameters are

$$k_1' = \frac{k_1}{k_1^*} = 4000 \text{ and } k_2' = \frac{k_2}{k_1^*} = 700.$$

The kinetic data provided above indicates that the unique ability of heparin to accelerate antithrombin action must be due either to a direct effect of the mucopolysaccharide upon the inhibitor (allosteric mechanism) or to interactions between free thrombin and mucopolysaccharide bound antithrombin (approximation mechanism).

The parameter k_1' represents the summation of all kinetic influences of the mucopolysaccharide on the above reaction. This would include contributions from the direct binding of heparin to antithrombin as well as those from the interaction between mucopolysaccharide bound to inhibitor and free thrombin. The parameter k_2' provides a minimal estimate of the kinetic results due to the direct binding of mucopolysaccharide to antithrombin. This interpretation is justified since "approximation" sites on the enzyme, if present, would be saturated with heparin and unable to function in a normal fashion. The kinetic importance of approximation phenomena can be calculated as either (k_1'/k_2') or $(k_1 - k_2')$, respectively. We favor the use of k_1'/k_2' based upon our belief that the approximation of thrombin via mucopolysaccharide bound to antithrombin and the assembly of enzyme-inhibitor complexes are likely to represent sequential events in the neutralization of this serine protease. If such is the case, our data would suggest that approximation phenomena are responsible for no more than 1 % of the direct effect of heparin upon antithrombin (15).

The relatively inactive heparin was examined in similar fashion to determine its effect upon the thrombin-antithrombin interaction. Several hundred fold higher concentrations of this molecular species are required to achieve a similar increase in the rate of thrombin interaction as compared to the highly active material. Furthermore, when sufficiently high levels of this mucopolysaccharide are employed, the maximal rate of enzyme inactivation is approximately 10 % of that achieved with the highly active heparin. These kinetic data are in complete accord with the presence of a small amount of active heparin (1-2 %) contaminating the relatively inactive fraction (9).

To extend our findings, we have analyzed the interactions of highly active low molecular weight heparin and antithrombin with factor IXa, factor Xa, as well as plasmin (15). In each instance, the binding of complex carbohydrate to the protease inhibitor correlated with the mucopolysaccharide dependent acceleration of enzyme neutralization. The kinetic parameters obtained during these studies also allowed us to examine the manner in which the mucopolysaccharide accelerates the inactivation of these enzymes by antithrombin (Table 1). Our data indicates that approximation phenomena are responsible for no more than 2 % of the direct effect of heparin upon antithrombin during the neutralization of factor IXa by the mucopolysaccharide-protease inhibitor complex. Furthermore, the latter mechanism is of no importance in the inactivation of factor Xa or plasmin by the heparin-antithrombin interaction product (15).

Table 1. Summary of Kinetic and Binding Parameters for Various Hemostatic Enzymes.

Kinetic or Binding Parameters	Thrombin	Factor IXa	Factor Xa	Plasmin
$k'_1 = \frac{k_1}{k^*_1}$	4000	10,200	1280	100
$k'_2 = \frac{k_2}{k^*_1}$	700	680	1280	100
H^{HE}_{DISS}	8.0×10^{-7}M/ 8.0×10^{-7}M	$2{,}58 \times 10^{-7}$M	8.73×10^{-6}M	-1.0×10^{-4}M

Structural Aspects of Heparin Species

Highly active and relatively inactive low molecular weight heparin species were analyzed with respect to uronic acid composition and sulfate group placement (Table 2) (16, 17, 18). Based upon molecular weight analysis, monosaccharide composition, and sulfate group distribution, we estimate that the highly active form has 1.1 additional residues of glucuronic acid per molecule and 1.5 fewer residues of N-sulfated glucosamine per molecule when compared to the relatively inactive species. High resolution nuclear magnetic resonance measurements indicate that the latter reduction in N-sulfated glucosamine is secondary to a concomitant increase in N-acetyl glucosamine. We suspected that the additional glucuronic acid and N-acetyl glucosamine residues might be located at adjacent sites on the highly active heparin polymer (16, 17, 18).

Table 2. Uronic Acid Composition and Sulfate Group Position

Heparin	Glucuronic Acid %*	Sulfate†/ Disaccharide	N-Sulfate†/ Disaccharide	O-Sulfate‡/ Disaccharide
Highly Active	30.7	2.26	0.70	1.56
Relatively Active	19.3	2.37	0.95	1.42

*Each value represents the mean derived from four separate determinations performed in triplicate. The iduronic acid value can be calculated by substracting the glucuronic acid value from 100 %.

†The values of total sulfate per disaccharide are expressed as molar ratios of a given parameter to glucosamine. Each value represents the mean of two separate determinations performed in triplicate.

‡This value was calculated by substracting column 3 from column 2.

To test this hypothesis, we individually subjected the two heparin species to nitrous acid cleavage, radiolabeled the newly formed reducing ends, separated the various components by paper chromatography and quantitated the respective peaks. Our analysis indicated that larger amounts of a specific oligosaccharide, *1B*, are found within the tetrasaccharide zone of highly active heparin as compared to a similar structure, isolated from relatively inactive mucopolysaccharide. Indeed, 1.1 *1B* oligosaccharide sequences per molecule, *1Ba*, are present within highly active heparin, whereas only 0.3 *1B* structures per molecule, *1Bi*, are found in the relatively inactive mucopolysaccharide.

Detailed chemical studies demonstrated that both oligosaccharides possess two uronic acid moieties per reducing end group, contain equimolar amounts of iduronic acid as well as glucuronic acid, and terminate in [^{3}H] anhydromannitol at the reducing end position. In addition, a complete destruction of all uronic acid residues resulted when *1Ba* was treated with 0.1 M sodium periodate (17, 18). Furthermore, the internal glucosamine residue of *1Ba* and *1Bi* appears to be N-acetylated, since the two components are completely resistant to cleavage with nitrous acid at varying pH (17, 18). Given the known alternating glucosamine-uronic acid structure of heparin, these experiments indicate that both *1Ba* and *1Bi* are tetrasaccharides with a monosaccharide sequence of uronic acid → N-acetyl glucosamine → uronic acid → [H^3] anhydromannitol.

Of course, *1Ba* and *1Bi* may be subtly different in structure. To elucidate these possible differences, we determined the type and degree of sulfation of the uronic acid residue present at the non-reducing end of these species. This was accomplished by employing purified exoglycosidases to remove single uronic acid residues from the non-reducing ends of these oligosaccharides. The reaction mixtures were subsequently filtered on columns of P2-polyacrylamide to determine the extent of enzymatic cleavage (Table 3).

Thus, highly active heparin possesses 1.1 *1B* tetrasaccharide per molecule. Careful examination of this nitrous acid fragment showed that 95 % of the non-reducing end group consists of non-sulfated iduronic acid, while 5.0 % may bear an ester sulfate substituent (Table 3). This minor degree of het-

Table 3. Summary of Data on 1*Ba* and 1*Bi* Tetrasaccharides

Heparin	1*Ba* or 1*Bi* Content	Uronic Acid Residue at the Non-Reducing End, %			1*Ba* Content	Anticoagulant Activity
		Glucuronic Acid	Sulfated Iduronic Acid	Non-Sulfated Iduronic Acid		Normalized to the Highly Active Fraction
Highly Active	1.1	0	0.05	0.95	1.05[b]	1.0
Relatively Inactive	0.3	0.29	0.625	0.085[a]	0.026[b]	0.03

[a] This value represents 12 % of the 71 % of the 1*Bi* tetrasaccharide possessing iduronic acid at the non-reducing end.

[b] This value represents column 1 multiplied by column 4.

erogeneity may be due to trace contamination of our sample with oligosaccharides such a 1 α tetrasaccharide that migrate close to 1*Ba* and contain sulfated iduronic acid as the predominant uronic acid residue. Furthermore, in very recent studies, Lindahl and his associates (19) utilizing a newly discovered exoglycosidase isolated by Leder (20) have made a very important observation that the N-sulfated glucosamine residue of the 1*Ba* tetrasaccharide contains a unique 3 sulfate moiety rather than the customary 6 sulfate group. These findings provide additional evidence of the special nature of the 1*Ba* tetrasaccharide and further suggest that it must represent a major portion of the antithrombin binding site of the mucopolysaccharide.

If the above data are utilized in conjunction with the uronic acid composition, electrophoretic mobility, periodate sensitivity, and high pH nitrous acid resistance of this 1*Ba* tetrasaccharide, it is possible to propose a structure for this component. On the basis of the available evidence, we conclude that 1*Ba* should be represented by the following monosaccharide sequence at the polymer level:

L-IDURONIC ACID	→	N-ACETYLATED-D-GLUCOSAMINE 6-SULFATE	→	D-GLUCURONIC ACID	→	N-SULFATED-D-GLUCOSAMINE 3-SULFATE

The relatively inactive mucopolysaccharide possesses 0.3 *Bi* fragments per molecule. Chemical and enzymatic analyses of this component indicate that only 2.6 % of the molecules present within the relatively inactive mucopolysaccharide can possess the unique 1*Ba* tetrasaccharide sequence found within each molecule of highly active heparin (Table 3). However, the preparations of relatively inactive mucopolysaccharide utilized in this study are not completely depleted of active species. Indeed, we estimate that these products contain 2-3 % of heparin components which exhibit anticoagulant activity (18).

The correlation between the relative abundance of the unique tetrasaccharide structure and the anticoagulant potency of these preparations strongly suggests that this critical sequence must represent a portion of the binding site on porcine heparin which is recognized by antithrombin. Our conclusion concerning the importance of this sequence is considerably strengthened by the invarient nature of this structure within the highly active heparin as well as the occurrence of two non-sulfated uronic acid moieties in close proximity and the presence of a N-sulfated glucosamine 3-sulfate group. It remains to be seen whether minor variations within the critical tetrasaccharide sequence, such as the replacement of the N-acetyl glucosamine-sulfate residue by an N-sulfated glucosamine-sulfate group, will alter the functional properties of highly active heparin. In addition, it may be necessary to position elements such as trisulfated iduronyl-glucosamine disaccharides on either side of the critical tetrasaccharide sequence in order to attain a complete protease-inhibitor binding site on the mucopolysaccharide. These structural features constitute 60-70 % of the chemical mass of the heparin molecule (21) (see below).

The presence of the 1*Ba* tetrasaccharide within the "active" fraction of porcine heparin and its absence within the relatively inactive mucopolysaccharide pool has been confirmed by Lindahl and his coworkers (22). These investigators have also demonstrated that this unique monosaccharide sequence is protected against the action of bacterial heparinase when the highly active heparin is in contact with the protease inhibitor. This provides additional evidence that the 1*Ba* tetrasaccharide must represent at least a portion of the antithrombin binding site of the mucopolysaccharide.

We next attempted to determine whether the ability of heparin to accelerate hemostatic enzyme-antithrombin interactions was solely dependent upon the tetrasaccharide sequence outlined above. To this end, anticoagulantly active heparin was randomly cleaved with limiting amounts of nitrous acid and dilute sulfuric acid. The resultant species were separated by P-10 gel filtration chromatography. The smallest fragments that exhibited a capacity to bind to antithrombin were found within the hexasaccharide, octasaccharide, and decasaccharide regions. These components were further purified by affinity fractionation employing equimolar amounts of the protease inhibitor (23).

Our studies revealed that the hexasaccharide, octasaccharide, and decasaccharide species bind to antithrombin with progressively increasing avidity. Indeed, the latter oligosaccharide exhibits a K_{DISS}^{H-A} which approaches that obtained when components of ~ 16 residues are employed (Table 4). Our investigations also demonstrated that the hexasaccharide, octasaccharide and decasaccharide species are able to catalyze factor Xa-antithrombin interactions at rates which range from 6.9 % (smallest component) to 60.9 % (largest component) of that obtained when heparin fragments of ~16 resides are utilized (Table 4). It should be emphasized that these components were assayed at virtually identical saturations of the protease inhibitor (~5 %). Thus the specific molar biologic activities observed for the various oligosaccharides represent the effect of equivalent numbers of mucopolysaccharide molecules bound to the protease inhibitor. The kinetic and binding parameters of the three mucopolysaccharide fragments suggest that the structures essential for accelerating factor Xa-antithrombin interactions are closely linked to those required for complexing with antithrombin. Chemical data obtained with these oligosaccharides indicate that this critical region is represented in large measure by the unique tetrasaccharide sequence previously described. Indeed, this monosaccharide sequence appears to be located at the non-reducing ends of the hexasaccharide, octasaccharide, and decasaccharide species (23). These observations are similar to those of other investigators concerning the partial structure of a heparin-derived octasaccharide which binds tightly to antithrombin (24, 25).

Given the above data, it was surprising to note that the three oligosaccharides had essentially no effect upon the rate of inactivation of thrombin by antithrombin (Table 4). These negative results are particularly impressive as sufficiently high concentrations of these components were utizlized to saturate the protease inhibitor (23).

We next attempted to define the smallest heparin fragment that is able to catalyze thrombin-antithrombin interactions. For this purpose, all components with an apparent molecular size greater than a dodecasaccharide were combined, concentrated, and fractionated by Sephadex G-50 gel filtration. The various components obtained by the above procedure were analyzed to determine their abilities to accelerate thrombin neutralization by antithrombin.

Table 4. The kinetic behavior and binding constants cf various mucopolysaccharide fragments

	Factor Xa Inhibitory Activity		Thrombin Inhibitory Activity		K_{DISS}^{H-A}
	Spec.Molar Act.* (units/µmol)	Final Conc.Used (M)	Spec.Molar Act.* (units/µmol)	Final Conc.Used (M)	(M)
Hexasaccharide	38.5	3.0×10^{-7}	<0.1	1.5×10^{-5}	5.5×10^{-6}
Octasaccharide	221	5.3×10^{-8}	<0.1	2.1×10^{-5}	8.0×10^{-7}
Decasaccharide	341	2.6×10^{-8}	<0.1	1.3×10^{-5}	2.9×10^{-7}
Heparin fragments of ~14 residues	460	2.3×10^{-8}	140	1.8×10^{-8}	2.8×10^{-7}
Heparin fragments of ~16 residues	560	2.1×10^{-8}	500	1.7×10^{-8}	2.4×10^{-7}

* Highly active heparin exhibits a factor Xa specific molar activity of 1840 units/µmol, a thrombin specific molar activity of 2750 units/µmol, and a K_{DISS}^{H-A} of 5.7×10^{-8} M. The larger affinity purified mucopolysaccharide fragments possess similarly designated kinetic and binding parameters that are three to five fold lower in magnitude. This phenomena may be secondary to the more selective separation schema utilized to isolate the highly active heparin.

The data reveals that mucopolysaccharide fragments of ~14 monosaccharide units exhibit this biologic property but that maximal specific activity is attained at 18-20 monosaccharide units (23).

The kinetic properties of comparison which catalyze thrombin-antithrombin interactions were examined in detail. For this purpose, heparin fragments of ~14 residues and heparin fragments of ~16 residues were affinity chromatographed as described earlier. Experimental results summarized in Table 4 indicate that the two affinity fractionated species are able to significantly accelerate thrombin-antithrombin as well as factor Xa-antithrombin interactions. However, heparin fragments of ~16 residues possess considerably greater activity than heparin fragments of ~14 residues with respect to thrombin inactivation. Data is also provided in Table 4 which reveals that the avidity of the larger component for antithrombin is slightly greater than that of the smaller species for the protease inhibitor (23). The detailed kinetics of thrombin neutralization were investigated with the two forms of mucopolysaccharide obtained above.

Initially, molecular species of the smallest possible dimensions (~14 residues) that are able to catalyze thrombin inactivation by antithrombin were examined (Fig. 6). The resultant fragments were shown to exhibit a k_1 of 4.6×10^{-7} $M^{-1}min^{-1}$. This kinetic parameter remains unchanged at high levels of mucopolysaccharide where potential approximation sites of the serine protease are saturated with complex carbohydrate. These experimental findings imply that the above component must possess the ability to accelerate thrombin-antithrombin interactions because of a direct effect on the protease inhibitor. Furthermore, this mucopolysaccharide species appears to lack the structural regions needed to approximate free enzyme with antithrombin (23).

Subsequently, heparin fragments of larger size (≅16 residues) were studied (Fig. 6). The resultant species exhibit a k_1 of 1.0×10^{8} $M^{-1}min^{-1}$. This kinetic paramter decreases significantly at high levels of complex carbohydrate but attains a constant value at heparin concentrations in excess of 1×10^{-6} M. Data obtained from the latter region allows us to calculate that the mucopolysaccharide exhibits a k_2 of 4.6×10^{-7} $M^{-1}min^{-1}$. The

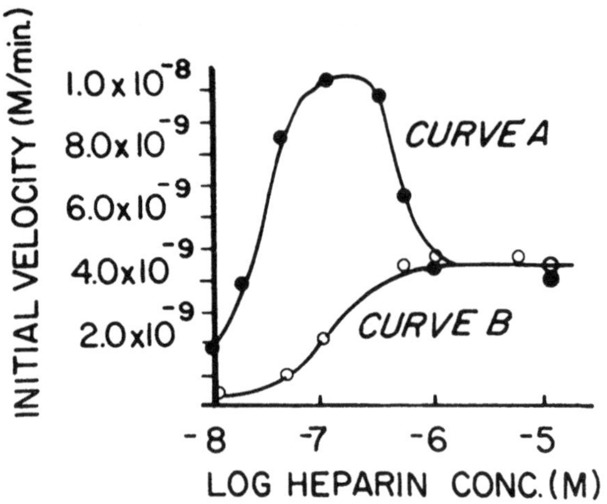

Fig. 6. The kinetic properties of heparin fragments that are able to accelerate thrombin-antithrombin interactions. The initial rates of enzyme inactivation by protease inhibitor were examined in the presence of heparin fragments of ~16 residues (curve A) (●—●) or ~14 residues (curve B) (o—o), respectively.

above estimate represents the rate of inactivation of heparin-thrombin interactions product by heparin-antithrombin complex. Given that potential approximation sites on the serine protease must be saturated with mucopolysaccharide under these conditions, k_2 provides a quantitative measure of the direct kinetics effect of heparin on antithrombin. This parameter is identical in magnitude to that of k_1 obtained for the smaller complex carbohydrate fragment. These findings suggest that the two forms of the mucopolysaccharide possess similar capacities to directly activate antithrombin with respect to thrombin neutralization. However, the larger species of heparin contains an additional disaccharide element that is required for approximating free enzyme with protease inhibitor. Therefore, this component is able to more rapidly accelerate the interaction of thrombin with antithrombin (23). In preliminary experiments, the heparin fragments of ~14 and ~16 residues have been degraded with a purified endoglucuronidase derived from human platelets. The data obtained suggest that the monosaccharide sequences responsible for activating antithrombin with respect to thrombin neutralization and for approximating free enzyme with protease inhibitor must lie on the non-reducing end of the critical tetrasaccharide (23).

These results suggest that heparin possesses multiple discrete structural domains which are responsible for its ability to complex with antithrombin and to modulate the biologic properties of the protease inhibitor. The absence or improper alignment of one or more of these regions within a heparin population would explain the previously reported differential actions of mucopolysaccharide preparations with regard to the neutralization of various hemostatic enzymes (25, 26).

References

1. Rosenberg, R. D., Damus, P. S. J. Biol. Chem. 248, 6490-6505 (1973).

2. Gitel, S. N.: Heparin: Structure, Function and Critical Implications. New York, Plenum Press. pp. 243-247 (1975).

3. Holmer, F., Soderstrom, G., Andersson, L.-O. Eur. J. Biochem. 93, 1-5 (1979).

4. Machovich, R. Biochim. Biophys. Acta 412, 13-17 (1975).

5. Smith, G. F., Craft, T. J. Biochem. Biophys. Res. Commun. 71, 738-745 (1976).

6. Griffith, M. J. J. Biol. Chem. 254, 3401-3406 (1979).

7. Griffith, M. J., Kingdon, H. S., Lundblad, R. L. Arch. Biochem. Biophys. 195, 378-384 (1979).

8. Rosenberg, R. D., Jordan, R. E., Favreau, L. V., Lam, L. H. Biochem. Biophys. Res. Commun. 86, 1319-1324 (1979).

9. Jordan, R. E., Beeler, D., Rosenberg, R. D. J. Biol. Chem. 254, 2902-2914 (1979).

10. Einarsson, R., Andersson, L.-O. Biochim. Biophys. Acta 490, 104-111 (1977).

11. Björk, I., Nordenman, B. Biochemistry 17, 3339-3344 (1978).

12. Jordan, R. E., Oosta, G. M., Gardner, W. T., Rosenberg, R. D. J. Biol. Chem. 255, 10073-10080 (1980).

13. Markwardt, F., Walsmann, P. Hoppe-Seyler Z. Physiol. Chem. 317, 64-77 (1959).

14. Henstell, H. H., Kligermann, M. Thromb. Diath. Haemorrh. 18, 167-178 (1968).

15. Jordan, R. E., Oosta, G. M., Gardner, W. T., Rosenberg, R. D. J. Biol. Chem. 255, 10081-10090 (1980).

16. Rosenberg, R. D., Armand, G., Lam, L. H. Proc. Natl. Acad. Sci. U.S.A. 75, 3065-3069 (1978).

17. Rosenberg, R. D. New York, Pergamon Press, pp. 353-368 (1978).

18. Rosenberg, R. D., Lam, L. H. Proc. Natl. Acad. Sci. U.S.A. 76, 1218-1222 (1979).

19. Lindahl, U., Bäckström, G., Thunberg, L., Leder, I. G. Proc. Natl. Acad. Sci. 77, 6551-6555 (1980).

20. Leder, I. G. Biochem. Biophys. Res. Commun. 94, 1183-1189 (1980).

21. Karapally, J. C., Dietrich, C. P. Can. J. Biochem. 48, 164-169 (1970).

22. Lindahl, U., Bäckström, G., Höök, M., Thunberg, I., Fransson, L.-Å. Proc. Natl. Acad. Sci. U.S.A. 76, 3198-3202 (1979).

23. Oosta, G. M., Gardner, W. T., Beeler, D. L., Rosenberg, R. D. Proc. Natl. Acad. Sci. U.S.A. 78, 829-833 (1981).

24. Thunberg, L., Bäckström, G., Grunberg, H., Riesenfeld, J., Lindahl, U. FEBSLetters 117, 203-206 (1980).

25. Choay, J., Lormeau, J. C., Petitou, M., Sinay, P., Casu, B., Oreste, P., Torri, G., Tatti, G. Thromb. Research 18, 573-578 (1980).

26. Thunberg, L., Lindahl, U., Tengblad, A., Laurent, T. C., Jackson, C. M. Biochem. J. 181, 241-243 (1979).

Discussion

Aronson remarked that *Rosenberg* has been working with that part of the heparin molecule which is biologically active, and actually the majority of the heparin is inactive. If one believes in the wisdom of nature, one should ascribe to the non-functional heparin also some function.

Perhaps one can extrapolate from the work of *Rosenberg* and conclude that even the part which is not functioning is important, for example for activating or binding something or helping the active part of the molecule to do something. He asked *Rosenberg* to speculate on this.

Rosenberg's comment was that one potential role of the inactive heparin fragments - which seem to have several roles - may be in a physiological mechanism which controls smooth muscle cell proliferation in atherogenesis. This may be a very principal and important mechanism in modulating smooth muscle cell proliferation within the arterial wall.

Aronson wondered about the recycling of heparin: if one adds protamine to the thrombin-antithrombin III-heparin complex, it is not possible to regenerate heparin. This is difficult to reconcile with recycling.

Rosenberg conjectered that there is a series of competing reactions in the catalytic mechanism, whether with platelet factor 4 or protamine. This really seems to be a mechanism for removing the heparin and preventing catalysis. There is a very fine balance between preventing and permitting catalysis. It is a rather complex mechanism which can be modulated at a variety of stages.

Lill said that the smalles oligosaccharide for thrombin inhibition has 14 residues; the mechanism is an allosteric one. Factor Xa is also inhibited by an allosteric mechanism, but for that, smaller oligosaccharides of about 4, 6, 8 or 10 residues can be used. It seems that oligosaccharides of various chain length can induce different allosteric effects at the antithrombin III molecule.

Rosenberg agreed that this must indeed be the case, but he thinks that it is even more complex. If one reflects upon the fact that thrombin, factor IXa and factor XIa react in different ways, one has to assume that antithrombin III is able to respond with various complicated conformational changes. These may bring up the arginine residues which are critical for the interaction and then expose a variety of secondary binding sites or perhaps another arginine residue.

In general, one must assume that the antithrombin III molecule may have multiple reactive sites. One also finds this on other inhibitors. Vegetable inhibitors, for instance trypsin inhibitors, have 3 to 4 binding sites even though they are small with a molecular weight of about 10,000.

These trypsin inhibitors from plants can be seen as prototypes for antithrombin III.

Up to now only one binding site is known on the antithrombin III molecule at the C-terminal part. It is possible that there are additional binding sites for other enzymes of the coagulation mechanism. That would make the inhibitor more versatile for the neutralization of serine proteases, which is a fascinating idea.

Róka pointed out that the last slide of the lecture showed that the heparin molecule binds to the antithrombin III molecule and at the same time to the thrombin molecule. He wanted to know if there is any evidence that a heparin molecule which only binds to thrombin can also change the rate of the reaction between antithrombin III and thrombin.

Rosenberg stated that on the basis of the evidence provided by the fractions that do not bind to antithrombin III (the waste fractions), there seems to be essentially no biological activity in this process. The binding to thrombin is not sufficient. If one takes the entire fraction, with the active and inactive portions, and performs kinetics using the appropriate properties of the inactive and active species, one can in essence explain the kinetics. So one finally has to conclude that the active material really has the prinicple biological effect.

Rosenberg mentioned an interesting report about a second heparin-cofactor, which has been actually well characterized from Majerus's laboratory. This appears to be a molecule which differs from antithrombin and does not seem to play a pharmacological role. It requires 5 units heparin per ml to be accelerated. *Rosenberg* thinks, however, that this molecule may well be the explanation for a variety of findings which are in some disagreement with known data. If one has that molecule within the preparation, the mechanism will not be the same as the mechanism of antithrombin III alone.

This new inhibitor is probably not of pharmacological importance in respect to heparin action.

Bhargava stated that inhibitory products of vegetable origin, for example SP 54, have in-vitro a rumbling effect on thrombin. Kinetics show that molecules with structural changes attack thrombin and by binding the thrombin produce a similar rate of inactivation as factor Xa does with antithrombin.

If they are both added one gets a very complex picture. Thrombin inactivation in a purified system need not be a property of heparin but may also be the porperty of another mucopolysaccharide of vegetable origin.

Rosenberg agreed to Bhargava's suggestion that one cannot rule out other potential mechanisms. One can invent mucopolysaccharides with approximation phenomena, which bind somewhat more strongly to thrombin than to antithrombin and subsequently get neutralisation from that kind of a mechanism.

Rosenberg thinks one should question the potency of that particular anticoagulant. Some work has been done with that particular molecule which suggests that it causes activity to be released within the circulation after injection.

Rosenberg, however, has never seen it after injecting the inactive fraction. So, if it is true, it must have some very different properties than heparin.

Witt asked if *Rosenberg* has already studied abnormal antithrombins.

Rosenberg replied that the "abnormal antithrombin III story" is becoming rather interesting. He pointed out that *Duckert* has a very interesting family whose antithrombin has a reduced affinity to heparin. It is a new type of abnormality.

Rosenberg has also found a fascinating new abnormality of antithrombin III in a rather extensive family.

Heparin binds to this abnormal antithrombin III a bit more tightly but can not activate it. It seems in essence to have a normal heparin binding site, at least in respect to its interaction with heparin, but the subsequent activation is not possible.

The members of this family have 30 - 40 % abnormal antithrombin III molecules. They suffer from profound thrombotic diseases.

Fussi asked if *Rosenberg* has found differences for different types of heparin (different organs, different species).

Rosenberg answered that most work concerning the function-structure relationship has been conducted with pig mucosal heparin. It is assumed from the work of various authors that there are no differences in the structure-function relationship for the different heparin types. The story will be similar if not identical.

Duckert asked *Rosenberg* why he had not mentioned factor VII or VII a.

Rosenberg said that this story is still emerging. It is too simple to assume that antithrombin III is the only inhibitor of the coagulation system. What one now sees are two facts:

1. Factor VII a is not inhibited by the antithrombin-heparin complex to a significant degree. This seems to be a real phenomenon that one has to accept.

2. A further interesting fact is the new inhibitor of activated protein C. The protein C is a serine protease related to the prothrombin family molecules. It is not inhibited by the antithrombin III-heparin complex. It has its own inhibitor, which is not yet purified. When this inhibitor is abnormal, the result is a decrease in factor V and VIII because of cleavage of these two molecules by the cofactor.

One will probably still find some more inhibitors which is still nothing known about.

The tight inhibitor of protein C controls a separate part of the coagulation mechanism and may be of additional importance. Not the whole coagulation system is really under the control of the antithrombin III mechanism.

Rosenberg believes that the particular importance which will turn up with the protein C molecule is its own inhibitory function.

He stressed the special importance of the protein C/protein C inhibitor system in relation to factor VIII and the connected platelet aggregation.

Wenzel referred to the different functions of antithrombin III when they are activated by the different compounds of heparin, as mentioned in *Rosenberg's* lecture.

He asked if *Rosenberg* has found differences in the rate of the velocity in the two dimensional immune electrophoresis, which depends on the heparin concentration, for antithrombin III alone and for the two types of heparin compounds when they are combined with antithrombin III.

Rosenberg believes that it should be possible to see differences in a purified system by crossed immune electrophoresis. He thinks it is a valuable technique.

Verstraete asked if the protein C inhibitor is a histidine rich protein.

Rosenberg pointed out that it is assumed to be a separate protease inhibitor with a large molecular size. Little work has been done on this new inhibitor up to now, but it seems to be turning out to be a very important system, which together with the antithrombin system may really be responsible for the regulation of all of the activities of the coagulation cascade.

Róka wanted to know if *Rosenberg* has investigated the inhibitory activity of the small fragments of heparin in vitro and in vivo, or if he had only measured the binding.

Rosenberg answered that the small fragments activate antithrombin III to factor Xa, but not to thrombin.

Róka wondered about the biological effect in patients.

Rosenberg said that there are studies going on.

Biosynthesis of Heparin

Johan Riesenfeld
Institute of Medical and Physiological Chemistry
Swedish University of Agricultural Sciences
Box 575
S-751 23 Uppsala, Sweden

Heparin, one of the connective-tissue polysaccharides or glycosaminoglycans, is well known for its blood-anticoagulant and lipolysis-stimulating properties. Produced by the mast cells, heparin, like most other glycosaminoglycans, is synthesized as a proteoglycan (1, 2). This proteoglycan is composed of a number of polysaccharide chains, molecular weight 60-100 x 10^3, covalently linked to a central protein core, thus forming a macromolecule with a molecular weight in the order of 10^6. The polypeptide core (or at least the polysaccharide-substituted portion of the core) has an unusual structure since it appears to consist of repeating serine and glycine residues only; at least two out of three of the serine residues are substituted with polysaccharide chains. The linkage to protein involves a specific oligosaccharide sequence characteristic of most connective tissue polysaccharides. This so-called *linkage-region* consists of a xylose residue O-glycosidically linked to serine, followed by two galactose and a glucuronic acid residue (3).

The relatively low-molecular, single-chain polysaccharide in commercial heparin preparations is formed by post-biosynthetic modification of the heparin proteoglycan. This process involves cleavage of the constituent polysaccharide chains by an endoglucuronidase, yielding shorter polymers with a molecular weight in the range of 5-20 x 10^3 (4, 5).

Heparin · New Biochemical and Medical Aspects

Printed in Germany

The heparin molecule consists of a heavily sulfated polysaccharide backbone of alternating hexuronic acid and glucosamine residues, joined by 1 → 4 linkages (see Fig. 1). The uronic acid component was initially believed to be D-glucuronic acid only; however, following the demonstration of its C-5 epimer, L-iduronic acid, in heparin preparations by Cifonelli and Dorfman in 1962 (6) this component was subsequently shown to be the major uronic acid constituent (for reviews on structure see Refs. 7-9). Sulfate substituents occur as ester linked (O-sulfate) groups at C-2 and C-6 of most of the iduronic acid and glucosamine residues, respectively. Furthermore, the majority of the glucosamine units carry sulfamido (N-sulfate) groups, this structural unit being unique to heparin and to the closely related glycosaminoglycan, heparan sulfate.

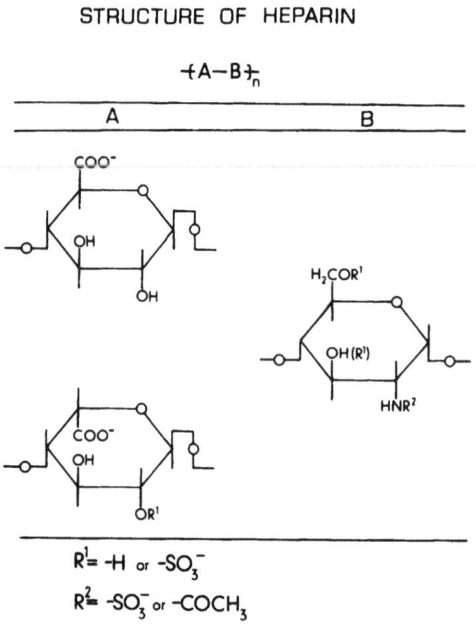

Fig. 1. Sugar components in the repeating disaccharide units (designated $\{A-B\}_n$ of heparin. The sugar unit A is either D-glucuronic acid (top) or L-iduronic acid (bottom). The former is linked by a β1 → 4, and the latter by an α1 → 4 glycosidic linkage to the unit B, D-glucosamine, which is, in turn, joined to the next uronic acid residue by an α1 → 4 linkage. The R1 substituent denotes an O-sulfate group or a hydrogen atom, whereas R2 is an N-sulfate or an N-acetyl group.

Glucosamine unites that are not N-sulfated are instead N-acetylated. Recently an additional O-sulfate group was discovered at C-3 of a small proportion of the glucosamine residues (10); this minor component appears to be closely associated with the antithrombin binding region of the heparin molecule. The variable sugar sequence and substitution pattern is reflected in the marked structural heterogeneity of the polysaccharide.

The biosynthesis of heparin has been investigated using microsomal fractions from transplantable mouse mastocytomas (for recent reviews, see 9, 11). Musch of the basic information from this system was provided by the early studies of Silbert (12-14). The earliest events in heparin proteoglycan biosynthesis, i. e. formation and initial glycosylation of the protein core, have not yet been subjected to experimental study. However, by analogy with the biosynthesis of the chondroitin sulfate proteoglycan, it may be assumed that polysaccharide chain formation is initiated by the transfer of a xylose residue from UDP-xylose to a serine unit in the preformed polypeptide core (catalyzed by xylosyl transferase), followed by addition of two galactose units and a glucuronic acid residue in an analogous manner. Chain elongation then proceeds by the stepwise transfer of N-acetyl-D-glucosamine and D-glucuronic acid residues from the corresponding UDP-sugars, catalyzed by N-acetylglucosaminyl and glucuronosyl transferase, respectively (9). After polymerization of about 100-150 disaccharide units, chain elongation is terminated in a hitherto unkown manner.

Conversion of this initial polymerization product of repeating glucuronic acid and N-acetylglucosamine residues into the biosynthetic end product, i. e. heparin, involves a series of a rapid and highly ordered, sequential manner, leading to the formation of a number of distinct biosynthetic intermediates, which have been isolated and characterized (15). Structural analysis of these polymeric intermediates indicated a sequence of reactions (Fig. 2), including (I) removal of N-acetyl groups from N-acetyl glucosamine residues (16), (II) N-sulfation of unsubstituted amino groups formed (15), (III) uronosyl C5-epimerization of D-glucuronic acid into L-iduronic acid residues (17-19), (IV) O-sulfation at C-2 iduronic acid residues and finally (V) O-sulfation at C-6 glucosamine units (20). In Fig. 2 the various reaction steps are illustrated by representative disaccharide units. The corresponding enzymes have all been studied in some detail. Assay procedures for most of the enzymes have thus been developed (16, 19, 21), and they have been solubilized from the microsomal membranes. The uronosyl C5-epimerase has been purified almost to homogeneity (22).

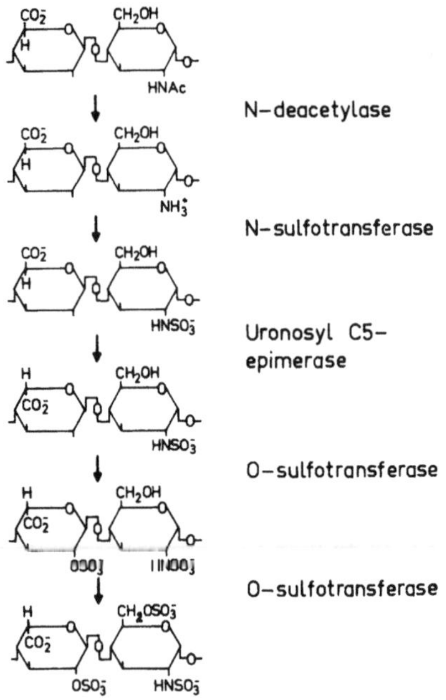

Fig. 2. Sequence of polymer modification reactions leading to formation of the predominant disaccharide unit in heparin.

The reaction sequence illustrated in Fig. 2 implies that the final product is invariably trisulfated disaccharide. A polysaccharide composed exclusively of such disaccharide units would have a homogeneous structure. The structural heterogeneity of heparin therefore indicates that the polymer-modification process is incomplete. Structural characterization of the biosynthetic intermediates has in fact revealed that only a fraction of the disaccharide units is involved in each step. Furthermore, studies on the substrate specificities of the polymer-modification enzymes indicated that the selection of target units is, at least partly, a nonrandom process (17-21). The introduction of N-sulfate groups (see Figs. 2 and 3) thus has a directory effect

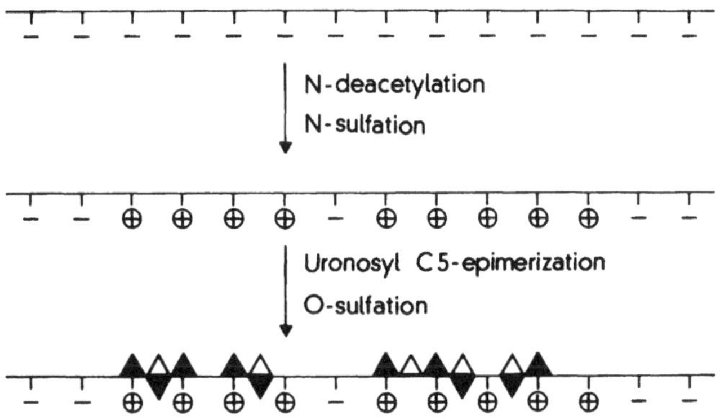

Fig. 3. Schematic representation of the polymer-modification process involved in the biosynthesis of heparin. The figure illustrates the incomplete course of the process; all disaccharide units available are not engaged in each modification reaction. Note the effect of N-deacetylation - N-sulfation on the structure of the biosynthetic end product. The continuous line denotes the initial polysaccharide chain of alternating glucuronic acid and N-acetylglucosamine residues, - N-acetyl groups, ⊕ N-sulfate groups, Δ iduronic acid residues, ▼ iduronic acid 2-O-sulfate groups and ▲ glucosamine 6-O-sulfate groups.

on the subsequent polymer-modification reactions, since both uronosyl C5-epimerization (and consequently 2-O-sulfation of iduronic acid) and 6-O-sulfation of glucosamine units occur, preferentially or exclusively in the N-sulfated regions of the polysaccharides (19, 20). A prerequisite to the introduction of these essential N-sulfate groups is the removal of N-acetyl groups. The initial modification reaction, N-deacetylation of glucosamine residues (16), therefore has a key role in the regulation of the overall polymer-modification process; the degree of N-deacetylation determines the degree of N-sulfation, which in turn affects the following modification steps. A schematic representation of these relationships is shown in Fig. 3. A polymer of repeating glucuronic acid - N-acetylglucosamine disaccharide units undergoes partial N-deacetylation, followed first by N-sulfation and then by uronosyl C5-epimerization and O-sulfation. In the final product, those regions that have become N-sulfated are also rich in iduronic acid and O-sulfate groups, whereas the N-acetylated regions remain essentially unmodified. The mechanism regulating the extent and distribution of N-deacetylation is at present unknown.

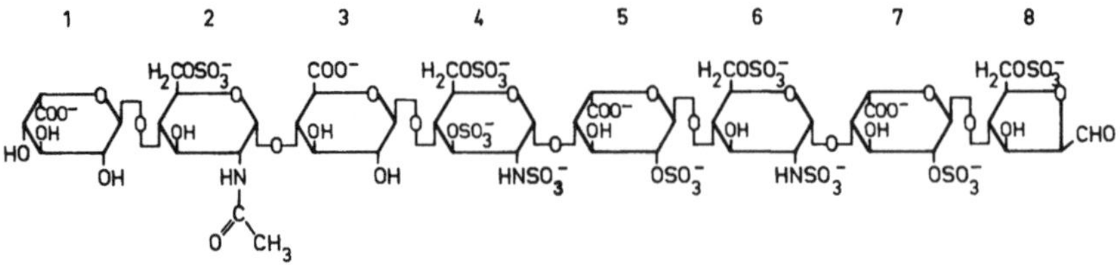

Fig. 4. Structure of the predominant antithrombin-binding octasaccharide fragment isolated after partial deaminative cleavage of pig mucosal heparin. The 2,5-anhydro-D-mannose residue in position 8 corresponds to an N-sulfated glucosamine unit in the intact polysaccharide.

As an illustration to the process of polymer modification, the structure shown in Fig. 4 may be considered. This structure represents the predominant antithrombin binding octasaccharide unit isolated after partial depolymerization of heparin with nitrous acid (10, 23-25; see also Refs. 26 and 27). Due to the remaining N-acetyl group in position 2 the trisaccharide sequence 1-3 remains low-sulfated. The glucuronic acid residue in position 3 is not recognized as a substrate by the uronosyl C5-epimerase and is therefore unable to epimerize into iduronic acid; nor is it a substrate for any O-sulfotransferase. The uronic acid unit in position 1 is converted into iduronic acid but remains nonsulfated. In contrast, the glucosamine residues in positions 4 and 6 become N-sulfated; subsequently, the glucuronic acid residues in positions 5 and 7 are largely converted into 2-O-sulfated iduronic acid units. The antithrombin-binding octasaccharide from heparin is thus composed of a poorly modified region (positions 1 to 3), centered around the N-acetylated glucosamine unit at position 2, and an extensively modified region (positions 4 to 8), containing N-sulfated glucosamine units. In addition, the 3-O-sulfate group at position 4 appears to be unique to the antithrombin-binding region in heparin and is probably essential to the anticoagulant activity. Other groups so far implicated as being of functional importance include the 6-O-sulfate group at position 2 (L. Thunberg, G. Bäckström, and U. Lindahl, unpublished results) and the two N-sulfate groups at positions 4 and 6 (25). Virtually nothing is known about the mechanisms that ascertain the appropriate positioning of these essential groups. It is obvious that the regulation of the polymer-modification reactions involved in the biosynthesis of heparin is of critical importance in relation to the biological activity of the polysaccharide.

Acknowledgements

I am grateful to Professor Ulf Lindahl for valuable criticism during the preparation of this manuscript. This work was supported by grants from the Swedish Medical Research Council (2309).

References

1. Horner, A. A.: J. Biol. Chem. 246, 231-239 (1971).
2. Robinson, H. C., Horner, A. A., Höök, M., Ögren, S. and Lindahl, U.: J. Biol. Chem. 253, 6687-6693 (1978).
3. Lindahl, U.: Biochim. Biophys. Acta 130, 368-382 (1966).
4. Ögren, S. and Lindahl, U.: J. Biol. Chem. 250, 2690-2697 (1975).
5. Ögren, S. and Lindahl, U.: Biochem. J. 154, 605-611 (1976).
6. Cifonelli, J. A. and Dorfman, A.: Biochem. Biophys. Res. Commun. 7, 41-45 (1962).
7. Lindahl, U. in: MTP International Reviews of Science: Organic Chemistry Series Two - Carbohydrate Chemistry (G. O. Aspinall, ed.), Vol. 7, p. 283-312, Butterworths, London (1976).
8. Lindahl, U. and Höök, M.: Ann. Rev. Biochem. 47, 385-417 (1978).
9. Rodén, L. in: The Biochemistry of Glycoproteins and Proteoglycans (W. J. Lennartz, ed.) p. 267-371, Plenum, New York (1980).
10. Lindahl, U., Bäckström, G., Thunberg, L. and Leder, I. G.: Proc. Natl. Acad. Sci. 77, 6551-6555 (1980).

11. Feingold, D., Rodén, L., Forsee, T., Jacobsson, I., Jensen, J., Lindahl, U., Malmström, A. and Prihar, H. in: Biology of Heparin (R. Lundblad, W. V. Brown, K. G. Mann and H. R. Roberts, eds.) p. 157-171, Elsevier/North-Holland, New York (1981).

12. Silbert, J. E.: J. Biol. Chem. 238, 3542-3546 (1963).

13. Silbert, J. E.: J. Biol. Chem. 242, 5146-5152 (1967).

14. Silbert, J. E.: J. Biol. Chem. 242, 5153-5157 (1967).

15. Höök, M., Lindahl, U., Hallén, A. and Bäckström, G.: J. Biol. Chem. 250, 6065-6071 (1975).

16. Riesenfeld, J., Höök, M. and Lindahl, U.: J. Biol. Chem. 255, 922-928 (1980).

17. Höök, M., Lindahl, U., Bäckström, G., Malmström, A. and Fransson, L.-Å.: J. Biol. Chem. 249, 3908-3915 (1974).

18. Lindahl, U., Jacobsson, I., Höök, M., Bäckström, G. and Feingold, D. S.: Biochem. Biophys. Res. Commun. 70, 492-499 (1977).

19. Jacobsson, I., Bäckström, G., Höök, M., Lindahl, U., Feingold, D. S., Malmström, A. and Rodén, L.: J. Biol. Chem. 254, 2975-2982 (1979).

20. Jacobsson, I. and Lindahl, U.: J. Biol. Chem. 255, 5094-5100 (1980).

21. Jansson, L., Höök, M., Wasteson, Å. and Lindahl, U.: Biochem. J. 149, 49-55 (1975).

22. Malmström, A., Rodén, L., Feingold, D. S., Jacobsson, I., Bäckström, G. and Lindahl, U.: J. Biol. Chem. 255, 3878-3883 (1980).

23. Lindahl, U., Bäckström, G., Höök, M., Thunberg, L., Fransson, L.-Å. and Linker, A.: Proc. Natl. Acad. Sci. USA 76, 3198-3202 (1979).

24. Thunberg, L., Bäckström, G., Grundberg, H., Riesenfeld, J. and Lindahl, U.: FEBS Lett. 117, 203-206 (1980).

25. Riesenfeld, J., Thunberg, L., Höök, M. and Lindahl, U.: J. Biol. Chem. 256, 2389-2394 (1981).

26. Rosenberg, R. D., Armand, G. and Lam, L.: Proc. Natl. Acad. Sci. USA 75, 3065-3069 (1978).

27. Rosenberg, R. D. and Lam, L.: Proc. Natl. Acad. Sci. USA 76, 1218-1222 (1979).

Discussion

Riesenfeld was asked by *Kakkar* for the analytical procedure which he used to elucidate the specific sequence of the antithrombin III binding site of heparin.

Riesenfeld described the details of his experiments and presented some special figures. *Riesenfeld's* explanation would go beyond the framework of this discussion and could not be understood without the figures.

The elucidation of the sequence of the binding site can be found in: J. Biol. Chem. 256, No. 5, 2389-2393 (1981) by J. Riesenfeld, L. Thunberg, M. Höök and U. Lindahl.

Lill raised the question if the whole biologically synthesized proteoglycan molecule has anticoagulatory activity or if there is evidence that specific hydrolases release polysaccharide chains which are active.

Riesenfeld said that there are preliminary data showing that the high affinity proteoglycan has a small but significant anticoagulatory activity.

Aronson asked if the whole synthesizing process takes place in the cytoplasm of the mast cells and if the products are then carried into the granules or if they are partially synthesized in the granules.

Riesenfeld answered that the investigations were not carried out at the subcellular level. The biosynthesis was studied in the 100 000 x g fraction. But the endoglucosidase which cleaves the macromolecule into shorter polymers is found mainly in the 20 000 x g fraction.

Aronson asked further if anything is known about the synthesis of heparan which forms the glycocalix and if this might resemble the synthesis of heparin.

Riesenfeld replied that there seems to be nothing known about this.

During the discussion on the mechanism of the attachement of the polysaccharide chains to the protein core, it was admitted that this has not yet been conclusively studied for heparin. But in analogy to chondroitin sulfate proteoglycan it is assumed that xylose is introduced into the preformed polypeptide core by a xylosyl transferase and that then the elongation of the polysaccharide chains proceeds. The possibility exists that the polysaccharide chains are preformed and attached as a whole to the protein core. But this is rather unlikely.

Physiological Heparin - its Function and Fate

Joan Dawes
MRC Immunoassay Team,
2, Forrest Road,
Edinburgh, EH1 2QW, UK.

What is physiological heparin? Although heparin as we use it therapeutically is derived from mammalian tissues, it may both have been altered by extraction procedures and changed by selection of a particular activity. Thus the official pharmacopoeias define heparin units in terms of the *in vitro* inhibition of coagulation systems, and certain manufacturing processes are based towards the production of heparin with high specific activity according to this limited definition - a definition which arose from the first recognised biological activity of heparin. It is now known that heparin has the potential for many different biological activities, some of which are listed in Table 1.

It is clear that such diverse activities offer considerable physiological potential. Moreover, it is most unusual for one substance to display such a range of acitivities; and here we come to two aspects of the structure of heparin which are central to this multiplicity of function. Heparin is a linear anionic polyelectrolyte (23), with a concentration of negative charge such that it is able to hydrogen bond to a wide range of molecules, not only those which are positively charged but even to proteins bearing an overall negative charge themselves. The distribution of charge along the backbone of the molecule maintains free heparin in an extended linear configuration, which may then fold to conform to the shape of any molecule to which heparin binds. The second important characteristic is too often forgotten. Heparin is not a molecule of single and defined structure; it is a type of carbohydrate, a class of molecules, each of which may have a unique primary sequence of monosaccharides. Moreover, heparin comprises a wide range of

Heparin · New Biochemical and Medical Aspects

molecular weights, from 3,000 to more than 40,000 in the case of commercial heparin (24), and to more than 1,000,000 for the so-called macromolecular heparin from such sources as rat skin (25), mouse mastocytoma (26) and human lung (27). Both the primary sequence and the molecular weight can influence the biological activity of each molecule. Thus the binding region for antithrombin III (ATIII) involves a 5-saccharide sequence, and the amount of heparin which binds to ATIII is a probability function for molecules containing one or more of these sequences (28). A high proportion of heparin molecules do not bind to ATIII at all, but fulfil other functions. In this context it is also important to remember that there are marked differences in heparins from different species and from different tissues.

In considering the physiological aspects of heparin, we must include not only its effects on those receiving commercial heparin as a drug, but also the contribution of endogenous heparin in the untreated individual. The two may differ in bias and in extent, and the degree of difference will reflect the closeness or otherwise of the structures included in the commercial material to those naturally present in the recipient. Herein lies the basis not only of differences in activity between commercial preparations, but also different effects on different species. Detailed conclusions drawn from animal experiments should be applied with caution to the human case. Moreover, a simplistic view of heparin action is further hindered by the presence of a broad spectrum of linear anionic polyelectrolytes *in vivo* (28). These are removed on processing in the preparation of commercial heparin (29), but it seems likely that they participate in many of the actions of endogenous heparin. The most important are probably the heparitins, or heparan sulphates, which are structurally closely related to heparin though they may be covalently linked to protein and occur naturally as proteoglycans (30). This will clearly influence their biological activity compared with the free chains of exogenous, and possibly also some endogenous, heparin. Nevertheless they are of particular interest as one of the most metabolically active constituents of plasma membranes (31).

The basis, then, for the diverse activities of heparin is the varying ability of the different chains to bind to other molecules, some of which are listed in Table 2. The spectrum of activities demonstrated by the different heparin

Table 1
Some of the potential biological actions of heparin

Anticoagulatory:

Bind to and activate antithrombin III, thereby inhibiting serine proteases (1).

Antithrombotic:

Bind to vascular wall, increasing its electronegative potential (2).

Inhibit proliferation of arterial cells (3, 4).

Neutralise proteins such as platelet factor 4, which may decrease the antithrombotic properties of the vascular endothelium (5).

Antiinflammatory and antiallergic:

Inhibit sensitivity reactions (6, 7, 8).
Block toxic bases (9, 10), particularly histamine (11).

In fat metabolism:

Reduce fat absorption from the intestine (12).
Liberate and activate lipoprotein lipase (13, 14).

In the ovarian cycle:

Modulate the response of follicles to hormonal stimulus (15).

Regulate a wide range of enzyme activities:

Activate e. g. brain tyrosine hydroxylase (16); pepsinogen (17); DNA polymerase (18).

Inhibit e. g. myosin ATPase (19); pyruvate kinase (20); RNA polymerases (21); pepsin (22).

Table 2
Substances which bind to heparins

Inorganic ions:

e. g. Na^+ (32); Ca^{2+} (33); SO_4^{2-} (34); PO_4^{3-} (35).

Dyes:

e. g. Methylene blue (36); Azure A (37); Neutral red (38); Acriflavin (38).

Alkylamines and alkaloids:

e. g. Cetylpyridinium chloride (39); Choline (23); Brucine (40).

Biogenic amines:

e. g. Histamine (41); Serotonin (41); Adrenalin (42).

Drugs:

e. g. Chloroquine (2); Neomycin (43); Streptomycin (44).

Basic proteins (45):

e. g. Protamines; Histones.

Plasma proteins (45, 46, 47):

e. g. Platelet factor 4; Fibrinogen; β-Lipoproteins; Antithrombin III; α-2-Globulin; γ-Globulins.

Viruses (48):

e. g. Tobacco mosaic virus; Tomato bushy stunt virus.

molecules in any one sample towards another substance makes such interactions particularly difficult to analyse. That about which most is known - the binding of heparin to ATIII which is the primary source of its anticoagulant activity - is described elsewhere in this volume, and detailed discussions of most other interactions must contain a speculative component. Some recent work (49, 50, 51) has, however, investigated the way in which heparin binds to platelet factor 4 (PF4). PF4 is a platelet-specific protein contained in the α-granules and released when platelets aggregate (52, 53). It is therefore probably highly significant in the complex balance which determines whether thrombosis will or will not occur. Here a distinction should be drawn between the anticoagulant activity of heparin and its clearly demonstrated ability to inhibit thrombus formation (54, 55). The two are frequently confused, but can be easily distinguished. This is the basis for the current use of *low dose heparin* in antithrombotic therapy, where a regimen is used which effectively lowers the risk of thrombus formation but does not measurably alter coagulation parameters (56).

PF4 is a tetramer of identical subunits of molecular weight 7,800 (57). It normally occurs as a complex with a chondroitin 4-sulphate proteoglycan (58), but has a very high affinity for heparin which displaces it from its proteoglycan carrier (59). Examination of the anisotropy of the fluorescence of dansylated PF4 on complexing with heparin (49, 50, 51) has revealed that the type of complex formed depends on the molecular weight of the heparin chains. Chains of less than 10,000 molecular weight showed increasing degrees of complexing with an increased PF4:heparin ratio until all the heparin binding sites were saturated. Larger heparin chains bound in a stepwise manner; initially a 1 : 1 complex with PF4 was formed, but as the amount of protein was increased more of it was bound until again the heparin binding sites were saturated and very large aggregates formed. Possible structures for the complexes are illustrated in Fig. 1; those of the large aggregates are undefined. These structures emphasise the change which can be imposed on the structure of heparin when it complexes with a protein.

Despite these careful physical studies, the mechanism of complex formation between heparin and PF4 is still incompletely understood. There does not seem to be a requirement for a particular carbohydrate sequence in the heparin chain as there is for binding to ATIII, for all heparin molecules, regardless of their primary sequence, bind to PF4. However, the interaction is probably not merely that of diffuse ionic bonding. Despite the high affinity of PF4 for heparin, the protein is not highly positively charged. It

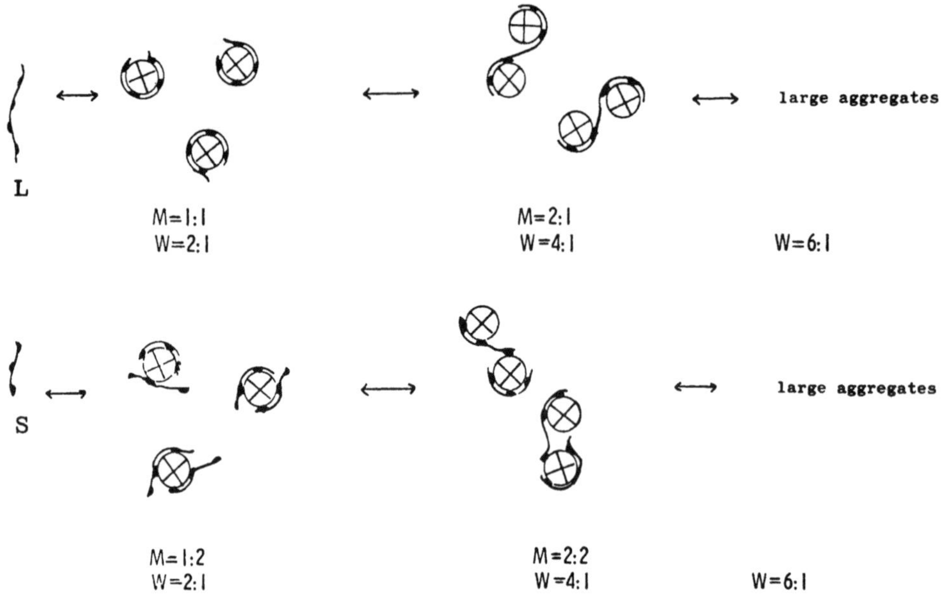

Fig. 1. Postulated models for the interaction of heparins with PF4.

possess a concentration of lysine residues at the COOH-terminus, however, and this is probably the most important site of the fairly precise interactions with heparin (60) which can give rise to the defined ionically stable intermediates described.

This work refers to interactions in solution, and although these may be important to the action of heparin - and are certainly easier to define than those occurring at an interface - it is likely that the major physiological functions of heparin are associated with the cell surface. It is now recognised that heparin administered by any route, but particularly subcutaneously or via the lung, is rapidly taken up by the cells of the reticuloendothelial system (61). The cellular heparin pool thus engendered or augmented acts as a source of plasma heparin for up to 3 weeks, but its immediate effects on the surfaces particularly of endothelial cells are at least equally important. Thus, after the injection of heparin its concentration in the endothelium can be more than 100 times that in plasma (62). The normal vascular endothelium carries heparin sulphate, which may be covalently bound to protein components of the plasma membrane or may be associated with a specific receptor. However, the heparan sulphate is retained, it contributes markedly to the overall electronegative cell surface charge. Thrombogenesis at the vascular wall is prevented by the maintenance of an electronegative charge of about 160 mV on the surface; this is derived from both biochemical processes and physical processes such as blood flow (63).

Clearly a reduction in the contribution of endogenous endothelial heparitins to this electronegative potential could precipitate thrombus formation, and such a reduction may occur in one of two ways. There may be a deficiency of endogenous heparitin, or the amount present may be normal, but its charge may be neutralised by binding of other molecules. Some plasma proteins, such as PF4, ATIII, lipoprotein lipase (LPL) or thrombin, have a high affinity for these anionic polyelectrolytes: others, including low density and very low density lipoproteins (LDL; VLDL), the thrombin-ATIII complex (T-AT), factor Xa and fibrinogen are of lower affinity but still bind sufficiently to mask the electronegative charge. The sequence of their affinities for heparin is indicated below.

$$\text{PF4} > \begin{matrix} \text{ATIII} \\ \\ \text{LPL} \end{matrix} > \text{thrombin} > \text{T-AT} > \text{LDL} > \text{VLDL} > \text{fibrinogen} > \text{Xa}$$

It is worth mentioning here that the existence of such a wide range of molecules which can be present in varying concentrations in plasma and bind to heparins must give rise to an extremely complex dynamic situation at the endothelial cell surface. Those with high affinity will displace those which bind less strongly; for example, Brown et al. found that PF4 inhibits the binding of LDL to its receptor on human fibroblasts (64). Thus an alteration in the plasma concentration of any one of these molecules will alter the distribution of those bound to the endothelial cell surface and, as a consequence, the plasma concentrations of the molecular species displaced. The endothelial cell surface is represented schematically in Fig. 2, I, and the effect of increasing the plasma concentration of PF4 by local platelet aggregation is indicated in Fig. 2, II. The balance of such interaction may be the basis not only for thrombogenesis or the prevention of thrombus formation, but also for the development, or not, of atheromatous plaque.

The administration of exogenous heparin results in a further dimension of complexity. If endogenous heparitins are deficient, this will rectify the deficiency. Even if they are not, heparin is taken up by the endothelial cell (65), perhaps because many of the heparitin receptors (R in Fig. 2) are free. Alternatively, commercial heparin, perhaps by reason of its higher charge density, may displace the endogenous material from its cell surface receptor. Kjellen et al. (66) found that heparin displaced two-thirds of the endogenous heparan sulphate from hepatocytes; this represents heparitin reversibly bound to receptors. The remaining one-third could only be released by protease treatment, being covalently bound to the cell membrane. It was calculated that there were about 4×10^6 heparitin receptors per cell. Heparins of high sulphate content and high molecular weight were the most efficient at displacing endogenous heparitins. *In vivo*, such displacement will both increase the negative charge on the endothelial surface and release into the circulation molecules with considerable biological activity of their own (Fig. 2, III). This is a possible mechanism whereby the apparent activity of a heparin or heparinoid may be different *in vivo* or *ex vivo* and *in vitro*, for the injected molecules are not those subsequently found in the blood. In this way heparinoids such as SP54 (67) and a semi-synthetic heparin analogue produced by Luitpold-Werk may display little or no anticoagulant activity *in vitro*, but are as effective as heparin after injection (68). The suggestion that the inactive molecules injected are metabolised to give active species (69) has not been experimentally verified, and a displacement mechanism is an attractive alternative.

The generally high affinity of commercial heparin compared with endogenous heparan sulphates will restore the electronegative potential of the endothelium in another way; it will remove molecules already bound to the endogenous heparitin (Fig. 2, III and IV). This is well illustrated by the effect of intravenous injections of heparin on the plasma PF4 concentration (70). Following the first of a series of injections PF4 was immediately released into the plasma (Fig. 3). The protein was not derived from the platelets and

I		II
R-heparitin-T-AT		R-heparitin-PF4 + T-AT
R		R
heparitin-LDL		heparitin-PF4 + LDL
R-heparitin$^-$	PF4 →	R-heparitin-PF4
R		R
heparitin$^-$		heparitin-PF4
R-heparitin-LPL		R-heparitin-LPL
R		R
↓ heparin		↓ heparin
R-heparin$^{=}$ + heparitin-T-AT		R-heparitin$^-$ + heparin-PF4
R-heparin$^{=}$		R-heparin$^{=}$
heparitin$^-$ + heparin-LDL		heparitin$^-$ + heparin-PF4
R-heparin$^{=}$ + heparitin		R-heparin$^{=}$ + heparitin-PF4
R-heparin$^{=}$		R-heparin$^{=}$
heparitin$^-$		heparitin$^-$ + heparin-PF4
R-heparitin$^-$ + heparin-LPL		R-heparitin$^-$ + heparin-LPL
R-heparin$^{=}$		R-heparin$^{=}$
III		IV

R: endothelial heparitin receptor

Fig. 2. Interactions at the endothelial cell surface.

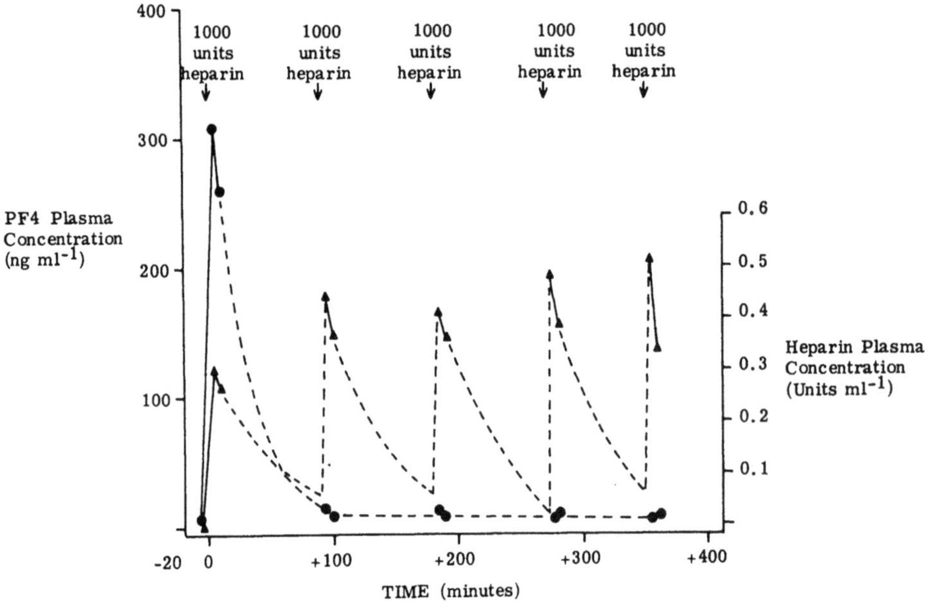

Fig. 3. The effect of multiple intravenous heparin injections on PF4 release.
● PF4, measured by radioimmunoassay (70)
▲ heparin, measured by anti-Xa assay (71)

was probably released from endothelial heparan sulphate (72). Subsequent injections did not have the same effect unless sufficient time - in this case several days - had elapsed for the endothelial reservoir to refill. The binding of PF4 to cultured human endothelial cells was examined by Busch et al. (59). Not only did PF4 bind specifically to the endothelial heparan sulphate, but it could be removed by other anionic polyelectrolytes of which the most effective was heparin. Similarly lipoprotein lipase is known to be released by heparin (13), and it may be postulated that most of the other bound proteins are returned to the circulation following heparin administration. The polyanions which contribute to the electronegative potential at the cell surface are thus *swept clean*, and the extent and duration of this effect will depend both upon the therapeutic regimen employed and the physiological state of the recipient.

Equally relevant to these considerations is the rate at which administered heparin is destroyed. As already mentioned, heparin is rapidly cleared from the circulation after intravenous injection, although because of its uptake on to the endothelial cell surface, clearance in this case cannot necessarily be equated with the termination of biological activity. Nevertheless, the activity expressed by heparin in solution may be different from that exerted as a component of the cell surface, and clearance must therefore be examined. Moreover, following clearance the heparin is ultimately catabolised and rendered biologically inactive, though this may not occur immediately.

Studies of heparin pharmacokinetics have mainly been based on coagulation tests on blood samples and the doses of intravenous heparin administered have often been high to compensate for the relative insensitivity of the assays used. The results have been confusing, probably because such doses swamp the primary biological mechanisms available for catabolising heparin. This view is supported by reports that the half-life of heparin varies with the dose (73), and by the continuous infusion studies of de Swart et al. (74). More definitive experiments have made use of radioactively labelled heparin. After the injection of $^{35}SO_4$-heparin into rats (75) or ^{125}I-heparin into humans (76), the label was rapidly taken up by the reticuloendothelial system and concentrated in the liver and spleen. In the human a macromolecular catabolite was subsequently released into the circulation; this did not bind to PF4, ATIII or protamine and was inactive in an anti-Xa assay. The results of this experiment are illustrated in Fig. 4. The biological activity, measured by anti-Xa assay, continued to decline, whereas a peak of released radioactive material appeared in the plasma by 160 minutes after the initial injection. This effect has not been described by other investigators for two reasons - much of the work on heparin catabolism has been carried out using animal models, in which the peak of released material is either very slight or absent, and the heparin used has been either tritiated or labelled with ^{35}S. Tritiated heparin is of low specific activity, and large amounts have been injected. Much of this is cleared directly through the kidneys and the peak of released material is masked. This peak is not detected when $^{35}SO_4^-$ is used because the macromolecular material released from the reticulo-endothelial system is markedly desulphated at both the N-

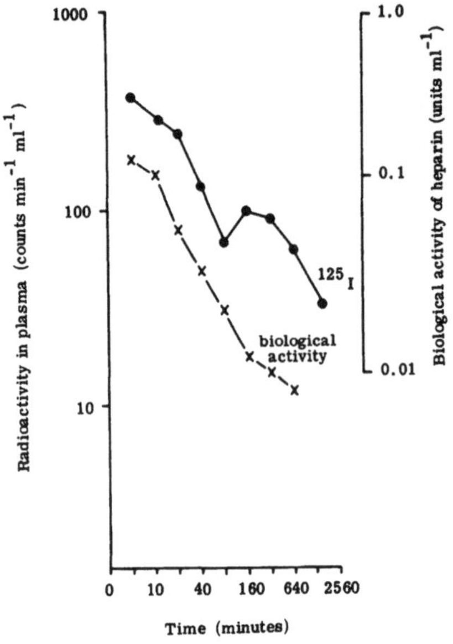

Fig. 4. Clearance of 1000 units of heparin after intravenous injection in man.

and O-positions; this accounts for its lack of biological activity. The enzymes responsible for heparin desulphation have yet to be clearly identified; a heparin N-desulphamidase has been demonstrated in various mammalian tissues (77), but O-desulphating activity has not been found. The heparitinase present in platelets (78) degrades sulphated material, and does not appear to be involved in the immediate catabolism of injected heparin. The desulphated macromolecular metabolite is not excreted as such, though a partially desulphated macromolecule known as uroheparin is found in the urine after administration of a high dose of heparin (79). The urinary end-products after injection of a low dose are small molecular weight fragments, probably produced by an endoglycosidase located in the kidney. The excretion of high-dose heparin in an intact form suggests that preliminary desulphation is essential for the action of this endoglycosidase.

It is not yet known how much of this catabolic mechanism is applicable to the endogenous heparitins. Using an assay involving competitive binding to protamine, we have recently been able to measure circulating heparitins in human plasma, and undegraded molecules in urine. These heparitins are not active in anticoagulant assays, but undoubtedly have important physiological functions which may be those discussed above, or may be different. We do not yet know whether the circulating heparitins are discarded from the endothelium - which does not appear to metabolise heparin to any significant extent (65) - or derived from another source. These, among other questions, remain to be answered, but the development of an assay which will measure the concentration of such molecules down to 10 ng/ml in biological fluids has opened up extensive new possibilities for the investigation of physiological heparin.

References

1. Rosenberg, R. D.: Seminars Hematol. 14, 427-440 (1977).

2. Jaques, L. B.: Progr. Med. Chem. 5, 139-198 (1967).

3. Clowes, A. W., Karnovsky, M. J.: Nature (London) 265, 625-626 (1977).

4. Eisenstein, R.: Artery 5, 207-221 (1979).

5. Jurgens, R.: Arch. für Pathol. und Pharmakol. 222, 107-111 (1954).

6. Ecker, E. E., Gross, P.: J. Infec. Dis. 44, 250-253 (1929).

7. Lecompte, J., Hughues, J.: Int. Arch. Allergy Appl. Immunol. 5, 367-373 (1954).

8. Miller, T. E., Page, A. R.: Fed. Proc. 22, 225 (1963).

9. Higginbotham, R. D.: Ann. N. Y. Acad. Sci. 73, 186-203 (1958).

10. Cobb, B., Nanson, E. M.: Ann. Surg. 151, 501-506 (1960).

11. Hartman, M. M.: Calif. Med. 98, 27 (1963).

12. Wollin, A., Jaques, L. B.: Can. J. Physiol. Pharmacol. 52, 760-762 (1974).

13. Brown, W. V., Shaw, W., Baginsky, M., Boberg, J., Augustin, J.: Lipoprotein Metabolism, ed. H. Greten, Springer Verlag, Berlin (1976).

14. Olivecrona, T., Bengsston, G., Marklund, V., Lindahl, U., Hook, M.: Fed. Proc. 36, 60-65 (1977).

15. Lindner, H. R., Amsterdam, A., Salomon, Y., Tsafriri, A., Nimrod. A., Lamprecht, S. A., Zor, U., Koch, Y.: J. Reprod. Fert. 51, 215-235 (1977).

16. Kuczenski, R. T., Mandell, A. J.: Neurochem. 19, 131-137 (1972).

17. Horowitz, I. M., Pamer, T., Glass, G. B. J.: Proc. Soc. Exp. Biol. Med. 133, 853-857 (1970).

18. Cook, R. T., Aikawa, M.: Exp. Cell Res. 78, 257-270 (1973).

19. Cruz, W. O., Dietrich, C. P.: Proc. Soc. Exp. Biol. Med. 126, 420-426 (1967).

20. Horn, H.-D., Bruns, F. H.: Deut. Ges. Inn. Med. 68, 407-410 (1959).

21. Scaffrath, D., Stuhlsatz, H. W., Greiling, H.: Physiol. Chem. 357, 499-508 (1976).

22. van Haeringen, N. J.: Thesis, Givan Solst, Amsterdam (1963).

23. Jaques, L. B.: Pharmacol. Rev. 31, 99-166 (1980).

24. Nader, H. B., McDuffie, N. M., Dietrich, C. P.: Biochem. Biophys. Res. Commun. 57, 488-493 (1974).

25. Horner, A. A.: J. Biol. Chem. 246, 231-239 (1971).

26. Ogren, S., Lindahl, U.: Biochem. J. 125, 1119-1129 (1971).

27. Horner, A. A.: Fed. Proc. 36, 35-39 (1977).

28. Jeanloz, R. W.: Arthritis Rheum. 3, 233-237 (1960).

29. Jorpes, J. E., Gardell, S.: J. Biol. Chem. 176, 276 (1948).

30. Lindahl, U., Höök, M.: Ann. Rev. Biochem. 47, 385-417 (1978).

31. McDuffie, N. M.: Heparin Structure, Cellular Functions and Clinical Applications, Academic Press, New York (1979).

32. Ascoli, F., Borte, C., Liquori, A. M.: J. Phys. Chem. 65, 1991-1992 (1961).

33. Lages, B., Stivala, S. S.: Biopolymers 12, 127-143 (1973).

34. Helbert, J. R., Marini, M. A.: Biochemistry 2, 1101-1106 (1963).

35. Otteson, R., Snellman, O.: Acta Chem. Scand. 13, 473-479 (1959).

36. Stone, A. L.: Fed. Proc. 36, 101-106 (1977).

37. Wollin, A., Jaques, L. B.: Thromb. Res. 2, 377-382 (1973).

38. Jaques, L. B., Bruce-Mitford, M., Ricker, A. G.: Rev. Can. Biol. 6, 740-754 (1947).

39. Scott, J. E.: Biochem. Soc. Trans 1, 787-806 (1973).

40. Schmitz, A., Fischer, A.: H. Z. Physiol. Chem. 216, 264-273 (1933).

41. Werle, E., Amann, R.: Naturwissenschaften 42, 583 (1955).

42. Kudryashov, B. A., Kalyshevskaya, T. M., Lyapina, L. A.: Vop. Med. Khim. 14, 277-283 (1969).

43. Higginbotham, R. D.: Texas Rep. Biol. Med. 18, 408-417 (1960).

44. Barlow, G. H., Sanderson, N. D., McNeill, P. D.: Arch Biochem. Biophys. 94, 518-525 (1961).

45. Jaques, L. B.: Biochem. J. 37, 189-195 (1943).

46. Bernfeld, P.: The Amino Sugars, ed. E. Balazs, R. Jeanloz, vol. IIB, Academic Press, New York (1966).

47. Fischer, A.: Biochem. Z. 278, 133-160 (1935).

48. Cohen, S. S.: J. Biol. Chem. 144, 353-361 (1942).

49. Bock, P. E., Luscombe, M., Marshall, S. E., Pepper, D. S., Holbrook, J. J.: Biochem. J. 191, 769-776 (1980).

50. Luscombe, M.; Marshall, S. E., Pepper, D. S., Holbrook, J. J.: In Press.

51. Marshall, S. E., Luscombe, M., Pepper, D. S., Holbrook, J. J.: In Press.

52. Weiss, H. J., Lages, B. A., Witte, L. D., Kaplan, K. L., Goodman, D. S., Nossel, H. L., Baumgartner, H. R.: Thromb. Haemostas. 38, 3 (1977).

53. Holmsen, H.: Biochemistry and Pharmacology of Platelets, Ciba Foundation Symposium 35, Elsevier/Excerpta Medica/North Holland (1975).

54. Solandt, D. Y., Best, C. H.: Lancet 1, 1042-1049 (1940).

55. Chin, H. M., Hirsh, J., Yung, W. L., Regoeczi, E., Gent, M.: Blood 49, 171-184 (1977).

56. Bruhn, H. D., Albert, J. P., Petermann, W.: Med. Klin. 72, 349-352 (1977).

57. Kurachi, K.: J. Biol. Chem. 253, 8301-8302 (1978).

58. Barber, A. J., Käser-Glanzmann, R., Jakabova, M., Luscher, E. F.: Biochim. Biophys. Acta 286, 312-329 (1972).

59. Busch, C., Dawes, J., Pepper, D. S., Wasteson, A.: Thromb. Res. 19, 129-137 (1980).

60. DeLamo, R., McCoy, L. E.: Fed. Proc. 37, 603 (1978).

61. Mahadoo, J., Hiebert, L., Jaques, L. B.: Thromb. Res. 12, 79-90 (1977).

62. Hiebert, L. M., Jaques, L. B.: Artery 2, 26-37 (1976).

63. Sawyer, P. N., Srinavasan, S.: Seventh European Conference on Microcirculation, Karger, Basel (1973).

64. Brown, M. S., Deuel, T. F., Basu, S. K., Goldstein, J. L.: J. Supramol. Structure 8, 223-234 (1978).

65. Glimelius, B., Busch, C., Höök, M.: Thromb. Res. 12, 773-782 (1978).

66. Kjellen, L., Oldberg, A., Höök, M.: J. Biol. Chem. 255, 10407-10413 (1980).

67. Benechemie, G. M. B. H.: SP54 Pentosan Polysulfat. Chemistry, Toxicology, Pharmacokinetics, München (1972).

68. Thomas, D. P., Barrowcliffe, T. W., Merton, R. E., Stocks, J., Dawes, J., Pepper, D. S.: Thromb. Res. 17, 831-840 (1980).

69. Levy, S. W., Jaques, L. B.: Thromb. Res. 13, 429-441 (1978).

70. Dawes, J., Smith, R. C., Pepper, D. S.: Thromb. Res. 12, 851-861 (1978).

71. Yin, E. T., Wessler, S., Butler, J. V.: J. Lab. Clin. Med. 81, 298-310 (1973).

72. Pumphrey, C. W., Pepper, D. S., Dawes, J.: Thromb. Haemostas. 42, 43 (1979).

73. Estes, J. W., Poulin, P. F.: Thromb. Diath, Haemorrh. 33, 26-27 (1974).

74. deSwart, C. A. M., Akkerman, J. W. N., Nijmeijer, A., Sixma, J. J.: Thromb. Haemostas. 38, 84 (1977).

75. Stan, T., Metz, J., Taugner, R.: Naunyn-Schmiedeberg's Arch. Pharmakol. Exp. Pathol. 280, 93-102 (1973).

76. Dawes, J., Pepper, D. S.: Thromb. Res. 14, 845-860 (1979).

77. Friedman, Y., Arsenis, S.: Biochem. J. 139, 699-708 (1974).

78. Oldberg, A., Heldin, C.-H., Wasteson, A., Busch, C., Hook, M.: Biochemistry 19, 5755-5762 (1980).

79. McAllister, B. M., Demis, D. J.: Nature, London 212, 293-294 (1966).

Discussion

Kakkar asked if the release of β-thromboglobulin and platelet factor 4 is heparin dose related.

Dawes explained that β-thromboglobulin is not released at all, only platelet factor 4. The release is dose related up to 2,500 U and then it plateaus. For these studies unfractionated heparin was used.

Kakkar pointed out that there is a different response after a second intravenous injection of heparin (5,000 APTT units, 90 min after the first injection) than when unfractionated or fractionated (low molecular weight) heparin is used. After the injection of unfractionated heparin no further release of platelet factor 4 is observed, whereas after fractionated, low molecular weight heparin, there is a further release of platelet factor 4, which seems to indicate either that the pool of platelet factor 4 was not exhausted or that it was regenerated quickly.

Róka reported on experiments which have shown that for the various proteins which bind to heparin, the heparin affinity is pH dependent except for in the case of thrombin, platelet factor 4 and protamine. A pH range from 9-5 was used.

Dawes confirmed these observations as far as platelet factor 4 and protamine are concerned and suggested that there is a much more specific binding involved in theses cases than one would expect.

In the other cases it is probably a matter of a more general electrostatic interaction. With protamine it is not very surprising but for platelet factor 4 it is a most unusual finding for a protein of such structure to bind to such an extent.

Vertstraete wanted to know what type of heparin was used for the binding studies.

Dawes answered that it was unfractionated pig mucosa heparin obtained from Sigma with a wide range of molecular weight. It had a very high specific activity.

Aronson said that there is a lacuna between the absorption of heparin on the endothelium and its appearance in the liver. He asked what happens after venous injection of heparin.

Dawes is of the opinion that it is a dynamic situation. It appears to be that the catabolic enzymes are located most specifically in the liver and in the spleen. The molecules which end up there are degraded and thus displaced from the equilibrium. The vascular endothelium in general does not appear to catabolize heparin to a considerable extent.

Schmitz-Hübner asked, what is the effect of the complex formation between platelet factor 4 and heparin fractions on their anticoagulatory activity in vitro. He wanted to know if low molecular weight heparin, for instance, is completely neutralized by platelet factor 4, or if it still has anti-Xa activity.

Dawes replied that it is neutralized and does not have anticoagulatory activity.

Rosenberg mentioned his experiments concerning the binding between heparin and platelet factor 4. He used radioactive labelled heparin derivatives to compare the binding of active and inactive fractions. It seems that actually platelet factor 4 does have specificity for the active fractions. The difference is 50 fold for active versus inactive fractions. The binding constant is very high and it seems that in the interaction platelet factor 4 acts on the active site.

Bhargava wanted to know what happens in vivo when platelet factor 4 is released from the endothelium after heparin injection.

Dawes explained that the endothelium becomes more negatively charged. Heparin releases platelet factor 4 from the endothelium and is also bound by platelet factor 4.

Bhargava asked why there is no influence on the thrombin time or APTT by the platelet factor 4 release after the injection of unfractionated heparin.

Dawes answered that there is no effect because only a very small portion of the injected heparin is bound to platelet factor 4. The greatest portion is left over and acts anticoagulatory.
Only about 400 ng of platelet factor 4 per ml plasma are released. Platelet factor 4 and heparin bind in a ratio of 1 : 1. There is plenty of heparin left over.

Schöndorf pointed out that after major operations the β-lipoprotein concentrations are decreased and the heparin concentrations are elevated compared to values before the operation. He asked if anything is known about the dependency of the heparin concentration in plasma on the β-lipoprotein concentration.
This question could not be answered.

Wenzel wondered if there is a rough relationship between the negative charge of the heparin and the platelet factor 4 release.

Dawes said that the density of negative charge is very important and that there is a strong relationship. Platelet factor 4 exhibits a preferential affinity to heparin molecules with the highest density of sulfation.

The second question of *Wenzel* was if it is possible that substances or activities similar to platelet factor 4 are liberated from leucocytes by heparin.

Dawes believes that it is possible, but that there is no evidence.

Duckert asked if after the infusion of inactive heparin it is possible that anticoagulatory active heparin is released from the endothelium.

Dawes thinks that this is possible.

Duckert further asked if *Dawes* thinks that there is heparin on the endothelium.

Dawes answered that as far as endogenous material is concerned, heparin and heparitin are more or less interchangeable. Exactly what it is is not known. There are not two distinct species of molecules but a continuous spectrum. That molecule is attached to the endothelium which has the highest affinity for the receptor. In cultures of endothelial cells, two third of endogenous heparitin can be displaced with heparin. The rest can be released by trypsin. That is the part which is bound covalently to the plasma membrane.

Verstraete asked for the evidence for the statement that platelet factor 4 after injection of heparin is released from the endothelium and not from the platelets.

The first reason *Dawes* mentioned was that after heparin injection platelet factor 4 appears immediately, and that therefore it has to be a contact phenomenon. β-thromboglobulin is not released.
A further reason is that she has been unable to release platelet factor 4 from platelets in vitro by using heparin.
She could show very recently by an immunofluoresence technique that platelet factor 4 is bound to the vascular endothelium and could demonstrate that this is released by heparin.

Verstraete asked for the situation in cell cultures and *Dawes* explained that endothelial cells in culture bind the added platelet factor 4 which can be released by heparin. If heparitin on the surface is destroyed by platelet heparinase, the cells can no longer bind platelet factor 4.
Platelet factor 4 is not synthesized by the endothelial cells. It is continuously released from the platelets and picked up by the endothelium.

Verstraete called this a dangerous idea!

Rosenberg pointed out that there is another potential possibility: platelet factor 4 must not necessarily be bound by normal endothelium but by defective endothelium in the form of a reservoir. This has been shown in animal experiments.

Dawes returned that an argument for the binding of platelet factor 4 to normal endothelium is the very remarkably consistent response of five normal subjects to the injection of heparin. Also three patients with atherosclerosis showed the same response concerning the release of platelet factor 4 as the healthy probands.
Duckert was curious whether turkeys, which develop atherosclerosis very easily, have heparin on the endothelium.

Dawes did not know.

Bhargava agreed that it is very difficult to reconcile that platelet factor 4 derives from the platelets, because it is only a very minute fraction of the amount which is in the platelets. If it really derives from the platelets, the second response to heparin should be observed.

Verstraete wished to know if *Dawes* had measured the platelet factor 4 levels after heparin injection in patients with thrombocytopenia. She said she had not. She had not yet got the patients.

Verstraete further asked if she had injected protamine in an individuum, perhaps Dr. *Pepper,* and subsequently injected heparin to see what happens. These chase experiments have not been performed!

Fabris reported that they have shown that in patients with thrombocytopenia, the release of platelet factor 4 after injection of heparin is very low.

Dawes replied that this could in fact mean either that it is coming from the platelets or that there is less on the endothelium, because there is less in the plasma.

Verstraete wondered about the effect on osteomodulin during long term heparin therapy which influences the calcification mechanism.

Dawes had not treated this aspect in her lecture because she had necessarily made a selection of the great number of possible effects. In addition many have only been shown in vitro.

Verstraete asked if low molecular weight heparin really binds on fibrinogen.

Dawes answered that she believes that in vivo low molecular weight heparin does not bind but only high molecular weight heparin, because there are so many other competing proteins of higher affinity.

Verstraete suggested colaboration with *Kakkar: Kakkar's* group has described that pyridoxal-5-phosphate compound which will prevent 5-hydroxy-tryptamine release. It would be interesting to study platelet factor 4 release in that system and also what would happen to platelet factor 4 release after heparin administration in individuals under long term therapy with this compound.

Kakkar stated that of the real plasma inhibitors (antithrombin III, α_2-macroblobulin and α_1-antitrypsin), antithrombin III has the lowest inhibitory capacity.
He said that one should look into the effect of heparin on the other inhibitors.

Kakkar thought that there is no work about the changes in the kinetics of the other inhibitors in presence of heparin in a purified system.

Rosenberg replied that there are essentially no effects on the other inhibitors in a purified system.

Mechanism of Heparin Rebound and Heparin-Protamine Interactions

Moshe Aronson, Ina Fabian, Ilan Bleiberg
Department of Histology and Cell Biology,
Sackler School of Medicine
Tel-Aviv University,
Ramat Aviv, Israel

Synopsis

Initially the ability of macrophages to degrade heparin was studied, whereupon it was found that both uptake and desulphation of heparin by macrophages were greatly enhanced in the presence of protamine. Next, the phenomenon of heparin-rebound was investigated, revealing that enzymic digestion of protamine occurred in the presence of plasma. Subsequent attempt to identify the plasma enzymes responsible for this proteolysis of protamine, demonstrated that plasmin-like enzymes were involved. Finally, the effect of protamine and other polycations on heparin uptake by macrophages was studied and shown to be largely dependent on charge neutralization. Gaps in the knowledge concerning the fate of heparin and heparin-protamine complexes in the body are discussed.

Introduction

The problem of heparin rebound was tackled at the suggestion of Dr. U. Seligsohn, who was briefed by us on our studies on heparin uptake by macrophages in the presence of protamine. These two avenues of research, namely heparin rebound and heparin uptake, at first ran in parallel but lately appear to be converging insofar as our findings with macrophages in tissue culture seem to shed some light on the mechanism of heparin rebound.

Heparin · New Biochemical and Medical Aspects

These two topics will be treated herein separately and not in a chronological order. Rather we shall attempt to delineate the germination rationale of our investigation, and then review our findings, evaluating in some depth the present status of our knowledge on the subject.

A. Uptake of Heparin by Macrophages in the Presence of Protamine and other Polycations

The present study was initiated as part of a systematic investigation of the interactions between eosinophils and mast cell components. Knowing that eosinophils tend to accumulate in large quantities wherever degranulation of mast cells takes place (1), we set out to ascertain whether eosinophils could possibly deactivate such components of mast cell granules, as histamine, serotonin and heparin. Although no such deactivation by eosinophils was observed (2, 3), we were fortunate in including other inflammatory cells for comparison purposes, because we found that (extracts of) macrophages, in particular, showed heparin desulphation activity (4).

This finding tied in with the fact that in areas of mast cell degranulation, not only eosinophils but also macrophages are abundant, and they, too, phagocytose the granules (1). We realized, however, that the release of a powerful agent like heparin may require a much faster neutralization action than can be achieved by uptake and desulphation alone. Aware that eosinophils possess a high amount of basic protein (5), we speculated whether this substance might rapidly neutralize the anticoagulatory action of heparin, while and in a second slower stage, the heparin would be desulphated by macrophages. Our investigation of this point indeed showed that the eosinophil basic protein greatly enhanced both the uptake and the desulphation of heparin by mouse macrophages. Various other basic proteins and polyaminoacids obviously including also protamine, were next investigated and the findings (6, 7) can be summarized as follows:

1. Protamine, histones (whether crude, arginine-rich, or lysine-rich), poly-DL-lysine, poly-L-ornithine, and the eosinophil basic protein - all greatly stimulated uptake of heparin by cultured macrophages.
2. The boost in uptake owing to the various polycations (as compared to

that of free heparin) ranged between 8-50 fold and occurred in the following order of decreasing uptake: L-ornithine = poly-DL-lysine > protamine > histones > eosinophil basic protein.

3. The monomers of the poly aminoacids, namely, L-ornithine and DL-lysine, enhanced heparin uptake only very slightly.

4. Serum interfered considerably with heparin uptake (as compared to that by macrophages maintained in M199 + lactate), which posed the question as to which serum proteins heparin was bound to *in vivo.*

5. The extent of desulphation was entirely unrelated to heparin uptake, the highest values being obtained by protamine and histone complexes (up to 60 % desulphation).

6. The foregoing findings are consistent with the hypothesis that heparin has to be dissociated from the polycation, presumably by lysosomal enzymes, prior to desulphation. This is supported also by our further finding that all the mentioned polycations inhibit the desulphation of heparin by macrophage extracts.

It has not been established from the summarized experiments whether heparin becomes internalized or rather both the binding and desulphation are restricted to the cell outer membrane.

The nature of the stimulus for the increased uptake effected by the polycations has yet to be clarified. Polycations are known to potentiate membrane activity (8, 9), but they could possibly enhance uptake also by neutralizing the negative charges of heparin.

B. Binding and Internalization of Heparin-Protamine by Mouse Macrophages

1. In this part of our study we investigated quantitative aspects of the enhancing effect of protamine (and other polycations) on heparin uptake. We conjectured that if the polycations exert their effects by stimulating membrane activity, then an excess of polycations over heparin should result in increased uptake. If, however, neutralization of heparin is the mechanism responsible, then to obtain maximal uptake there should be for any given

concentration of heparin a corresponding concentration of polycation, while the effect of polycation excess should be rather minimal. The relationship should thus be linear, meaning that a doubling or quadrupling of the heparin concentration should require doubling or quadrupling the polycation, with consequent doubling or quadrupling of the uptake.

2. Another question investigated was the possible internalization of the drug, that is whether the heparin is indeed taken up and undergoes desulphation within the cell.

This was studied by chasing experiments whereby an excess of *cold* heparin was added to macrophages pretreated with the *hot* agent. The chasing experiments were conducted both with free- and polycation-complexed heparin. In all cases chasing was done both at 37 °C as well as at 4 °C, because at the latter temperature only electrostatic binding of heparin can occur, with no uptake dependent on metabolic reactions.

3. Also tackled by us were methodological considerations as, for instance, the effect of heparin precipitates. Insofar as some of the polycations form insoluble complexes with heparin, it is conceivable that uptake of heparin by macrophages could entail mainly the phagocytosis of such precipitate particles. This possibility was investigated both directly as well as by a preparative technique wihich mostly prevented the formation of precipitates. Use was made of the fact that heparin and histones form soluble complexes at low and insoluble complexes at high concentrations. The chasing experiments were consequently conducted with both these types of histone complexes. Results of these experiments (10) can be summarized as follows:

a) The various polycations (protamine, histones, poly-DL-lysine, polyornithine) do exert small, specific effects, but charge neutralization seems to be mainly responsible for the enhancement of heparin uptake by macrophages. Once an *optimal ratio* between heparin and a polycation is ascertained, it becomes possible to predict quite accurately the extent of uptake expected on increase of the one, the other or both reactants. Supplementary electrophoretic studies showed that at the *optimal ratio* very little heparin migrated from the application point, whereas at half the optimal amount of protamine, about 60-70 % of the heparin migrated along the gel.

b) Most of the heparin, whether free or polycation-bound, can be removed by chasing, provided that its exposure to the cells has taken place in the cold. In marked contrast, with cells which had been incubated with the labelled heparin at 37 °C, only a minute part of the heparin could be exchanged by chasing.

c) Results of the chasing experiments with soluble and insoluble forms of heparin histones, although not consistently identical, were nonetheless in the same general direction. There was certainly no need to postulate that uptake is mediated via phagocytosis of particles (albeit the possibility that precipitates are formed on the cells' membrane cannot be easily excluded experimentally).

The outlined results suggest that at least two stages occur in the uptake of heparin by macrophages. These entail:

(1) A rapid stage which takes place in the cold, is reversible, and is based on electrostatic binding of the free or complexed heparin to the cell membranes; and

(2) a slow stage requiring active metabolism and resulting in heparin internalization.

C. Heparin Rebound

The phenomenon of heparin rebound has been familiar for the past 25 years (11). Clinicians administering protamine to patients pretreated with heparin in order to neutralize the drug, observed that while initially the blood behaved in its *pre-heparin* manner, it occasionally reverted to a hypocoagulable state. This effect has been ascribed to the re-appearance of free heparin and occurs several hours after the protamine injection, but opinions differ widely concerning its etiology, thus reflecting our basic ignorance of the fate of heparin and heparin-protamine complexes in the body. The following mechanisms as compiled by Ellison et al. (12) have been proposed to explain the phenomenon: Heparin is released by erythrocytic breakdown (13); heparin escapes from the circulation into the extra-vascular space and returns via the lymphatics following protamine clearance (14); heparin is neutralized by an unknown endogenous antagonist, which eventually is cleared from the blood (15); and finally, protamine may be removed by metabolism (16).

At the start of our investigation we were not aware that Frick and Brogli (17) had already reproduced the phenomenon under *in vitro* conditions and that they even speculated, albeit without experimental proof, that the protamine was inactivated or destroyed by a plasma enzyme. Hence we initially again demonstrated that the phenomenon can be obtained *in vitro*, and thereafter proceeded to establish (18) that:

1. Upon incubation of protamine (whether free or complexed with heparin) with plasma at 37 °C, the neutralizing activity is largely abolished (the incubation mixture contained 400 µg protamine and 4 U heparin/ml).
2. Incubation of the above mixture in the presence of the known proteinase inhibitor diisopropyl fluorophosphate (DFP) prevented the abrogation of the neutralizing ability of protamine.
3. On electrophoresis the protamine spot disappeared following incubation of protamine in plasma at 37 °C, with DFP again exerting an interfering effect.

These results suggested that heparin rebound is caused by resurgence of free heparin in the circulation following the enzymic degradation of protamine. They also pointed to the advisability of using relatively high concentrations of protamine in clinical application for neutralizing heparin. Indeed, Ellison et al. (12) have already shown that at low dose protamine (average protamine: heparine ratio 0.56), there were occasional cases of heparin rebound, whereas patients receiving higher doses (average ratio - 1.15) did not exhibit this phenomenon. One should bear in mind, however, that protamine excess in itself may be toxic and cause a state of hypocoagulability.

Our study left several important questions unanswered, to wit: which plasma enzymes acted on the protamine; whether protamine could be supplanted by other neutralizing agents, and whether protamine could possibly be fractionated so that one of the fractions would be more suitable for neutralization.

D. Possible Protamine Substitutes

As already mentioned, our search for protamine substitutes stemmed from the requirement for a very precise neutralization of heparin by protamine in which either too little or too much protamine proves detrimental. An additional incitement was the fact that patients with a history of allergy to fish may become hypersensitive to protamine (19). Our previous work evinced the possibility that histones may prove to be good protamine substitutes. We also investigated poly-DL-lysine and poly-L-ornithine as representing synthetic polymers (despite their putative unsuitability owing to toxicity and precipitability, respectively).

Our results (20) can be summarized as follows:

1. So far as neutralization is concerned, histones were found to neutralize the anticoagulatory action of heparin, but larger quantities of these compounds were needed than of protamine.
2. Administered in excess, histones also exerted an anticoagulatory effect.
3. Under conditions extant during clinical work, the binding and desulphation of heparin by macrophages proceeded much better in the presence of protamine than of histone.
4. As for heparin rebound, this was obtained also with histones, which were degraded by incubation with plasma.
5. Poly-DL-lysin showed a wider neutralization range than did protamine.

While these results indicate the superiority of protamine over histones on every count, they nevertheless show promise that the search for synthetic polymers, as protamine substitutes, may ultimately prove rewarding.

E. Fractionation of Protamine

Protamine comprise a family of closely related peptides, and it was thought worthwhile to explore the possibility that one of the fractions may present a better neutralization profile. Recently we obtained (B. Moav, I. Fabian and M. Aronson - unpublished results) four fractions by employing Ando and Watanebe's technique (21), which relies on CM-Sephadex C-25 columns.

The four fractions were tested for heparin neutralization by the APTT test, but since all behaved indentically in respect to heparin neutralization, this approach was deemed unprofitable.

F. Characterization of the Plasma Enzyme(s) Involved in Protamine Degradation

We have recently commenced studying the protaminolysis which takes place in the plasma, attempting to identify the enzyme(s) involved. Our previous finding that protamine degradation is inhibited by DFP tended to implicate trypsin-like enzyme(s) with an active serine group. By use of several specific inhibitors and through a screening of potential candidates in the plasma, we were able to obtain a rough preliminary characterization of the enzyme(s). As this study is not yet completed (D. Benayahu and M. Aronson - unpublished results) our conclusions are perforce partial and tentative. Nonetheless, results so far may be summarized as follows:

1. There is considerable difference in the protaminolytic activity of plasma from various healthy donors. (One plasma specimen was practically devoid of this activity.) We are now trying to correlate protaminolytic activity with the known clinical condition of patients.
2. Kinetics of protamine degradation *in vitro*, under conditions resembling the clinical situation, were determined both by electrophoresis and by the APTT test. Surprisingly enough the results were similar, the neutralizing ability of protamine disappearing within 5-17 hours.
3. Treatment of the plasma with celite, which removes from it both factor XI and factor XII (22), did not alter its ability to degrade protamine.
4. Three specific inhibitors, namely, N-p-tosyl-L-lysine chloromethylketone HC1 (TLCK); trans-4-(amino methyl cyclohexane carboxylic acid (AMCH); and E-amino caproic acid (EACA) were evaluated for their effect on protamine digestion. The first is a known inhibitor of trypsin-like enzymes, while the latter two are specific for both trypsin and plasma. Our evaluation revealed a much stronger inhibition by TLCK than by the other two inhibitors. However, TLCK did not exert the same degree of inhibition in all the tested plasmas. These results are interpreted by us as follows:

a) several plasma enzymes can degrade protamine and they seem to exist in varying proportions in healthy individuals.

b) Plasmin is not the main protaminolytic enzyme.

c) In surgical cases plasmin supplements the factor existing in normal plasma.

It should be noted in this connection that the conclusion that plasmin is not the main plasma factor responsible for protamine degradation has already been reached by Amris in 1962 (23). This author, who investigated protaminase activity of serum and plasma (without relating to the heparin rebound problem) presented solid evidence against plasmin being important in the protaminolytic system in that he found very little plasmin activity in normal plasma, and little difference in protaminase activity between plasma and serum. Recently, I. Blass and associates (personal communication) have provided good experimental evidence that the protaminase activity of plasma can be ascribed, at least in the first hours of incubation, to carboxy-peptidase N - an enzyme described by Erdös et al. (24).

G. Fate of Heparin and Heparin-Protamine in the Body: A Precautionary Note

In the course of our investigation, we came to realize that in order to gain full insight on the heparin rebound phenomenon, we must first elucidate the fate of heparin and heparin-protamine in the body. Search in the literature for studies on the pharmacokinetics of heparin in the body yielded but few useful conclusions. In a recent comprehensive review, Jaques (25) enumerates the difficulties which hamper our understanding of what really happens to heparin in the body. One of the main difficulties is that the measurement of radioactivity is not necessarily consonant with measurement of heparin. Lately, Shanberge's group described *in vivo* effect of protamine administration on heparin clearance in rats (26).

Recently, we (H. Allon, I. Bleiberg, I. Fabian and M. Aronson - unpublished results) started a pilot study in which heparin clearance from the blood stream of mice was compared in the absence and presence of protamine (the latter agent injected one minute after the first). Results showed that:

1. Following i. v. injection of tagged heparin, there was a rapid clearance of radioactivity from the blood.

2. Clearance in the presence of protamine was faster.

3. Accumulation of radioactivity in the liver was faster in the presence of protamine.

4. A heparin rebound effect was obtained in the protamine-injected animals within several hours after the protamine injection.

The above experiments were carried out with mice which were bled only onec because we feared that successive withdrawal of blood from a small animal might affect the blood volume and distort the results. Subsequently, and for economic reasons, we did bleed our animals 4 times in the course of each experiment, and obtained different results from the afore-described. Furthermore, there were considerable differences between mice of the same group. It seems that the repeated wounding of the animals resulted not only in blood volume effects but also in the appearance of coagulation factors. Conceivably the cumulative effect of 4 woundings in an animal of small blood volume (2 ml) is not inconsiderable (from the standpoint of coagulatory and fibrinolytic factors). As, unfortunately, in Shanberge's article (26) the fluctuation of results within the same group is not given, it is not clear whether these workers encountered the same problem.

At this stage two conclusions are inevitable, namely:

1. That the significance of heparin and protamine titration is closely tied to an understanding of the specific conditions prevailing in the patient (or animal).

2. That interpretation of clearance data must be undertaken with utmost caution.

Discussion

Is it possible to integrate all the available data on heparin rebound and heparin-protamine interaction into a coherent working hypothesis? The answer, unfortunately, is no, because a formidable gap still exists in our understanding of the pharmacokinetics and clearance of heparin and heparin-protamine in the body. The half-life of heparin in the bloodstream is about 90 minutes, and it is known to become bound both the endothelial cells and to the RES. The exterior of cells onto which heparin binds has negative charge, as for instance the heparan sulphate of the endothelium and of the glycocalyx of many cells. It is even claimed that heparin may replace some of this endothelial heparin (27). The glomerular basement membrane which serves as the filtration barrier in the kidney, also contains numerous heparan sulphate groups, whose role is to repel electrostatically the plasma proteins (28), the majority of which are negatively charged. It would be reasonable to assume that heparin associates with certain plasma proteins in order to transport or bind to cells, or to cross the glomerular filter. It is not yet known which plasma proteins serve as heparin carriers (29). Although antithrombin III has a high affinity for heparin, it was shown not to be the heparin-binding protein of plasma (30). It is quite possible, however, that with the appearance of coagulation factors in the plasma, heparin becomes bound to the antithrombin III-thrombin complex. In this connection it is of interest that Rosenberg and Damus (31) have shown that heparin is not regenerated by its neutralization with protamine. Additionally we believe that in our experiments on the elimination of heparin and heparin-protamine from the bloodstream of mice, the discrepancy in results between animals bled only once and those bled 4 times is quite pertinent. Work is now in progress in our laboratory on heparin uptake by mouse macrophages in the presence of antithrombin III and antithrombin III-thrombin complex.

As for the rebound phenomenon, assumedly we are dealing both with circulating heparin and with that part of the cell bound heparin that can return to the circulation (although we are quite ignorant of why, where, and when the latter event occurs). A further assumption is that our *in vitro* experiments with mouse macrophages can be taken at face value as representing the *in vivo* situation of the RES in man.

Having made these two assumptions, we are now in a position to suggest several possible explanations which independently or perhaps cooperatively may shed light on what happens when protamine is injected into heparin-treated patients. We belive that any or all of the following takes place:

1. The protamine brings back cell-bound heparin into the circulation.

2. The protamine stimulates heparin ingestion by the RES cells.

3. The protamine is first adsorbed on the negatively-charged glycocalyx and then it binds the circulating heparin, thus forming a bridge between the two SO_4^{--} containing polyanions. Following digestion of the protamine by the plasma enzymes (and also by plasmin in the appropriate cases), heparin is released once more into the circulation.

It would be difficult to visually confirm the second possibility insofar as it entails uptake of protamine-heparin, digestion of the former and exocytosis of the latter without desulphation (which results in loss of the anticoagulatory activity).

We know from the clinical data that heparin rebound may occur when insufficient amount of protamine is given, but never when present in excess (12). This seems to rule out the first possibility, because more protamine should re-introduce even more heparin.

It is conceivable that with lower concentrations of protamine, an extracellular bridge is formed, which binds the heparin, albeit only temporarily - until the protamine is digested. With higher protamine concentrations the heparin is taken up intracellularly and is desulphated. This conjecture is also consistent with our finding that uptake into macrophages is comprised of 2 steps: adherence and internalization. Since the internalization stage is a slow one, protamine should be available in sufficient excess to serve both for charge neutralization and for replenishment of that part which is digested before internalization is completed.

References

1. Mann, P. R.: J. Path. 98, 183-187 (1969).

2. Fabian, I., Aronson, M.: J. Reticuloendothel. Soc. 17, 145-150 (1975).

3. Fabian, I., Aronson, M.: Biochem. Pharmacol. 27, 1909-1911 (1978).

4. Fabian, I., Bleiberg, I., Aronson, M.: Biochem. Biophys. Acta 437, 122-128 (1976).

5. Gleich, G. J., Loeyering, D. A., Maldonado, I. E.: J. Exp. Med. 137, 1459-1471 (1973).

6. Fabian, I., Bleiberg, I., Aronson, M.: Biochem. Biophys. Acta 544, 69-76 (1978).

7. Fabian, I., Bleiberg, I., Aronson, M.: In: Macrophages and Lymphocytes Part A. Edited by M. Escobar and H. Friedman, Plenum Publ. Corp., 175-182 (1980).

8. De Vries, A., Salgo, Y., Matoth, A., Nevo, A., Katchalski, E.: Arch. Int. Pharmacodyn. 104, 1-8 (1955).

9. Ryser, H. J. P., Hancock, R.: Science 150, 501-503 (1965).

10. Bleiberg, I., Fabian, I., Aronson, M.: Biochem. Biophys Acta 674, 345-353 (1981).

11. Kalff, W. J., Effler, D. B., Groves, L. K. et al.: Clev. Clin. Q. 23, 69-78 (1956).

12. Ellison, N., Beatty, P. C., Blake, D. R., Wurzel, H. A., Mac Vaugh III, H.: J. Thor. Cardiovasc. Surg. 67, 723-729 (1974).

13. Dodrill, F. D., Marshall, N., Nyboer, J., Hughes, C. H., Derbyshine, A. S., Stearns, A. B.: J. Thorac. Surg. 33, 60-70 (1957).

14. Schreiner, R.: Discussion of Nakamoto, S. and Holmes, J. H.: Our experience in regional heparinization. Trans. Am. Soc. Artif. Intern. Organs 4, 36-37 (1958).

15. Perkins, H. A., Acra, D. I., Rolfs, M. R.: Blood 18, 807-815 (1961).

16. Hyun, B. H., Pence, R. E., Davila, J. C., Butcher, J., Custer, R. P.: Surg. Gynecol. Obst. 115, 191-198 (1962).

17. Frick, P. G., Brögli, H.: Surgery 59, 721-726 (1966).

18. Fabian, I., Aronson, M.: Thromb. Res. 18, 535-542 (1980).

19. Caplan, S. N., Berkaman, E. M.: New Engl. J. Med. 295, 172-173 (1976).

20. Fabian, I., Aronson, M.: Thromb. Res. 17, 239-247 (1980).

21. Ando, T., Watanabe, S.: Int. J. Prot. Res. 1, 221-224 (1969).

22. Nossel, H. L., Niemetz, J., Mibashan, R. S., Schulze, W. G.: Brit. J. Haematol. 12, 133-144 (1966).

23. Amris, C. J.: Scand. J. Clin. Lab. Invest. 14, 105-116 (1962).

24. Erdös, E. G., Sloane, E. M., Wohler, J. R.: Biochem. Pharm. 13, 893-905 (1964).

25. Jaques, L. B.: Pharmacol. Rev. 31, 99-167 (1979).

26. Kitani, T., Nagarajan, S. C., Shanberge, J. N.: Thromb. Res. 17, 375-382 (1980).

27. Mahadoo, J., Jaques, L. B.: Med. Hypot. 5, 835-841 (1979).

28. Kanwar, Y. S., Farquhar, M. G.: Proc. Natl. Acad. Sci 76, 4493-4497 (1979).

29. Takeda, Y., Kobayashi, N.: Thrombos. Haemos. 38, 685-695 (1977).

30. Marciniak, E.: J. Lab. Clin. Med. 84, 344-356 (1974).

31. Rosenberg, R. D., Damus, P. S.: J. Biol. Chem. 248, 6490-6505 (1973).

Discussion

Rosenberg wonders about the statement that carboxypeptidase is the enzyme which degrades protamine and thus breakes the binding to heparin. Carboxypeptidase only cleaves a few amino acid residues from the C-terminal end of the molecule and thus makes this interaction less likely. It seems curious because that would imply that the binding site is in the C-terminal region. Might there be an analogy to the C-terminal part of platelet factor 4?

Aronson replied that he had not conducted the work himself but had quoted the studies of Erdös, which presented evidence in favour of this enzyme.

The studies of Erdös were performed at 30 °C and those of Aronson at 37 °C. This should not make a difference, but there might be one.

A convincing argument for carboxypeptidase is also that a great amount of arginine is split off.

Duckert mentioned that Frick and coworkers (Zurich) had already suggested some time ago that there is a digesting enzyme in plasma.

During the discussion it was pointed out that the rebound phenomenon is only observed with protamine sulfate and not with protamine chloride. The function of protamine sulfate is quite different from that of protamine chloride.

This does not reconcile with the observations of Aronson. He is of the opinion that it may not be the difference between sulfate and chloride but a difference in the source of the protamines used.

Duckert reported on experiments with protamines of the same source, in which only perotamine sulfate showed the rebound phenomenon.

Aronson would not believe these differences.

Duckert mentioned that his opinion is also proven by the clinical observations that using protamine chloride, there is no rebound.

Aronson replied that it might be a question of quantity.

Duckert said that in haemodialysis it is difficult to neutralize heparin by protamine sulfate, because heparin appears again. Using the same amount of protamine chloride there are no problems at all.

Verstraete confirmed Duckert's observations and told that they used protamine of the same source as chloride and sulfate and could not reconcile the hypothesis of Aronson with protamine chloride. They in addition have the same clinical experience as Duckert.

Verstraete raised the following point: The clinicians have observed that in patients with acidosis the rebound phenomenon much more readily occurs. It might be that the dissociation of protamine and heparin is more rapid in an acidotic milieu.

Witt suggested that there may be pH-dependency of the catabolizing enzyme. *Verstraete* confirmed this suggestion.

Kakkar reported about a paper in Lancet (T. K. Day, Nov. 10, 1979) some months ago which described the fractionation of protamine. Two fractions were obtained which behaved differently. One fraction had a definite anticoagulatory activity.

Wenzel asked about the heparin uptake stimulating factor of histones, if it is again a question of the charge.

Aronson agreed.

Wenzel mentioned experiments of his laboratory with histones and basic proteins from the nuclei of leucocytes. There were differences in the action between arginine- and lysine-rich fractions.

Aronson confirmed that they found differences between arginine- and lysine-rich fragments in former experiments. In his later experiments he employed only crude histone fractions so that from these experiments he cannot say anything about differences of the fractions concerning charge neutralization.

Spaethe reported that in cases with open heart surgery, there was no rebound if the heparin was neutralized with a large amount of protamine. When only small amounts of protamine were given, rebound was seen beginning about three hours after operation. Then heparin could be measured again. So the conclusion must be that one has to give large amounts of protamine. On the other hand there is an inhibitory influence of protamine on coagulation. He wonders if it is possible that protamine has an influence on the antithrombin-thrombin binding capacity. This has been claimed in the literature. Also an influence on the fibrin polymerisation has been described.

Aronson said that his point was that one has to neutralize heparin very carefully, too much or too little protamine is not good.

Róka raised the question concerning the cellular pool of heparin. He wanted to know about binding of heparin to laminine. He had heard that laminine has a high affinity to heparin and asked if this could be some kind of heparin pool in the cell which can regulate the amount of heparin available in plasma.

Aronson replied that one can find laminine in the basement membrane. The fact that one finds so many heparin sulfate groups in the kidney speaks for this hypothesis.

Verstraete reported Motulsky's results that if the heparin effect is measured by the inhibition of factor Xa, 20 % of this activity cannot be neutralized by protamine. This could explain some of the bleedings that are seen although the in vitro tests seem to satisfy the requirements.

Aronson did not comment directly on this problem. His group is trying with their system to see whether one can have uptake of heparin in the cells, perhaps on antithrombin-thrombin. They intend also to consider other factors which are involved in heparin uptake to find out which of the plasma proteins heparin actually binds to naturally.

II. Methods for the Determination of Heparin

Overview on Methods for the Determination of Heparin

Irene Witt
Biochemisches Labor
Kinderklinik der Universität Freiburg i. Br.

After the discovery of heparin in 1916 by McLean (1) and the demonstration of its anticoagulatory effect by Howell in 1918 (2), it was introduced for routine clinical use as an anticoagulant in the 1930s.

The first methods for measuring the heparin content of preparations were established in 1924 by Howell (3). They were based on the inhibition of the coagulation of fresh whole blood.

A modification of this whole blood method in which the blood is preserved by sodium sulfate and bovine brain thromboplastin is added to the assay was later accepted as the official method of the British Pharmacopoeia.

This modification allows the blood to be stored below +4 °C for several weeks, and the addition of thromboplastin reduces the coagulation time considerably and makes the end-point sharper.

Also citrated or oxalated blood or plasma was used to determine the influence of heparin. The method of Reinert and Winterstein, who in 1938 (4) used citrated sheep plasma to measure the influence of heparin on the coagulation time after recalcification, was finally accepted as the official method of the US Pharmacopoeia.

The methods using fresh whole blood may well reflect the biological activity of heparin. They are said to have a very good reproducibility, but they are not at all suited for routine assays.

Heparin · New Biochemical and Medical Aspects

Printed in Germany

Today the most common assays for measuring the influence of heparin are the activated partial thromboplastin time (APTT) and the Thrombin Time (TT).

The APTT method belongs to the assays which measure the overall influence of the anticoagulant on whole blood or plasma. The APTT was first introduced by Langdell in 1953 (5). The test was later modified by the addition of an activator, such as kaolin or celite, which accelerates the partial thromboplastin time.

The principle of the test is as follows: The addition of partial thromboplastin, calcium-ions and an activator such as kaolin to the plasma sample activates the intrinsic system. The APTT depends on the activity of factor XII, factor XI, IX, X, V, VIII and prothrombin. At present, the APTT seems to be the best suited clotting method for monitoring heparin therapy.

Because wide differences exist between different partial thromboplastins in their sensitivity to the anticoagulant effect of heparin, only standardised reagents with good heparin sensitivity should be used. The disadvantage of the APTT is that it is influenced by fibrinogen degradation products (FDP), by activity changes in clotting factors not caused by heparin and the impossibility of distinguishing between the action of heparin and that of oral anticoagulants. In addition the APTT cannot differentiate in the regions of very low and very high heparin concentrations.

The thrombin time belongs to the type of tests which measure the inactivation rate of specific clotting proteases. Thrombin methods were first introduced in 1941 by Jaques and Charles (6). Later many modifications were employed. The principle is that thrombin is added to the plasma to be analysed and the clotting time is measured.

The thrombin time has proven a useful test for monitoring heparin. One criticism of the test is that its relationship to heparin level is only linear over a small heparin dosage range. In addition the thrombin time is not only influenced by heparin but also to a considerable degree by FDP.

Further methods for measuring the specific inactivation of a single protease were introduced in 1973 by Denson and Bonnar (7) and also by Yin et al. (8): the anti-Xa assay. Two modifications exist. Both are two stage assays, which are very sensitive even at low heparin concentrations.

But they are also affected by the presence of high levels of FDP. They are very time consuming and expensive and therefore not suited for routine analysis.

The possibility of neutralizing heparin with protamine was first described in 1938 by Chargaff and Olson (9).

In 1953 Preston and Parker (10) introduced polybrene as a heparin neutralizer.

There are many modifications of the titration assays. The residual heparin, after the addition of protamine or polybrene to the test system, can be measured either by the thrombin clotting time of the APTT.

Although in 1980 a new variation has been described by Talstad (11) using the estimation of residual heparin by a photometric assay with S-2222, these methods ar too cumbersome for routine use. In addition they are very imprecise.

The first method for the photometric determination of heparin with a chromogenic substrate was described by Teien in 1976 (12).

At present three photometric heparin assays are commercially available.

The Kabi Coatest is a development from the method of Teien. The principle is the measurement of the inhibitory action of the antithrombin-heparin-complex against factor Xa. In this method exogenous antithrombin is added to the test system. In general this principle is said to measure the heparin concentration of a plasma sample.

The Boehringer test kit for the determination of heparin was developed by Bartl and Lill in 1979 (13). The principle of this system is the measurement of the inhibitory action of the antithrombin-heparin-complex against thrombin.

In this method no exogenous antithrombin is added to the test system. Therefore the heparin measured strongly depends on the antithrombin concentration in the analysed plasma sample and actually measures the heparin activated antithrombin.

The heparin assay of Merz and Dade, which was developed by Mitchell et al. in 1978 (14) follows the principle of the other tests, but instead of a chromogenic substrate a fluorogenic substrate is used. The inhibitory action of the antithrombin-heparin-complex against thrombin is measured. Exogenous antithrombin is added to the test system.

A great advantage of the photometric tests is their specificity in measuring the influence of heparin, but they still have difficulties.

Some of the problems of the photometric test systems are that standard curves have to be performed daily, that for standards the same heparin preparation should be used as for the treatment of the patient and that for low and high concentration ranges different standard curves are needed.

Although many techniques for the evaluation of the therapeutic action of heparin have been described, the ideal test hast not yet been found.

Possibilities for Measuring Heparin

1. General Clotting Assays

   Fresh Whole Blood Clotting Time

   Modification: Preservation by sodium sulfate and addition of bovine brain thromboplastin → British Pharmacopoeia (B.P.)

   Whole Blood or Plasma Recalcification Time

   Citrated sheep plasma → US Pharmacopoeia (U.S.P.)

   (Activated) Partial Thromboplastin Time

2. Specific Protease Inactivation Assays

   Anti-activated Factor X Assay

   Thrombin Time

3. Titration Assays

   Protamine Titration Assay

   Polybrene Titration Assay

4. Photometric Assays with Chromogenic or Fluorogenic Substrates

   Inactivation of Factor X a with Addition of Antithrombin

   Inactivation of Thrombin without Addition of Antithrombin

References

1. McLean, J., Amer. J. Physiol. 41, 250 (1916)
2. Howell, W. H., Holt, E., Amer. J. Physiol. 47, 328 (1918)
3. Howell, W. H., Amer. J. Physiol. 71, 553 (1924)
4. Reinert, M., Winterstein, A., Arch. Int. Pharmacodyn. 62, 47 (1939)
5. Langdell, R. D., Wagner, R. H., Brinkhaus, K. M., J. Lab. Clin. Med. 41, 637 (1953)
6. Jacques, L. B., Charles, A. F., Quart. J. Pharm. Pharmacol. 14, 1 (1941)
7. Denson, K. W. E., Bonnar, J., Thromb. Diath. haemorrhag. 30, 471 (1973)
8. Yin, E. T., Wessler, S., Butler, J., J. Lab. Clin. Med. 81, 298 (1973)
9. Chargaff, G., Olson, K. B., J. Biol. Chem. 122, 1958 (1938)
10. Preston, F. W., Parker, R. P., Arch. Surg. 66, 545 (1953)
11. Talstad, J., Thromb. Res. 18, 485 (1980)
12. Teien, A. N., Lie, M., Abildgaard, U., Thromb. Res. 8, 413 (1976)
13. Bartl., K., Dorsch, E., Lill, H., Ziegenhorn, J., Thrombos. Haemostas. 42, 1446 (1979)
14. Mitchell, G. A., Gargiulo, R. J., Huseby, R. M., Lawson, D. E., Pochron, S. P., Sehuanes, J. A., Thromb. Res. 13, 47 (1978)

Control of Heparin Therapy by Measurement of the Antithrombin III-Heparin-Complex

Properties of the Boehringer Mannheim Heparin Assay.

Helmut Lill
Beoehringer Mannheim GmbH
Biochemical Research Center Tutzing
D-8132 Tutzing, Germany

Summary

A method for determining the biological activity of heparin in plasma using thrombin and the substrate Tos-Gly-Pro-Arg-pNA (chromozym® TH) is described. The procedure is based on the photometric determination of the inactivation of thrombin after incubation with the plasma sample. In other assays, heparin concentration in plasma is measured with excess AT III added to the sample. Contrary to those methods, in our assay system the addition of pooled plasma or of purified AT III is omitted. This results in heparin exerting its inhibitory effect only via the amount of AT III already present in the sample. As can be shown, heparin-induced thrombin inhibition depends strongly on the antithrombin III level present in the plasma.

Introduction

A variety of different methods exists for the measurement of heparin in plasma. Whether factor Xa or thrombin are used with chromogenic peptide substrates (Teien et al., 1976; Witt, 1977; Bartl et al., 1979), however, the main difference between all methods is whether exogenous antithrombin III (AT III) is added to the assay or not.

Heparin · New Biochemical and Medical Aspects

Thus if purified AT III or pooled plasma containing AT III are added to the system, the rate of thrombin- or Xa-inhibition becomes independent of the AT III-concentration in the plasma sample. In this way only the heparin concentration will be measured, and no reference to the in vivo formation of AT III · heparin-complex can be obtained.

The heparin assay presented here does not use exogenous AT III. Therefore not simply heparin concentration, but the actual AT III · heparin-complex in its in vivo state is measured. As AT III is the basis for the heparin-induced anticoagulant potential of the blood, AT III · heparin-complex must be considered the main parameter of interest in the monitoring of heparin therapy.

Properties of the Boehringer Mannheim Heparin Assay

[AT-III · heparin] + thrombin (excess) → [AT-III · heparin · thrombin] + residual thrombin

Tos-Gly-Pro-Arg-pNA + H_2O $\xrightarrow{\text{thrombin}}$ Tos-Gly-Pro-Arg-OH + p-nitroaniline

Fig. 1. Measurement of the AT III · heparin-complex; principle

AT III · heparin-complex already present in the plasma sample reacts with bovine thrombin, which is added in excess. Residual thrombin activity is measured at 405 nm, using the substrate chromozym®TH.

The testcombination consists of three agents (Fig. 2). These are tris-buffer (pH 7.5) containing sodium chloride and an inhibitor preventing the action of other plasma proteases, secondly thrombin of bovine origin, and thirdly the substrate chromozym®TH. At the beginning of the assay, a mixture of buffer and thrombin has to be set up.

	Initial concentrations of solutions:
1 Buffer	
tris-buffer	200 mmol/l, pH 7.5
sodium chloride	70 mmol/l
aprotinine	6.5 IU/ml
2 Thrombin	3.13 U/ml
3 Chromozym®TH (Tos-Gly-Pro-Arg-pNA · AcOH)	1.5 mmol/l
4 Mixture of 1 and 2 (reagent mixture)	
tris-buffer	198 mmol/l
sodium chloride	69 mmol/l
aprotinine	6.4 IU/ml
thrombin	0.03 U/ml

Fig. 2. Reagents of the Boehringer Mannheim testcombination heparin

Pipette into plastic cuvettes:		
	Blank (B)	Sample (S)
reagent mixture redist. water sample or standard	2.00 ml 0.02 ml –	2.00 ml – 0.02 ml
Mix immediately, start stopwatch simultaneously, and incubate for exactly 3 min at 25°C. Add:		
solution 3 (chromozym TH)	0.20 ml	0.20 ml
Mix and determine the absorbance change △A/min up to the end of the 2nd minute.		

$$\frac{\Delta A/\min_{(S)} \times 100}{\Delta A/\min_{(B)}} = \text{residual thrombin activity (\%)}$$

Fig. 3. Assay protocol and calculation

Thrombin and the undiluted plasma sample have to be incubated for exactly 3 minutes (Fig. 3). After this incubation period substrate is added and the absorbance change at 405 nm is followed. Residual thrombin activity is measured and is calculated in percent of the thrombin blank reaction. At least one thrombin blank must be measured per test-series.

In principle the term "percent of residual thrombin activity" should be sufficient as the sole parameter in control of heparin therapy. But for the time being, unfortunately the therapeutic range using this parameter alone is not yet known. For this reason, "percent of residual thrombin activity" needs to be translated into terms people are familiar with, e. g. heparin units.

Therefore heparin standards are used to correlate "percent of residual thrombin activity" with heparin units. After measurement of four heparin standards a calibration curve is set up by plotting "percent of residual thrombin activity" versus the heparin concentration of the standards (Fig. 4).

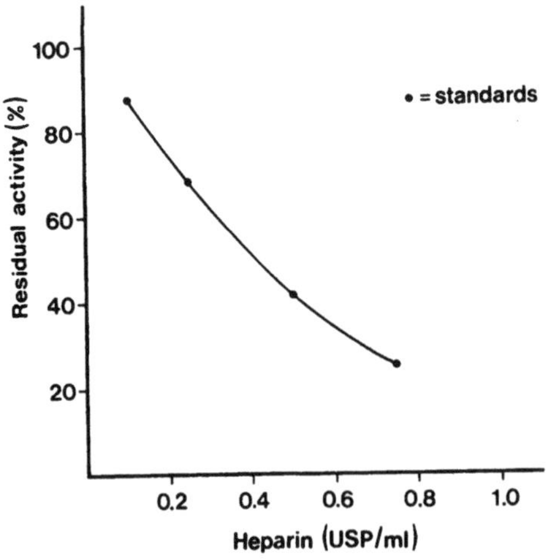

Fig. 4. Standard curve of the manual heparin assay (25 °C)

In order to overcome the inconvenience of a non-linear standard curve a computer program was worked out. The shape of the standard curve can be described mathematically by the hyperbolic function $y = \frac{A}{1 + BX} + C$. We found that this function fits the experimental values very well (Fig. 5).

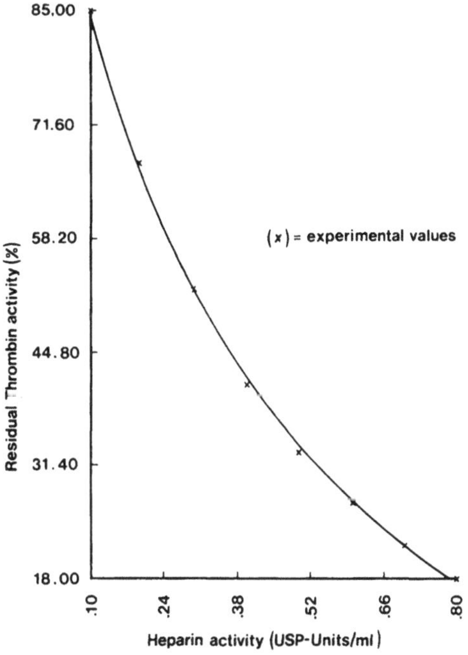

Fig. 5. Computer fitted standard curve

For the understanding of the results (heparin units/ml plasma) some additional interpretation is necessary. From the standard curve, heparin units can be read for normal AT III concentrations. With plasma samples of varying AT III-contents but with constant heparin concentration it can be shown that thrombin inhibition by heparin depends strongly on the AT III-level present in the plasma sample (Fig. 6).

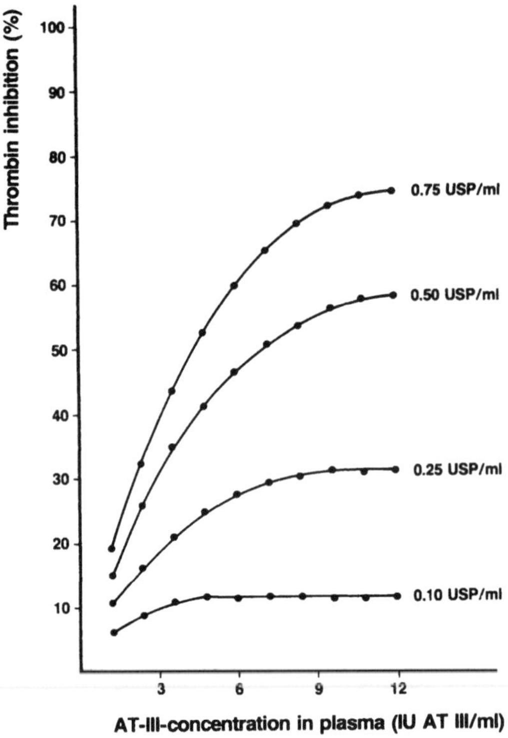

Fig. 6. Dependence of heparin action on AT III concentration in the plasma sample

Each curve in Fig. 6 represents a different but constant heparin concentration. This dependence is what we actually wanted to measure using this assay. If at normal heparin dosage abnormally low heparin values are observed in a patient, one should first see if the patient's AT III level is low, before other possible explanations are checked. The following conclusions can be drawn from our findings:

1. This heparin assay indicates the biological activity of heparin via plasma AT III; it does not indicate real heparin concentrations.

2. In this way a valuable parameter for the heparin-induced anticoagulative potential of the plasma during therapy is obtained.

3. This assay is a convincing concept for monitoring heparin therapy.

Acknowledgements

We are grateful to Dr. D. Markowetz for working out the computer program.

References

1. Bartl, K., Dorsch, E., Lill, H., Ziegenhorn, J.: Determination of the Biological Activity of Heparin by Use of a Chromogenic Substrate. Thrombosis and Haemostasis 42, 1446. (1979).

2. Teien, A. N., Lie, M., Abildgaard, U.: Assay of Heparin in Plasma Using a Chromogenic Substrate for Activated Factor X. Thrombosis Research 8, 413. (1976).

3. Witt, I.: Neue Methoden der Gerinnungsanalyse mit chromogenen Substraten. Journal of Clinical Chemistry and Clinical Biochemistry 15, 239 (1979).

Determination of Heparin by a Fluorogenic Synthetic Substrate

Reiner Spaethe, Margot Naumann, Joan Strauß
Medical-scientific Department
American Hospital Supply Deutschland GmbH
D-8000 München

During the last 35 years the use of heparin for therapy has increased. Heparin is given in a high dosage of more than 0.2 U/ml plasma for the following treatments: thrombophlebitis, thromboembolism, patients with acute and chronic disseminated intravascular coagulation and during extracorporal circulation in open heart surgery and renal dialysis.

For prophylaxis plasma levels lower than 0.15 U/ml plasma are desired. This prophylactic administration of heparin has very much decreased the postoperative thrombosis after surgical intervention (1-8).

The big difference between in vivo concentrations of heparin lower than 0.15 U/ml plasma and very high values of over 1.0 U/ml during an extracorporal circulation makes it necessary to control the heparin level with high sensitivity, spread over a wide therapeutical range with exact and reproducible results. Correct results only can be expected if the test system used is not disturbed by other parameters.

A measure of heparin effect should reflect the in vivo balance between the direct action of the drug on blood clotting and the ability of other components to potentiate or antagonize heparin. There are wide variations in individual response to heparin and also in the same patients from one day to another. Injected heparin becomes bound to endothelium; direct measurement shows that the concentration in the endothelium is more than 100 times that in the plasma (9). It has a high affinity to lipoprotein lipase and displaces this enzyme. Together AT III and heparin inhibit accumulation of platelets.

Heparin · New Biochemical and Medical Aspects

It activates AT III to inhibit serine proteases. It has a high affinity to platelet factor 4 and lipoproteins. Elevation of heparin antagonists as discerned may increase the heparin resistance as well as a fluctuation in AT III levels. In consequence individual response to heparin is the most likely explanation of ineffective treatment in some and excessive bleeding in others. Such individual variation in the response to heparin influences the different test systems for monitoring.

More problems can arise when there is a disturbance of hemostasis like DIC or an oral anticoagulant treatment. Well established methods for monitoring heparin therapy like the APTT and the thrombin time are more or less sensitive to factor deficiencies, the presence of fibrin degradation products and other anticoagulants.

The choice of methods of laboratory control of heparin therapy is dependent on the dosage given to the patient. *Low dose* prophylaxis and high dosage therapy cannot be monitored routinely with thrombin time or APTT. Vinazzer (10) found that by measurement of heparin concentration with thrombin time reliable values are obtained above 0.2 U/ml plasma and with APTT above 0.1 U/ml. High heparin concentrations result in unmeasurable clotting times. The relationship of thrombin time to heparin level is only linear over a small heparin dosage range. The APTT gives an overall reflection of the clinical affect of heparin activity. It is undoubtedly a sensitive screening test for diagnosis of defects of the intrinsic system. But APTT too is influenced by preexisting coagulation disorders. It is now well accepted that monitoring of heparin in these critical cases of low dose and high dose heparin therapy should be done better enzymatically by synthetic substrates.

Tilsner published (11) results of low dose heparin prophylaxis with different therapeutic regimens. He could demonstrate that this prophylaxis was ameliorated by individual dosage of heparin. Only with synthetic substrates is a sensitive and accurate monitoring of heparin possible in these cases.

The measurement of plasma heparin concentration in evaluating the high heparin levels during extracorporal circulation is helpful for calculation of the amount of protamine sulfate required for neutralization. Heparin levels in coagulation disorders can also be measured better by synthetic substrates. Mitchell and coworkers (12) published in 1978 a specific sensitive heparin assay using a synthetic fluorogenic substrate. The assay measures the rate of fluorescent tag release which results from thrombin proteolysis of a synthetic peptide substrate which mimics fibrinogen. The advantage of using this fluorogenic substrate in comparison to other amidolytic methods was seen in its great sensitivity to thrombin. The test system for our heparin assay is seen in Fig. 1.

Heparin $\xrightarrow{\textbf{Excess AT III}}$ **AT III · Heparin**
(COMPLEX)

AT III · Heparin + Thrombin ⟶
(COMPLEX)
AT III · Heparin · Thrombin + Residual Thrombin
(COMPLEX)

Residual Thrombin + D-Phe-Pro-Arg-AIE ⟶ **D-Phe-Pro-Arg + AIE**

Fig. 1. The Theory of the Fluorogenic Substrate Assay for Heparin

Heparin in the patients sample first reacts with excess antithrombin III to form the heparin-AT-III-complex. This complex is then measured by its ability to inhibit purified thrombin. Any thrombin not neutralized is free to react with substrate, thus producing fluorescence. As a substrate we use D-phenylalanine-proline-arginine-5-amidoisophethalic-acid, dimethylester, diacetate (AIE) (Fig. 2). The substrate is very sensitive to the detection of thrombin allowing the use of small amounts of thrombin (0.05 NIH U) and non defibrinated plasma without clotting interference during the determination. The peptide has a very good water solubility.

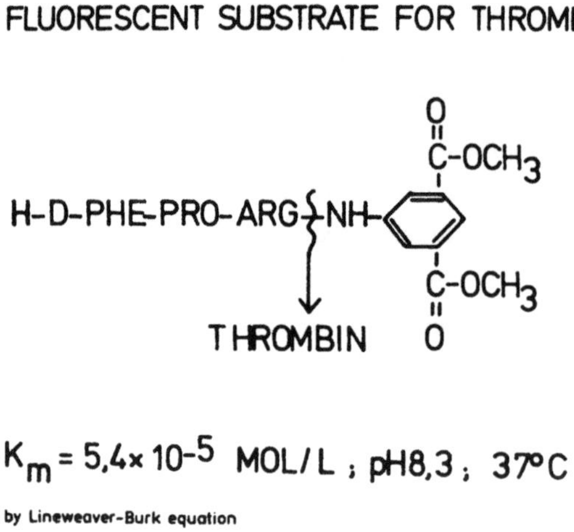

Fig. 2.

The two-step-test procedure can be seen in Fig. 3.

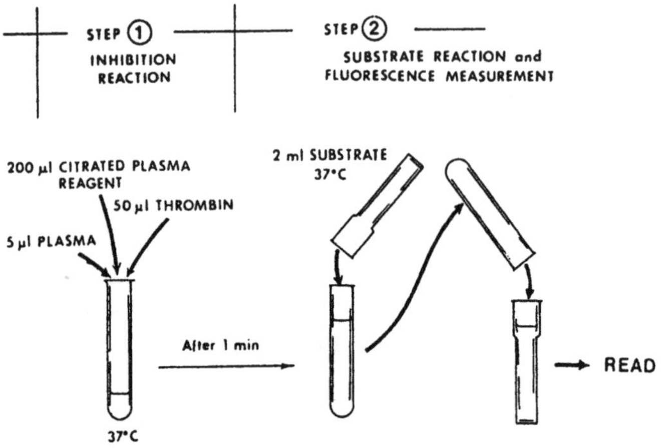

Fig. 3. Test Procedure for the Fluorogenic Substrate Assay of Heparin

In step 1, 200 µl of 1:40 diluted buffered normal citrated plasma as source of AT III is mixed with 5 µl of heparin containing test sample; then 50 µl of 1 NIH U/ml human thrombin is added. The mixture is incubated for 60 seconds at 37 °C when mucosa-heparin is used. For the measurement of lung heparin the sample should be incubated for 120 seconds to reach a similar sensitivity of the heparin curve. In our assays we have detected a small but significant blank value for determinations performed with normal plasma in the absence of heparin (12). This blank is probably contributed by the other clotting inhibitors. Therefore, we prefer a pooled normal plasma instead of purified AT III to equalize all of the inhibitory factors.

In step 2 the test mixture is transferred to a single use cuvette containing 0.3 micromoles of substrate, and the uninhibited thrombin is determined by kinetic measurement of the released AIE in a fluorometer (Fig. 4).

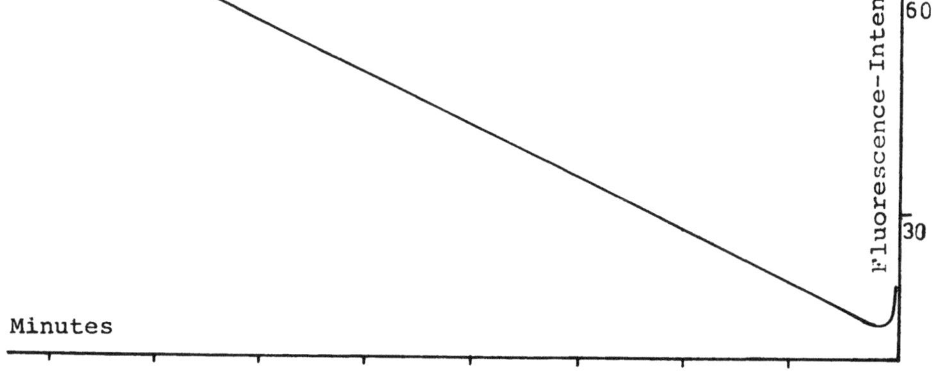

Fig. 4. Kinetic of Substrate-Splitting during a Heparintest with Protopath-System (78 % Residual Thrombin)

The test is available as a reagent kit* containing the diluted buffered normal citrated plasma, a lyophilised human thrombin of 1 NIH U/ml, the substrate cuvettes and a heparin control. To ameliorate the test results and to allow a quick measurement we designed a special fluorometer. The equipment calibration establishes a reading of 100 % thrombin activity when no detectable heparin is present, and standard curves are prepared to represent decreases in fluorescence caused by thrombin inhibition due to increased levels of heparin.

The instrument directly expresses the results in percent residual thrombin, and the heparin concentration of unknown samples is determined by use of a standard curve.

Fig. 5 shows 3 different curves representing results obtained on 3 different heparin preparations. The commercial preparation gives a standard curve which is less sensitive and varies from the other curves by about 20 %. Based on such findings we suggested the need to prepare standard calibration curves with the same heparin used for patient treatment. It is our experience that the heparins of the manufacturers are internally more or less consistant but that differences between manufacturers do exist.

In Fig. 6 the assay precision of the method is shown. Both within day and day-to-day results show coefficients of variation of less than 5 % when working at the lower concentration. At values near 0.8 U/ml, precision is usually more than 10 % depending on the heparin preparation used and low residual thrombin. At high concentrations better results are to be reached by dilution of the sample.

---

*Protopath TM Proteolytic Enzyme Detection System
American Dade, Division of American Hospital Supply Corporation, Miami, Florida, USA

In Germany: American Hospital Supply Deutschland GmbH
München, Abteilung Merz + Dade

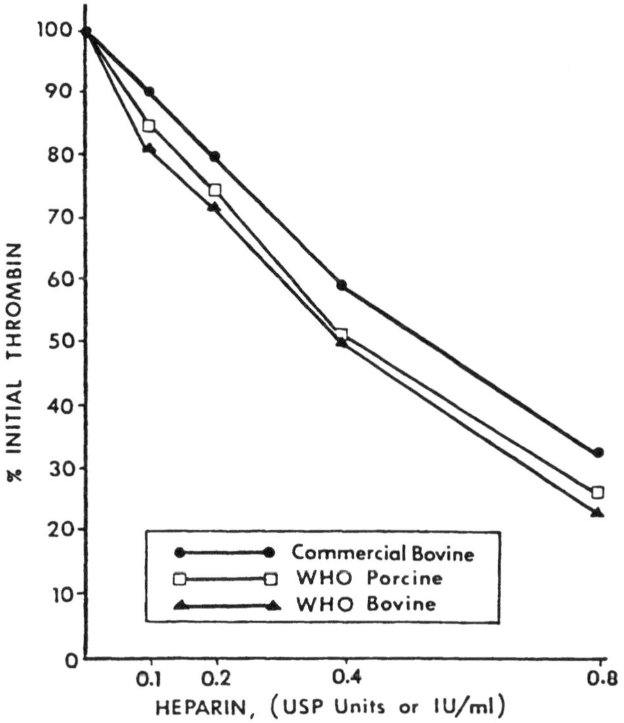

Fig. 5. Standard Curves for the Fluorogenic Substrate Assay of Heparin

ASSAY PRECISION FOR STANDARD HEPARIN DETERMINATIONS

WITHIN-DAY, N = 4

HEPARIN, U.S.P. U/ML	MEAN % INITIAL THROMBIN	COEFFICIENT OF VARIATION, %
0.1	93.4	1.5
0.2	83.0	3.6
0.4	61.3	4.4
0.8	28.0	10.4
DAY-TO-DAY, N = 5		
0.1	91.1	2.9
0.2	79.8	3.3
0.4	59.6	3.1
0.8	30.2	11.8

Fig. 6. Assay Precision for Standard Heparin Determinations

As discussed above, in coagulation physiology there is more and more of a demand to measure heparin concentrations even below 0.1 U/ml; therefore fore we made a continuous calibration curve with more measuring points between 0 and 0.15 U/ml (Fig. 7).

With this heparin it is already shown that a good discrimination below 0.1 U/ml became possible. Because of the high sensitivity of fluorometric measurement, this range seemed to be ameliorable; increasing the amount of plasma volume we received a wider spread of the calibration curve (Fig. 8).

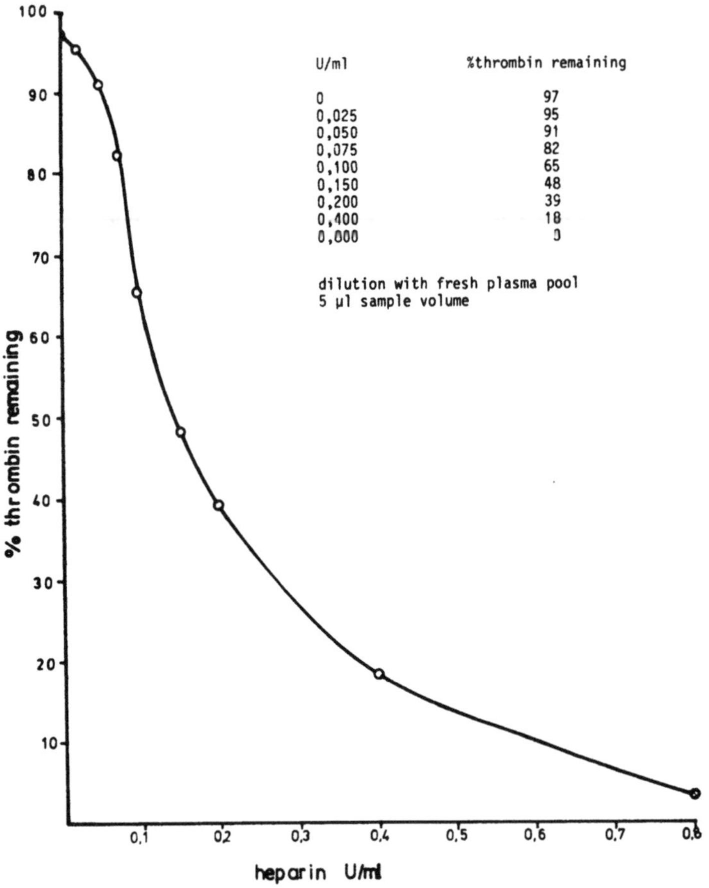

Fig. 7. Heparin Calibration Curve (normal procedure)

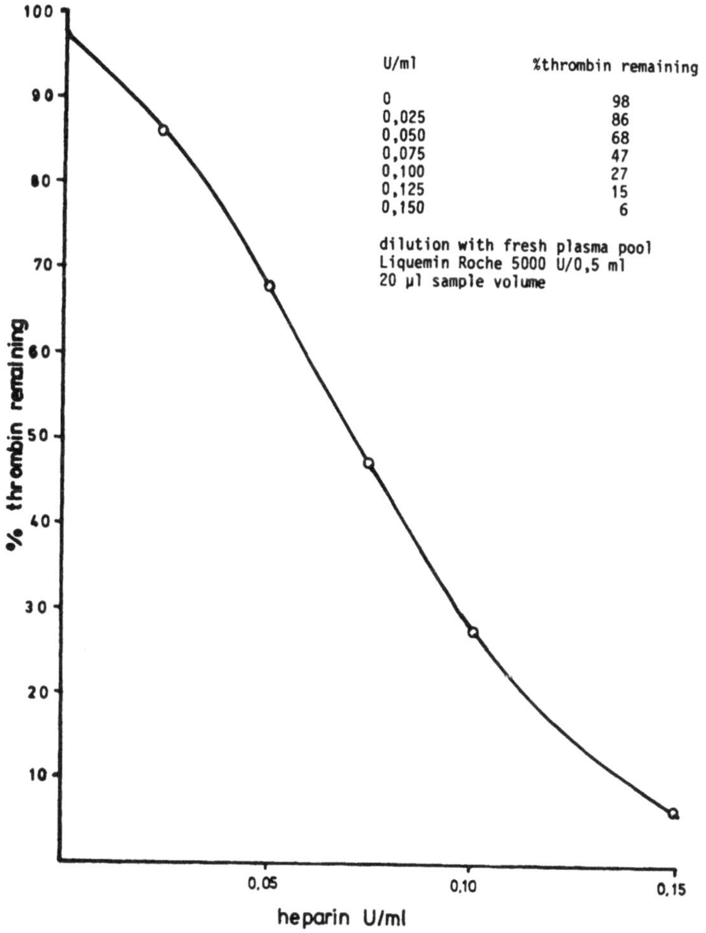

Fig. 8. Heparin Calibration Curve for low Heparin Levels < 0.15 U/ml

Plotting a calibration curve beside the correct dilution of the heparin, it is important to prepare a poolplasma which is as free from platelets as possible. Centrifugation of 15-20 minutes at 1250-2000 g is recommended. Fig. 9. shows a measurement of heparin standards in the plasma with a low platelet count of 75900/µl, once measured immediately and once after deep freezing.

EFFECT OF FREEZING AND THAWING PLASMA WITH A LOW PLATELET COUNT, 75.900/µL, ON STANDARD HEPARIN VALUES

HEPARIN U/ML	ASSAY VALUES % RESIDUAL THROMBIN	
	FRESH PLASMA	FROZEN PLASMA
0,1	88,1	95,0
0,2	77,2	85,5
0,4	54,0	65,6
0,8	26,2	38,9

Fig. 9. Effect of Freezing and Thawing Plasma with a low Platelet Count, 75 900/µl, on Standard Heparin Values

It is now evident that heparin was bound on platelet factor 4 after deep-freezing, resulting in a higher amount of residual thrombin. Obviously the same criteria are important for aptient plasma which must be taken off very carefully because it should contain as few platelet factors as possible.

Fig. 10 shows the influence of the pool plasma on calibration curves. The same heparin dilution was always used.

Curve 1 shows a fresh plasma pool, curve 2 and 3 a lyophilised normal plasma. With plasma 1, incorrectly collected, remarkably more heparin was bound, so that the amount of residual thrombin remained higher. The heparin control, effected similarly, shows a good accuracy at an assay value of 78 % (66-90 %) residual thrombin with values between 73 % and 76 %.

At the moment two different methods are discussed: either to measure the total free heparin concentration by adjustment of the antithrombin deviation in the sample by addition of AT III to the patient plasma - or to see whether the measurement of biologically effective activities offers more advantages. Using this method (13) the AT III level of the patients sample is not corrected. In this case heparin can perform its inhibitory activity on thrombin exclusively by means of the amount of AT III in the sample.

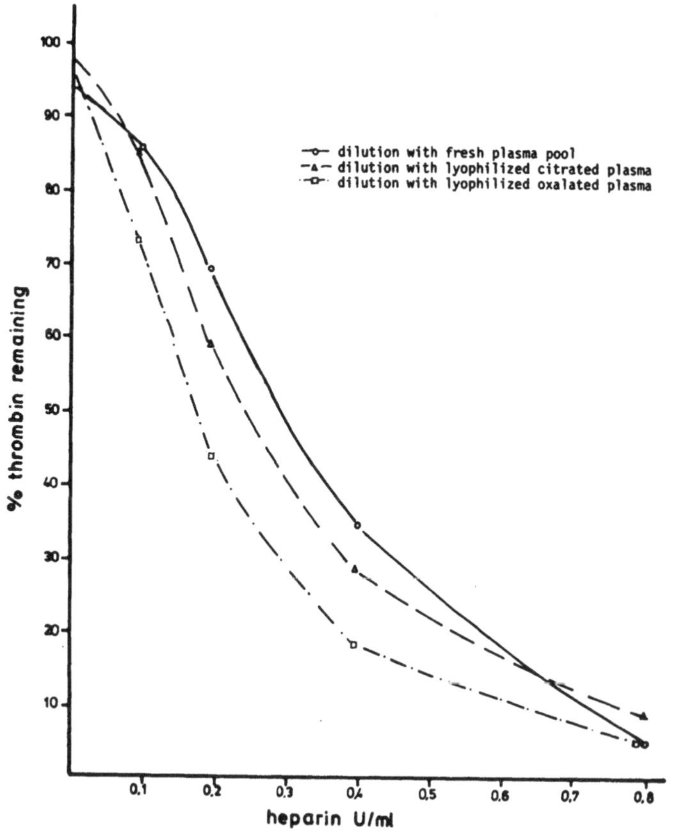

Fig. 10. Influence of Plasma Pools on Calibration Curves

Fig. 11 shows the calibration curve of heparin dilutions in a plasma pool. The values of curve 1 were obtained by adding AT III derived from the buffered citrated plasma included into the kit. For curve 2 instead of citrated plasma a buffer was added. Otherwise the method of the test kit was unchanged.

With the presented method the biologically active heparin and also the heparin concentration can be measured simply, with great sensitivity and exactly. Considering the reaction of heparin in view of the first results of the new possibilities for therapy with AT III - perhaps in combination with heparin - both methods of heparin measurement (biologically effective activities and total free concentration) may be very important in the future.

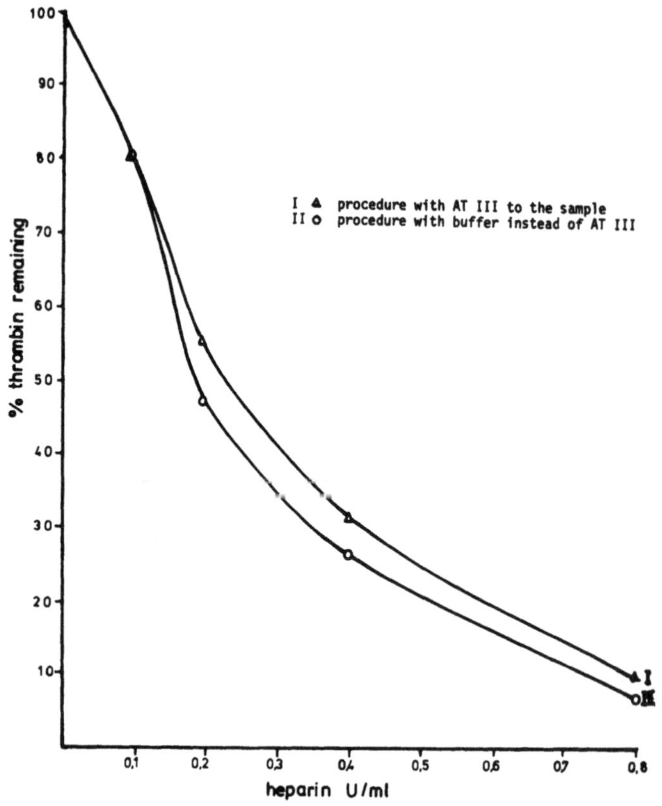

Fig. 11. Calibration Curves with different Methods of Heparin Measurement

Acknowledgement

We thank Dr. Robert Bishop, Dr. Georg Mitchell and coworkers for some of the results they have given to this paper.

References

1. Wessler, S., Gitel, S. N.: Heparin: New Concepts Relevant to Clinical Use. Blood 53, 525 (1979).

2. Kakkar, W. et al.: Efficacy of Low Doses of Heparin in Prevention of Deep-Vein Thrombosis after Major Surgery. Lancet 101 (1972/2).

3. Turpie, A. G. G., Hirsch, J.: Prophylaxis and Therapy of Venous Thrombo-Embolism. CRC Critical Reviews in Clin. Lab. Sci. 247, April (1979).

4. Nicolaides, A. N., Desai, S. et al.: Small Doses of Subcutaneous Sodium Heparin in Preventing Deep Venous Thrombosis after Major Surgery. Lancet 890 (1972/2).

5. Sagar, S., Stamatakis, J. D., Higgins, A. F. et al.: Efficacy of Low-Dose Heparin in Prevention of Extensive Deep-Vein Thrombosis in Patients Undergoing Total Hip Replacement. Lancet 1154 (1976).

6. Biel, R. C., Wagner, U., Wesler, R. et al.: Heparin Levels Using Chromogenic Substrate S-2222 During Low-Dose Heparin and Low Dose Heparin-Dihydroergotamin Prophylaxis After Gynecological Surgery. Thromb. Haemost. 42, 380 (1979).

7. Mc Carthy, S. T., Robertson, D., Turner, J. J. et al.: Low Dose Heparin as Prophylaxis Against Deep Vein Thrombosis After Acute Stroke. Lancet 800 (1977).

8. Rathaus, M., Bernheim, J., Sara, K.: Low Dose Heparin in Rapidly progressive Glomerulonephritis. Arch. Intern. Med. 139, 251 (1979).

9. Jaques, L. B.: Heparin: An Old Drug with a New Paradigm. Science 206, 528 (1979).

10. Vinazzer, H.: Zur Bestimmung von Heparin im Plasma. Qualitätsvergleich verschiedener Methoden. Anaesthesist 28, 299 (1979).

11. Tilsner, V., Müller, U., Reuter, H., Raedler, A.: Results of Low Dose Heparin Prophylaxis of Venous Thrombosis Considering Plasma Heparin and Antithrombin III Concentration. Thrombosis Research 17, 519 (1980).

12. Mitchell, G. A., Gargiulo, R. J., Huseby, R. M., Lawson, D. E., Pochron, S. P., Sehuanes, J. A.: Assay for Plasma Heparin Using a Synthetic Peptide Substrate for Thrombin: Introduction of the Fluorophore Aminoisophthalic Acid, Dimethylester. Thrombosis Research 13, 47 (1978).

13. Barth, K., Dorsch, E., Ziegenhorn, J.: Bestimmung der biologischen Aktivität von Heparin mit einem Chromogenen Substrat. a) 23. Tagung der Deutschen Arbeitsgemeinschaft f. Blutgerinnungsforschung, Heidelberg 1979, b) Lab. med. 4, 46 (1980).

Properties of the Coatest® Heparin Assay

Petter Friberger
Kabi AB, Peptide Research
S-43122 Mölndal, Sweden

Summary

In the presence of antithrombin, heparin possesses a potent anticoagulant activity. This activity is directed against several coagulation factors among which thrombin and Factor X_a are best characterized. It has therefore been rather natural that these enzymes have been used to measure the activity of heparin. To avoid the release of heparin antagonists from the platelets, blood is sampled on ice.

The plasma sample and extra antithrombin, added in order to decrease the influence of this protein on the assay, is diluted 1:10 in buffer. The rate at which added Factor X_a is inhibited is dependent on the heparin activity. This is measured by using a chromogenic substrate for Factor X_a. The choice of standard is discussed.

Heparin has usually been assayed by its activity in a recalcification or an APTT system. Such a system is extremely complex which makes it difficult to standardize. When selective chromogenic substrates were introduced, it was possible to design a more simple system where heparin is measured by its potency to accelerate the reaction between a suitable protease and antithrombin (AT).

As Factor X has a central position in the coagulation system (Fig. 1) and is available in a purified and activated form, it was chosen for heparin assay. The choice of enzyme is probably critical in several respects. Activated Factor X (FX_a) does not interfere with fibrionogen or platelets and does not activate prothrombin in a diluted Ca^{2+} free system. It has recently been shown by Holmer et al. (1) that heparin of different molecular weight influences differently on the inhibition of e. g. FX_a and thrombin (Fig. 2). High molecular weight heparin also seems to be more readily neutralized by

Heparin · New Biochemical and Medical Aspects

heparin antagonists, e. g. platelet factor 4 (PF 4). That may imply that heparin, active in a thrombin inhibitory system, is consumed but that there is sill a substantial anti FX_a effect of low MW heparin.

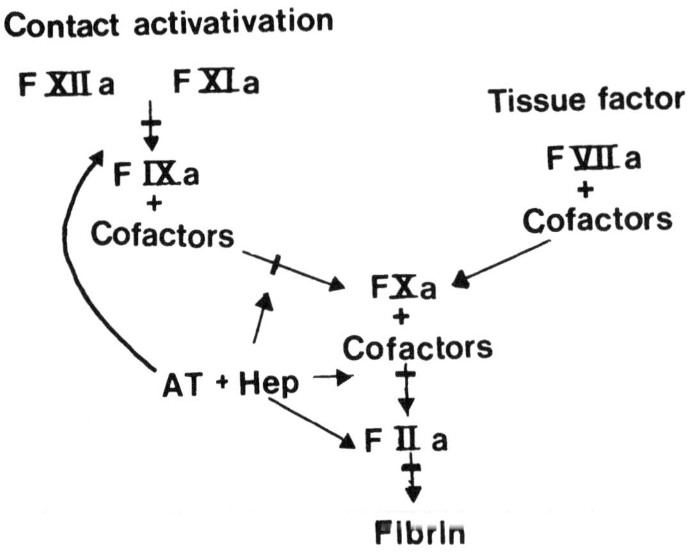

Fig. 1. A schematic sketch of the coagulation system which shows the central position of Factor X_a and what factors are most sensitive to the inhibition by antithrombin (AT) and heparin (Hep).

The assay has been designed in such a way that the potentiating effect of the heparin on the inhibition of FX_a is determined. This can be an effect of a small amount (concentration) of high affinity heparin or a considerably higher amount of unfractionated heparin. Thus, the assay does not give the total concentration of heparin but rather its activity in an important function of heparin.

The platelets present in blood can release the potent heparin antagonist PF4. Theoretically about 20 IU of heparin can be neutralized by totally released platelets in one ml of blood. For platelet poor plasma (20,000 platelets/µl) the corresponding figure is 1 IU of heparin. That means that more than 5 % of the total release in platelet poor plasma would be unacceptable.

If the blood is cooled down when drawn, or immmediately thereafter, the risk of the PF4 release is very much reduced although the platelets are known to aggregate under such conditions. These things have been extensively studied by Teien et al. (3, 4).

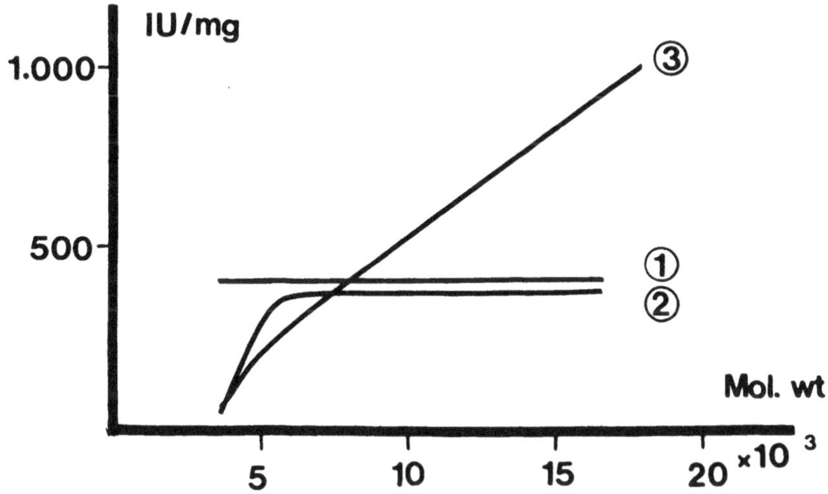

Fig. 2. The potency of heparin of different molecular weight to inhibit different bovine enzymes in the presence of antithrombin 1) Typical relation for FX_a, $FXII_a$, and plasma kallikrein, 2) Typical relation for thrombin and FIX_a and 3) Typical relation for FXI_a.

Method

The method which was worked out by Teien et al. (3, 4) is described in Table 1. The reaction between FX_a and the heparin - AT complex is rapid under optimal conditions. The bovine enzyme reacts about twice as fast as the human. The FX_a concentration is of the same order as that which theoretically can be activated in the sample plasma.

Table 1. Method description for the Coatest® heparin assay

Plasma dilution 1 : 10 with 100 % extra AT (37 °C)		µl 200
F X a (25 °C)		µl 100
Incubate for	exactly sec	30
Substrate, 1mM S-2222 (37 °C)		µl 200
Read A/min <u>or</u> incubate for	exactly sec	180
Acetic acid 50 %		µl 300

The mechanism of FX_a inhibition in our system is shown in Fig. 3. An optimal amount of AT is needed. That means that the heparin, to be assayed, should be bound as completely as possible to AT (Fig. 4). However, at high AT concentrations, a significant amount of enzyme is inhibited by AT that is not bound to heparin.

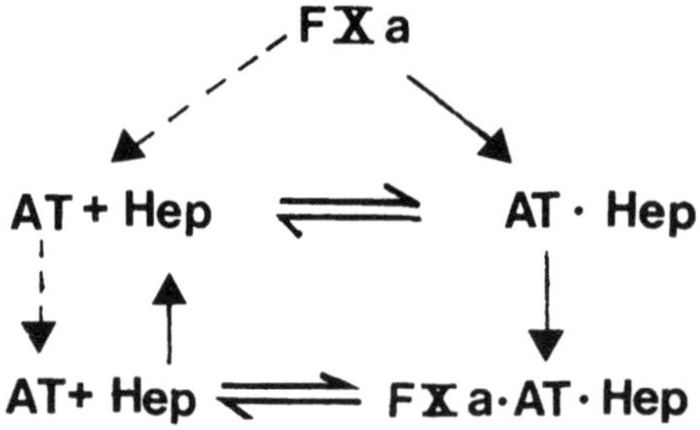

Fig. 3. Reaction pathways in the heparin assay

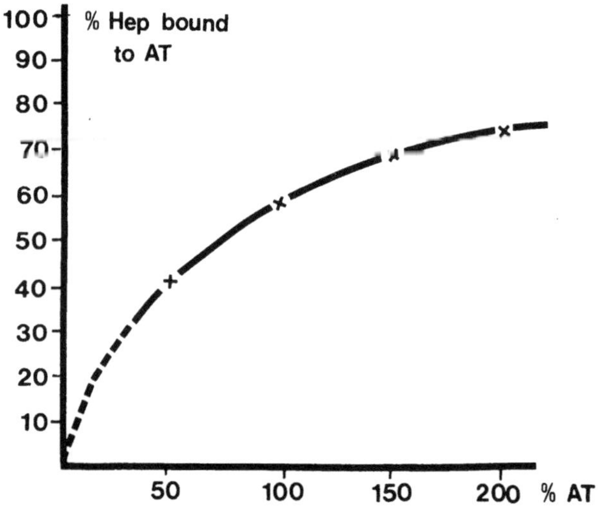

Fig. 4. The calculated amount of heparin bound and its dependence on the antithrombin concentration (K_d = 100 nmol/l and AT in plasma = 2.2 µmol/l were used). The dependence on the amount of heparin in the range 0.05 - 0.8 IU/ml is less than 2 %.

When the substrate is added to reach a concentration of approximately K_m, reducing the concentration of the reactants by the dilution, the rate of inhibition is decreased significantly (to less than 20 % of the original value). The inhibition reaction would be stopped more effectively and the substrate reaction would proceed more linearly (10 - 35 % of the substrate is hydrolyzed) if a higher substrate concentration was used. However, when this was tested practically, no significant improvement was found. When an initial rate assay is to be used, an accurate reading from the recorder graph is not possible at the present substrate concentration. The double concentration is then recommended. A typical standard curve in the range expected for effective heparin treatment is shown in Fig. 5.

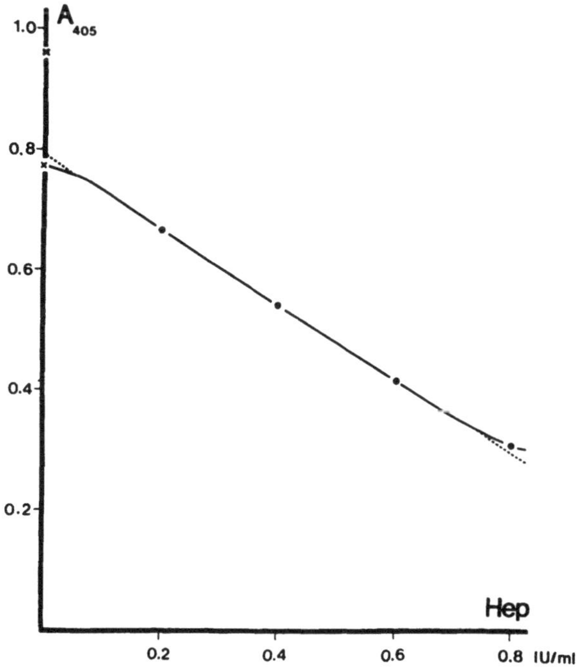

Fig. 5. Standard curve for heparin (KabiVitrum batch 326114). The x at A_{405} = 0.95 is the activity of the FX_a without plasma and antithrombin and the x at A_{405} = 0.77 is the activity when no heparin is added. The difference between the extrapolated curve and the lower x is the effect of heparin antagonist (PF4) on the standard curve - a parallel displacement upwards.

By using a prolonged incubation time (180 seconds) for the inhibition stage, heparin in the range 0.05 to 0.20 IU/ml plasma (concentration obtained after subcutaneous administration) can be determined. In this range the lyophilized plasma in the kit cannot be used because it may contain up to 0.05 IU/ml of heparin antagonist (Fig. 5). It is probably just the existence of antagonists that put a limit to the sensitivity of a heparin assay of this type.

Standardization

A standard curve is made by using the same batch of heparin as used in the patient. That means that the units given on the label by the producer is used. The results are comparable with those of other assays using the same type of standardization procedure. The activity left in the blood a certain time after administration is measured.

Another possible way of standardization is to use WHO standards or national standards. It would, however, be much more attractive to use a "high affinity heparin" eluted from matrix bound AT under standardized conditions also having a well standardized MW distribution.

Stability and accuracy

Kit reagents used for several years have been tested according to the specifications. The results are accounted for in Table 2. The rather low AT activities found depend on some losses during lyophilization. This was not detected by using an immunochemical technique in the production.

All reagents have shown a good stability. In a few cases losses in AT activity have been reported.

By using five different kits on five different occasions within one month, a day to day CV of 3.5 was obtained. The corresponding kit to kit CV was 1.9. The day to day CV mainly depends on differences in temperature and equipment used.

Clinical use

The Coatest® heparin assay is thus very simple and reliable which makes it suitable for clinical use. Like most chromogenic assays, it is also suitable for automation. When the conditions for an optimal heparin treatment are established, it can finally be decided whether it is necessary to assay the

Table 2.
Quality control of the kit and kit reagents.

Reagent or parameter	Value according to specification Mean	Range	Obtained data Mean ± SD	No of batches
FXa	71 nkat	61-81	76 ± 6	10
AT	~10 PEU	-	8.4 ± 1.1	8
S-2222	15 mg	14-17	16.0 ± 0.5	6
Standard curve:				
Correlation coefficient		≥0.990	0.997 ± 0.002	10
Slope	0.654 A/IU	0.499-0.809	0.627 ± 0.063	"
Intercept	0.843 A	0.658-1.028	0.795 ± 0.060	"

heparin activity routinely or not and on what occasions heparin shall be assayed. Holm et al. (5) and others have used the chromogenic heparin assay successfully.

References

1. Holmer, E. et al. Biochem. J., 193, 395 (1981).
2. Andersson, L.-O. et al. Thromb. Res. 15, 531 (1979).
3. Teien, A. et al. Thromb. Res. 8, 413 (1976)
4. Teien, A. et al. Thromb. Res. 10, 399 (1977).
5. Holm, H. et al. Synthetic Substances in Clinical Blood Coagulation Assays. Eds. Lijnen, Collen & Verstraete. p 63, Martinus Nijhoff Publ. (1980).

Discussion

Concerning the dependence of the heparin determination on the antithrombin III concentration in the plasma sample to be analyzed. *Witt* presented the following experimental results:

Different amounts of heparin (Liquemin) were added to plasma samples containing varying amounts of antithrombin III. These plasma samples were assayed for heparin with both the Boehringer test and the Kabi Coatest. The findings show (see table) that the heparin determination with the Kabi Coatest is also dependent upon the antithrombin III concentration in the plasma sample even though excess antithrombin III is added to the test system. This indicates that it is the heparin activity rather than the heparin concentration which is being measured by the Kabi Coatest.

	Heparin found (USP/ml)			
	Boehringer Test		Coatest	
Heparin added (USP/ml)	AT III 12 U/ml	AT III 27 U/ml	AT III 12 U/ml	AT III 27 U/ml
0.10			0.1	0.45
0.20	0.18	0.28	0.24	0.58
0.40	0.34	0.58	0.52	0.79
0.70	0.62	> 0.70		

Witt explained in answer to *Friberger*'s question concerning the value "27 U of antithrombin III" that these are inhibitor units per ml plasma and that this is nearly twice the amount of the normal plasma concentration.

Friberger stressed that when *Teien* constructed the test system, the intention was to provide the possibility by adding antithrombin to recover exactly the amount of heparin in the plasma sample irrespective of the antithrombin concentration in the plasma.

In the discussion there was no consensus concerning the question of the dependency of the Coatest on the antithrombin III concentration in the plasma sample.

Spaethe pointed out that it is necessary to have a test system by which the biological activity of heparin in dependency on the antithrombin III concentration in the plasma sample can be measured and also a system by which the concentration of heparin can be measured when excess antithrombin III is added to the test system.

Lill asked which standard curves Witt had used for the measurements.

Witt answered that for the measurements the standard curves were performed according to the instructions of the commercial test kits.

Wenzel mentioned that he had done the same experiments as Witt some time ago and that he came to the same conclusions. He repeated that for the treatment of patients one needs values which reflect both clinically important states:

1. the non-responsiveness to the administered heparin dosage and
2. the decrease of antithrombin III.

He is convinced that we have to use two test systems which are working under optimal conditions, that means one system for the measurement of functional antithrombin III which contains high concentrations of heparin so that all of the antithrombin III is converted to an active form and also a second system which demonstrates how much antithrombin III is activated by the administered heparin.

Witt stressed that there is no test system available up to now which measures the total heparin concentration in a plasma sample and that it is not correct to speak of heparin "concentration". One argument for this is that she has never found diverging differences between the two test systems (Boehringer and Coatest) which would have to be the case if the Coatest measures the heparin concentration and the Boehringer test the heparin activity, that is the heparin activated antithrombin.

Duckert thought that the Coatest calls for so much antithrombin III that the saturation point of heparin should be reached and that the heparin concentration is measured.

Duckert further made a comment concerning the statement of Witt that for controlling the therapy of a patient the same heparin should be used for the standard curve as that which was administered to the patient.

He reported on a conference in Avignon where the same problems were discussed. Dr. Juan from Marseille had said that it is not necessary to use the same heparin because the heparin measured in the patient's plasma is no longer the same as that administered. In her experiments she could demonstrate that she gets the same results for a patient's plasma using different types of heparin for the standard curves.

The question was raised if anybody knows at what antithrombin III concentration the heparin effect is diminished or lost when the patient's antithrombin III decreases.

The question could not be answered.

A Sensitive Competitive Binding Assay for Heparin

Joan Dawes
MRC Immunoassay Team,
2, Forrest Road,
Edinburgh, EH1 2QW, UK.

Introduction

The heparin assays currently available are of two types: chemical methods, which measure all heparin molecules but are very insensitive and require purified material as substrate, and biological assays. The latter are relatively sensitive and can be used on biological fluids, but are subject to interference from other components of such complex mixtures. Moreover, a biological assay only detects those heparin molecules which are active in that assay. Although this may be an advantage under some circumstances, the use of a biological assay presupposes a knowledge of the relevant biological activity. In the case of heparin, which can display a wide range of biological activities, it is not yet clear which are and which are not particularly important *in vivo*. For example, it is possible that one of the main antithrombotic functions of heparin is the maintenance of an electronegative charge at the endothelial cell surface; all heparin molecules can contribute to this charge, not only the restricted populations detected in the conventional anticoagulant assays. There is therefore an urgent need for a simple, sensitive assay system which is independent of specific biological activities and detects the whole heparin population in complex mixtures such as plasma and urine.

We have developed such an assay, in which heparins in the sample compete with ^{125}I-labelled heparin for binding to protamine which has been covalently linked to Sepharose 4B.

Heparin · New Biochemical and Medical Aspects

Printed in Germany

Methods

Protamine-Sepharose 4B. Sepharose 4B (Pharmacia) (75 g) was suspended in water (150 ml) and cyanogen bromide (5 g) was added at room temperature with continuous mixing. The pH was maintained at 10.6 by addition of 2M NaOH. After 30 min., when the reaction was complete, the mixture was filtered on a sintered glass funnel and washed thoroughly with $NaHCO_3$ (0.1M), followed by citrate buffer (0.1M, pH 6.0). The activated Sepharose was resuspended in 150 ml citrate buffer; 5 µl of a 1M solution of phenylmethylsulphonylfluoride in dimethylsulphoxide was added, followed by a solution of 0.5 mg protamine sulphate (salmon; Sigma) in 10 ml water. The suspension was mixed at room temperature for 18 h. The coupled protamine-Sepharose was then thoroughly washed with citrate buffer (0.1M, pH 6.0) followed by phosphate buffer (0.05M, pH 7.4). It was resuspended in phosphate buffer (0.05M, pH 7.4) containing 1 % Tween 20 and 30 µM phenylmethylsulphonylfluoride and stored at 4 °C. This reagent was stable for about 6 months.

^{125}I-Heparin. Porcine mucosal heparin (Sigma; Batch No. 79B-1510) was iodinated to a specific activity of 25-35 µCi μg^{-1} as described by Dawes and Pepper (1). Its shelf life was about 6 weeks, but could be extended by the removal of low molecular weight iodinated material in a Sephadex G50 column.

Assay. The assay mixture contained 50 µl protamine-Sepharose suspension, 50 µl ^{125}I-heparin (12.5 ng ml^{-1}), 50 µl standard heparin or sample and 0.05M phosphate buffer pH 7.4 containing 1 % Tween 20 to a final volume of 300 µl. The concentration of protamine-Sepharose which bound 50 % of the tracer in the absence of unlabelled heparin was used. This was normally a 1/25-1/50 dilution of the solid phase; higher dilutions gave poor reproducibility due to difficulties in dispensing this type of suspension. The standard heparin (Sigma or Evans) solution contained 1 µg ml^{-1} and was serially diluted to 2 ng ml^{-1}.

Assay tubes were shaken at room temperature for 16 h. The protamine-Sepharose was then washed twice with the assay buffer and the solid phase counted in a gamma counter.

Preparation of biological samples. Biological samples were incubated with pronase (*Streptomyces griseus*; Sigma) at a final enzyme concentration of 5 mg ml^{-1}, at 37 °C for 16 h. They were then capped and boiled for 15 min, and finally mixed well before assay.

Results

This assay measured commercial heparin down to a concentration of 10 ng ml^{-1} of sample, a sensitivity considerably greater than those of the biological assays available. The range of the standard curve was 10-400 ng ml^{-1}. This sensitivity was obtained only by incubating for 16 h; although it was possible to use a more rapid assay, sensitivity was lost under these conditions. The assay was relatively independent of pH, being unaffected over the pH range 5.5-9.0, but it was sensitive to ionic strength. If possible, the assay should be conducted at an ionic strength below 0.4; salt concentrations higher than this can be used as long as the standard curve is constructed at the same ionic strength, but at some cost to the sensitivity and precision of the assay. Above an ionic strength of 0.6 the assay did not function. Most divalent cations at a concentration of 5 mM had no effect on the standard curve, but 2.5 mM^{2+} did depress binding.

The assay also detected other sulphated polysaccharides, but the affinity of heparin for protamine was higher than that of related natural polymers, in some cases by several orders of magnitude. The concentrations of various sulphated polysaccharides required to inhibit binding of the heparin tracer by 50 % (50 % inhibn.) are given in Table 1. It can be seen from these data that the most important characteristic in determining the affinity of a molecule for protamine is its degree of sulphation. Thus a heparan sulphate containing 16.3 % sulphate bound 270 times less strongly to protamine than an isolate containing 30 % sulphate; the affinity of this heparan was close to that of Sigma heparin, which contained 31 % sulphate. The only compounds which had higher affinities than heparin were synthetic sulphated polysaccharides such as dextran sulphate and pentosan sulphate, which had higher sulphate contents than any of the naturally occuring molecules. Interestingly, the position of the sulphate residues also affected affinity. Chondroitin 4-

Table 1

Relative affinities of acidic polysaccharides for protamine

Substance	Source	Batch	Mean molecular weight	% SO_4	50 % inhibn. (µg/tube)
Hyaluronic acid [1]	Human umbilical cord	-	230,000	0	» 1,000
Keratan sulphate [1]	Human costal cartilage	-	~ 20,000	21.0	560
Chondroitin 6-sulphate [1]	River sturgeon cranial cartilage	-	29,000	16.8	480
Chondroitin 4-sulphate [1]	River sturgeon notochord	-	15,000	16.3	33
Dermatan sulphate [2]	Porcine	-	25,000	19.0	9.3
Heparan sulphate [1]	Bovine lung	-	30,000	16.3	8.0
Heparan sulphate [2]	Porcine	Type II	8,000	30.0	0.030
Heparin [3]	Porcine mucosal	793-1510	12,000	31.0	0.012
Pentosan sulphate [4]	-	SP54-N7	3,000	48.0	0.0030
Dextran sulphate [3]	-	48C-0241	40,000	53.7	0.0037

Fractions were obtained from: [1]M. B. Mathews, University of Chicago; [2]E. Johnson, National Institute of Biological Standards and Control, London; [3]Sigma Chem. Comp. Ltd.; [4]Benechemie GMBH, Munich sulphate bound 15 times more strongly than chondroitin 6-sulphate, from which it differs only by the position of sulphate substitution.

The molecular weight of the sulphated polysaccharides must also be taken into account in assessing the binding data. Table 2 illustrates the effect of molecular weight very clearly. When expressed in weight terms, a high molecular weight proteoglycan containing heparin chains attached to a peptide backbone was of apparently lower affinity than its constituent acidic polysaccharide, derived by proteolysis of the parent molecule. Similarly, dextran sulphate of molecular weight 500,000 seemed to be of lower affinity than a preparation of molecular weight 40,000. These apparent differences vanished when the amounts of sulphated polysaccharide were expressed in molar terms. It seems that each molecule of protamine binds one molecule of acidic polysaccharide, irrespective of molecular weight. As protamine is small (mol. wt. ~ 5,000) and most sulphated polysaccharides are considerably larger, this is a not unexpected conclusion. It is conceivable that a protamine molecule may bind more than one small heparin fragment, but the affinity of such fragments was found to be low. Thus a decasaccharide containing the antithrombin III-binding sequence had an affinity for protamine 17-fold less on a weight basis, more than 100-fold less on a molar basis, than the heparin from which it was derived. This result emphasises that the competitive binding assay is completely independent of particular biological activities.

Clearly, as the affinity of the sulphated polysaccharides for protamine varies, it is not possible to express the results of the assay of an incompletely defined unknown in weight terms. Using Sigma heparin as a standard, the units adopted were ng equivalents of heparin ml^{-1}; Evans heparin gave the same standard values.

The competitive binding assay was subject to interference from a variety of proteins, so that it was not possible to assay untreated biological fluids. Precipitation of proteins by a range of methods was unsuccessful; using ^{125}I-heparin as a tracer, it was found that coprecipitation of up to 80 % of the heparin in the sample invariably occurred. However, predigestion of serum, plasma, urine and other biological fluids with pronase yielded material

Table 2

The effect of molecular weight on the apparent affinity of sulphated polysaccharides for protamine

Substance	Source/batch	Mean molecular weight	% SO_4	50 % inhibn. (µg/tube)	50 % inhibn. (pmoles/tube)
Proteoglycan[1]	Rat skin	1,000,000	34.0	0.210	0.210
Heparin chains from proteoglycan[1]	Rat skin	70,000	33.7	0.015	0.214
Dextran sulphate[2]	48C-0241	40,000	53.7	0.0037	0.093
Dextran sulphate[3]	2909	500,000	52.0	0.040	0.080

Fractions were obtained from: [1]A. Horner, University of Toronto; [2]Sigma Chem. Comp. Ltd.; [3]Pharmacia Fine Chemicals AB.

Table 3
The concentrations of heparin-like materials in some biological fluids

Species	Fluid	No. of Samples	Heparin/heparan sulphate (ng equiv. heparin ml^{-1})
Rabbit	Serum	3	120-150
Human	Serum	15	2,200-5,600
Human	Urine	5	510-860
Pig	Follicular fluid	6	25,000-35,000

which was readily assayed. When doubling dilutions of the test sample gave a curve prallel to the standard curve, it was judged that interference from molecules other than sulphated polysaccharides had been effectively removed. Characteristic concentrations of heparin-like materials are given in Table 3; these were obtained after treatment of the sample with chondroitinase ABC (*Proteus vulgaris*: Sigma) as well as pronase. Chondroitinase ABC did not affect the values obtained with serum and urine samples, but did reduce the measured concentration of acidic polysaccharides in follicular fluids. Clearly, follicular fluids contain high concentrations of chondroitins, but the concentrations in other biological fluids are too low to interfere with the measurement of heparin and heparan sulphate.

Using this assay it has been possible to purify the endogenous heparin-like polysaccharide from human cryosupernatant. Purification of larger quantities will enable fuller characterisation of this material.

Conclusion

The properties of this new type of competitive binding assay for heparin and related sulphated polysaccharides can be summarised thus:

Disadvantages:
(1) Response depends on the structure of the polysaccharide.
(2) Biological fluids require pretreatment with pronase.

Advantages:
(1) Sensitive (measures 10 ng ml^{-1}).
(2) Independent of biological activity.
(3) Versatile.
(4) Inexpensive.

When used in conjunction with the available biological assays, this method should yield valuable information about the distribution and function of heparins on cultured cells *in vitro*, and *in vivo* both in the normal individual and in various disease states. It may be useful in monitoring heparin therapy.

Reference

Dawes, J., Pepper, D. S.: Thromb. Res. 14, 845-860 (1979).

Acknowledgements

I would like to express our gratitude to Drs. D. Lane, A. Horner, E. Johnson and M. B. Mathews, who provided us with valuable standards and fractions of sulphated polysaccharides. Dr. Johnson also determined some of the molecular weights and sulphate contents for us. Without their help we could not have attempted this work.

Discussion

Heene asked if there is any possibility to stimulate the endogeneous heparin excretion.

Dawes replied that there probably is, but that this is very new. There are no measurements up to now.

Róka wanted to know how the level in the urine increases after exogeneous heparin administration.

Dawes said that the level increases within 30 min and that a peak is reached after one hour.

Aronson raised the question as to how much endogeneous heparin is synthesized in the body within 24 hours.

Dawes inferred that considering the amount of heparin excreted, there must be a high turnover and a lot of heparin must be synthesized.
Studies with endothelial cells indicate that heparin sulfate is one of the most metabolic reactive constituents, so the turnover is probably quite high. But there are not yet any data.

Duckert stated that there are several metabolites of heparin excreted in urine and wanted to know if they have the same affinity in her test system as heparin.

Dawes explained that urinary heparin is partially desulfated, particularly in the N-position. The N-sulfation is quite important for the affinity; therefore the amount of urinary heparin will be underestimated because of the N-desulfation.

Experiments with labelled heparin have shown that after administration of 5000 units heparin intravenously, a reasonable percentage is excreted intact.

Róka asked if the labelled heparin and the sample are added to the test system at the same time and how long it takes until equilibrium is reached.

Dawes replied that the assay can be run for a range of times. If one needs a very sensitive assay, down to the nanogram level, then one has to run it overnight. High levels can be measured in one hour. The drawback at the moment, as far as time is concerned, is the pronase treatment, which has to be done with biological samples.

Róka asked if it is necessary to remove the pronase.

Dawes answered that it is necessary and that they boil it.

Determination of Low Dose Heparin Activities in Plasma

Ladislaus Róka
Institut für Klinische Chemie und Pathobiochemie
an den Universitätskliniken der Justus Liebig-Universität Gießen
D-6300 Gießen

Heparin is administered for the prophylaxis and therapy of thrombotic disease. However, effective prophylactic and therapeutic plasma levels of heparin are not accurately defined. The assumption that prophylactic low dose heparin administration provides a permanent protection against thrombosis can only be tested by measuring antithrombotic active heparin. Detection of minute amounts of heparin may be important to decide whether patients treated with subcutaneous heparin (5,000 units every 8 hours) are adequately anticoagulated between injections. The anticoagulatory effective heparin is due to heparin-activated antithrombin III (AT). An assay for this anticoagulatory effective heparin must therefore differentiate between progressive AT and heparin-activated AT in a plasma sample.

The speed by which AT inactivates thrombin varies with the relative amounts of thrombin and AT present. With constant amounts of thrombin and plasma, the reaction speed is proportional to the AT contained in the sample (Fig. 1). When the reaction constant K is known and AT is normal, the inactivation rate of thrombin by progressive AT can be predicted. If under these conditions the reaction speed is higher than calculated, the presence of heparin-activated AT has to be assumed. If AT is completely heparin-activated, the reaction rate is limited by the amounts of total AT and thrombin, respectively. Any reaction speed between maximal and progressive can be correlated to a certain concentration of heparin-activated AT. If AT is completely heparin activated, thrombin inactivation is complete within a few seconds at 37 °C. If at the same thrombin to AT-ratio AT is purely progressive, the reaction is much slower and takes several

Heparin · New Biochemical and Medical Aspects

hours. If for practical reasons a short reaction time is chosen, only a very small fraction of progressive AT contained in plasma reacts with thrombin.

The influence of heparin-activated AT on the reaction rate was determined in the following way: Plasma samples containing either progressive or only heparin-activated AT were mixed in different proportions (Fig. 2). When

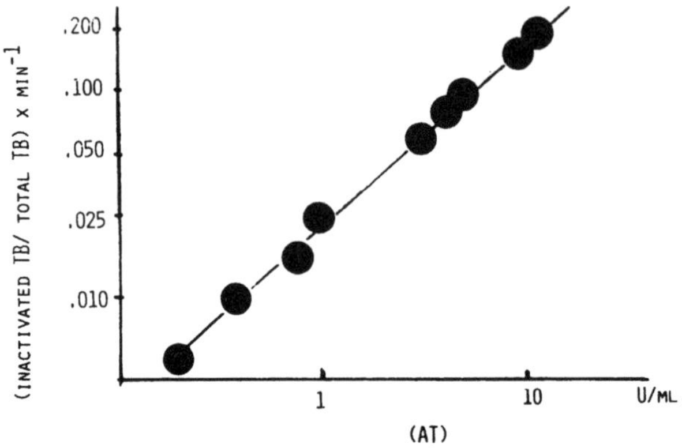

Fig. 1. Initial reaction rate dependent on AT-concentration

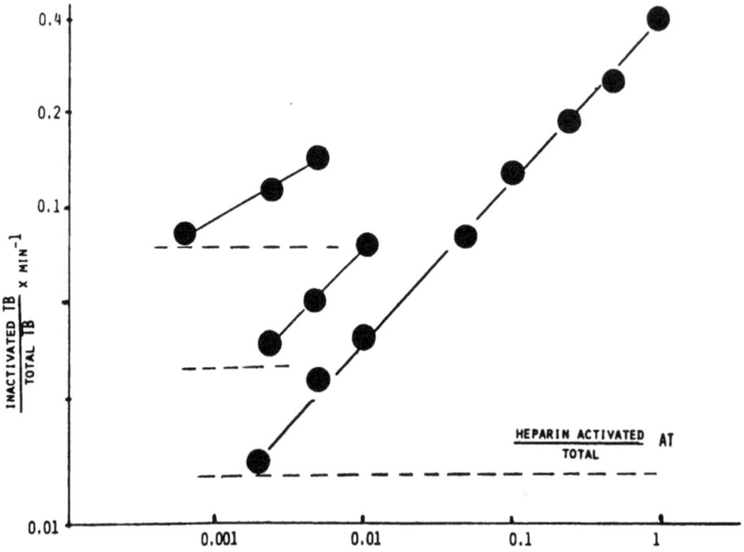

Fig. 2. Reaction rate of different ratios of heparin-activated to total AT at three different levels of total AT

measuring these different mixtures, it turned out that the sensitivity of the heparin assay can be improved by adding more AT to the reaction mixture. With the larger sample volumes, progressive AT reacts faster too. Differences in reaction rates between heparin-activated AT and progressive AT become larger if increasing concentrations of AT are added to the reaction mixture.

The marginal concentration of heparin-activated AT in the reaction mixture was calculated to be 5×10^{-4} inhibitor units. This amount can be measured in the presence of a 3,000 fold excess of progressive antithrombin, if a difference method is used. Employing the difference method the sample is measured in two reaction mixtures, one without and the other with added platelet factor 4 (Fig. 3). Platelet factor 4 neutralises all the heparin in the sample, thus converting all the heparin-activated AT into progressive AT. Platelet factor 4 is used either in purified form or derived from the platelet concentrate of the sample. After centrifuging 1 ml of platelet rich plasma and discarding 900 µl of supernatent, 100 µl of platelet concentrate are obtained, in which progressive AT activity is measured after liberation of platelet factor 4. The amount of PF 4 contained in this concentrate is able to neutralize one unit of heparin (Fig. 4).

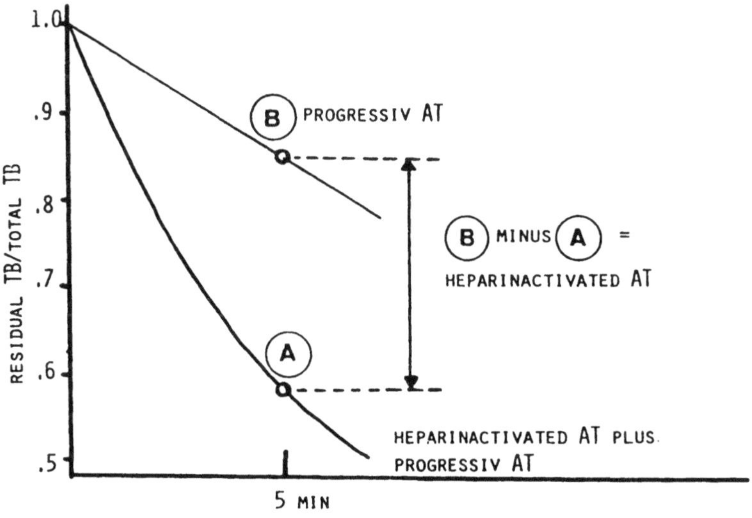

Fig. 3. Difference method for estimation of heparin-activated AT

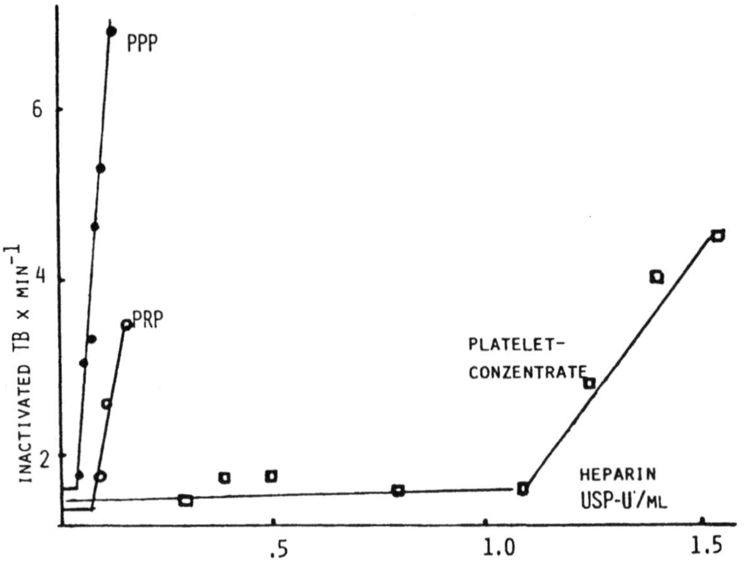

Fig. 4. Neutralisation of heparin by platelet poor plasma (PPP), platelet rich plasma (PRP) and platelet concentrate

Discussion

Friberger asked if polybrene could be used instead of platelet factor 4.

Róka said that he tried polybrene and protamine, but platelet factor 4 works best. The other two components had to be used in rather high concentrations.

Thaler was curious about disease states with high concentrations of α_2-macroglobulin. He asked if this disturbs the calculation.

Róka replied that it does not.

Duckert inquired if one gets the same curve by

1. measuring the residual thrombin without adding heparin and
2. after adding heparin and neutralization with platelet factor 4.

Róka replied in the affirmative explaining that the platelet factor 4 by itself does not change the amount of thrombin consumed, even if added as a crude preparation.

Lill asked if the amount of the plasma sample used in the assay influences the method.

Róka replied that the difference between the amount of thrombin inactivated in the presence or absence of heparin depends to a certain extent on the amount of plasma in the reaction mixture.

One can increase this difference by using more plasma in the reaction mixture.

The extent of inactivation can be increased by using more thrombin, but the amount of activated antithrombin III which is measured is not influenced.

Zimmer suggested that the same information can be obtained by measuring the whole antithrombin III concentration in the heparinized plasma and by measuring also the heparin activated antithrombin III with the Boehringer test kit.

Róka agreed but said that there are some difficulties. From the total amount of antithrombin III, conclusions as to the progressive activity of antithrombin III should be possible. But it has to be taken into consideration that for measuring total antithrombin III and heparin activated antithrombin III, different amounts of plasma are used within the assays. For this reason the results are difficult to compare. Thus the proposed differential measurement is more accurate.

Bender raised a question concerning the handling of the platelet concentrate after sonification. He wanted to know which amount of the concentrate was used, and how long it was incubated.

Róka explained the procedure: the platelet rich plasma is prepared from the blood sample and used to prepare the platelet concentrate. The supernatant is used for the measurement of the heparin activated antithrombin III together with the progressive antithrombin III. The remaining 100 µl of sonicated platelet concentrate can be used for measuring the progressive antithrombin III activity. For that 20 or 40 µl are used so that there is enough material to repeat this measurement and also that of the heparin activated antithrombin III. The sonificated platelet suspension can be kept for a whole day.

Verstraete wanted to know if one can find out precisely with this method what the patient needs in terms of heparin.

Róka replied that only the clinicians can find this out.

Verstraete agreed, but he believes that the differential test will help to find out more exactly the amount of heparin which is needed. He asked if *Róka* considers the platelet count of the patient's plasma from which he prepares the platelet poor plasma, because it is from these platelets that platelet factor 4 will be released in the plasma.

Róka stated that the aim should really be to find out which amount of heparin activated antithrombin III is needed for a given purpose in a given patient. Under certain prophylactic conditions this level may be lower than for therapeutic purposes. But the exact optimal level can only be found out by measuring the level exactly and correlating it with the outcome of the patients (if the patients are protected or not). This cannot be predicted only from the heparin level measured. It has to be correlated with the clinical fate of the patient.

This level will not be constant when intermittent application of heparin is used. What one wants to learn is if and how much the heparin activated antithrombin III level is allowed to decline between injections. There is still nothing known.

In addition, nothing is still known about the correlation between the heparin level and its therapeutic effect.

Verstraete agreed but felt that the real question is what part of the injected heparin is biologically, functionally active.

Róka affirmed that this is his aim. One finds that if one administers the same amount of heparin per kg of body weight to different patients, one does not get the same amount of heparin activated antithrombin III, because part of the heparin goes to other places. That is why it is necessary to determine the therapeutic level of heparin activated antithrombin III.

Verstraete feared that *Róka's* method disregards the haematocrit and also the endogenous platelet factor 4.

Róka replied that he does calculate the haematocrit, but it has to be regarded only when it differs too much from normal.

Concerning the amount of platelet factor 4 in the plasma, *Róka* said that in the circulating plasma there is always a certain amount of free platelet factor 4. If one adds heparin to a plasma sample a certain amount of heparin is bound to heparin-binding substances other than antithrombin III. When they are saturated, heparin activated antithrombin III can be found. A considerable portion of the heparin neutralizing material is platelet factor 4, because by adding platelet factor 4 one can elevate the non-antithrombin III-binding capacity of the plasma. In the plasma of a patient who has not received any heparin, no activated antithrombin III can be measured. If heparin is added to the same plasma sample the formation of heparin activated antithrombin III has a lag phase because heparin is first bound to other compounds than antithrombin III. This lag phase is different for various plasma samples. One can imitate this by adding platelet factor 4 to the plasma sample.

Concerning the liberation of platelet factor 4 during the preparation, *Róka* explained that one cannot liberate platelet factor 4 by contrifuging platelet rich plasma. This only happens after the addition of thrombin to the platelets.

Rosenberg proposed looking at the problem of heparin determination in two separate ways: first as a kinetic system and second in a more practical way.

Seen kinetically, all these methods basically give the same values, which is some measure of the so called heparin activated antithrombin III. This is the measurement of a complex, of the heparin-antithrombin III interaction product, and also a measurement of the recycling time of heparin which actually occurs. In plasma it is a combination of measuring the concentration of the heparin-antithrombin III complex and the heparin recycling time. The measurements are some Δ/time.

These measurements can be effected in a variety of ways. There will be no important interaction by platelet factor 4, because the concentration in plasma is very low. More likely are whole host of other interactions which will slow down the recycling time and hence effect the concentration of the complex.

The real point is that what we are not observing is what is the effect of that effective concentration of the heparin-antithrombin III complex in the individual patient. Theoretically it would be necessary to measure all of the different enzymes of the coagulation cascade as they are activated in the vascular system and determine whether each of them has turned up specifically and at what level for the various products within the heparin preparations.

That is in principle what we really need. That goes to the central point. There are data available which suggest that various patients, who have been heparinized, even with higher doses than usual, are really not heparinized.

There are reasonable data from *Nossel* which show that some patients have fibrinopeptides, although they have received 10,000 units heparin as a single bolus. They should have adequate amounts of activated antithrombin III, but fibrinopeptide evolution has not been quenched.

When *Rosenberg* measured the prothrombin activation fragments in such patients, he found the same thing; they are not quenched. One can show in vitro that the patient's plasma is able to inactivate added factor Xa or thrombin, but in the patient's vascular system the enzymes are not quenched.

The question really is if those chemical examinations are pertinent to the final result. Rosenberg suspects that they are to some degree. The kind of assays are needed from which one can really say if it makes a difference if we see protected enzymes in the vascular system which clinically turn out to be active against fibrinogen.

Róka agreed with *Rosenberg*. The only important thing is to learn if the heparin therapy was of any use for the patient or not. This can be done if one can find out if some heparin-protease complex has been formed, because only in these cases, where proteases are activated, do we need heparin activated antithrombin III. We can only say if the patient has formed activated enzymes if protease-antithrombin III complexes can be found.

We should look for methods which can measure these complexes. One way of doing this might be the detection of neoantigens in these complexes.

Róka then stated his opinion concerning heparin recycling. When antithrombin III and thrombin or factor Xa have complexed, then heparin will be liberated. This is necessary to keep the reaction going. This can be shown by an experiment.

At low pH heparin does not leave the complex. When we have low levels of heparin in a sample and measure the reaction between antithrombin and thrombin at acidic pH, the reaction is fast at the beginning, then stops and continues in a progressive way. This indicates that heparin is used up and non longer liberated from the complex.

When the pH, for instance after one hour, is changed to normal, then the reaction explodes because now the heparin is liberated and the reaction starts again with full speed. Under these experimental conditions *Róka* assumes that heparin is recycling.

Rosenberg conjectered that *Róka* assumes an infinite recycling rate for his assay conditions, which is probably not true. Presumably what is being measured is an average residence time of heparin on the antithrombin III molecule. He suggested that these measurements do not reflect the real in vivo conditions.

Dawes pointed out that many people have shown by radioimmunoassay that it is extremely difficult to stop platelets releasing platelet factor 4. She assumes that *Róka* must have a release of platelet factor 4 in his platelet preparations. She suspects that he has used an insensitive method of detecting platelet factor 4.

Róka explained that he had only wanted to show that platelet factor 4 was not being released in this biological system in amounts which could inactivate heparin.

Dawes stressed that one should not believe that no platelet factor 4 at all is released.

Characterization of Heparin Preparations in Vivo by Different Test Systems*

Job Harenberg, Fernando Fussi**, Werner Junker, Kurt Mattes,
Ellen Weber, Rainer Zimmermann
Abteilung Klinische Pharmakologie
Innere Medizin I und II der
Medizinischen Klinik der Universität Heidelberg
Bergheimer Straße 58
D-6900 Heidelberg
**Hepar Industries
Franklin, Ohio, USA

Summary

Unfractionated (UF) and low molecular weight (LMW) heparin was applied subcutaneously at three different doses to a group of six volunteers. The ex vivo effect on the aPTT, anti-Xa activity and thrombin clotting time (anti-IIa activity) was measured over a period of 6 - 9 hours. The data show that LMW heparin has a more pronounced anticoagulant activity at lower doses than UF heparin. This effect is even twice as high in respect to the anti-Xa activity. It is concluded that LMW heparin has a higher affinity to antithrombin III than UF heparin and that the LMW heparin-antithrombin III complex has a higher affinity to factor Xa than to other coagulation factors in vivo.

*Supported by grants from the Deutsche Forschungsgemeinschaft

Heparin · New Biochemical and Medical Aspects

Introduction

The fate of heparin in vivo can be characterized only by using radiolabeled material (1, 2) or by determination of the pharmacodynamic effects on different enzyme systems (3-5). Regarding the hemostatic system, effects of heparin preparations with a high and low molecular weight have been described in vitro (6-8) and ex vivo (9-10). However, the most important point has always been to determine which of the parameters is the most appropriate or sensitive one for controlling the anticoagulant effect (11-12).

Furthermore, different affinities of heparin preparations to antithrombin III and different affinities of the different heparin-antithrombin III complexes to the coagulation factors IIa and Xa have been assumed in vivo from ex vivo studies (13-15).

We now report on the effect of UF and LMW heparin administered at three different doses subcutaneously in healthy volunteers on the aPTT, IIa and Xa activity ex vivo in order to obtain information on the affinities and binding sites of the two heparin preparations to antithrombin III and of the two heparin-antithrombin III complexes to coagulation factors.

Materials and Methods

Six healthy volunteers agreed to take part in the study after having given their informed consent. UF heparin from pig mucosa (mean MW 12,000, no. 714) and LMW heparin from the same source (mean MW 6,000, no. 1539) prepared by chemical depolymerization in presence of peroxides (16) were used.

On the basis of USP standardization, specific potencies in IU of 1 mg dry substance were 150 IU for the UF heparin and 155 IU for the LMW heparin in the anti-Xa assay and 150 IU (UF heparin) and 90 IU (LMW heparin) in the aPTT assay respectively (17). Of each heparin, 100, 50 and 25 USP/kg body weight were subcutaneously administered into the volunteers at weekly intervals thus providing intraindividual control. Blood samples were withdrawn before injection and after 0.5, 1.5, 2, 2.5, 3, 3.5, 4, 4.5, 5 (25 USP/kg), 6, 7 (50 USP/kg), 8 and 9 hours (100 USP/kg).

The effects on the a PTT, anti-IIa activity (thrombin clotting time) and anti-Xa activity (chromogenic substrate S 2222) were determined as described previously with commercially available reagents (13, 14).

For statistical analyses, the area under the curve of the results obtained was calculated for each volunteer. These data were then subjected to the Wilcoxon pair test for dependent variables. The required level of significance was 5 %.

Results

The UF heparin showed a marked anticoagulant effect ex vivo on the aPTT, thrombin clotting time and anti-Xa activity after the subcutaneous application of 100 USP/kg body weight. The ex vivo effect decreased substantially in all test systems when 50 USP/kg had been applied subcutaneously (Fig. 1, 2). After 25 USP/kg body weight, a significant effect could no longer be observed either on the aPTT, the thrombin clotting time or on the anti-Xa activity (Fig. 1, 2, 3).

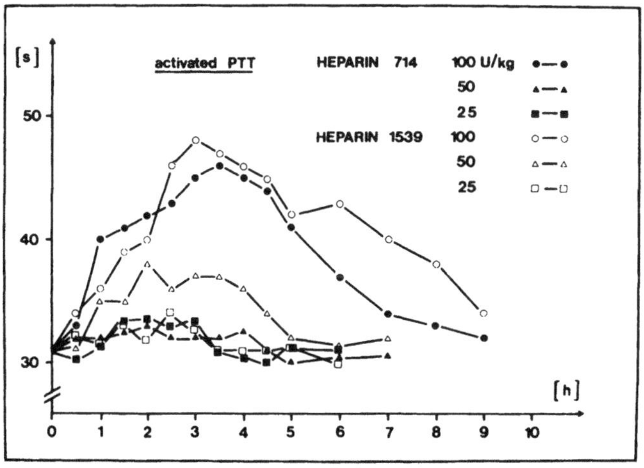

Fig. 1. The ex vivo effect of UF heparin (714) and LMW heparin (1539) on the aPTT (ordinate, sec) is shown (mean values) before and after s.c. application (abscissa, hours) of three doses (100, 50 and 25 USP/kg body weight)

The effect of the LMW heparin ex vivo on the aPTT and thrombin clotting time was within the same range as that of the UF heparin at 100 USP/kg body weight (Fig. 1, 2). The anti-Xa activity, however, was significantly higher at this dose ($p < 0.05$, Fig. 3) than the effect of the UF heparin.

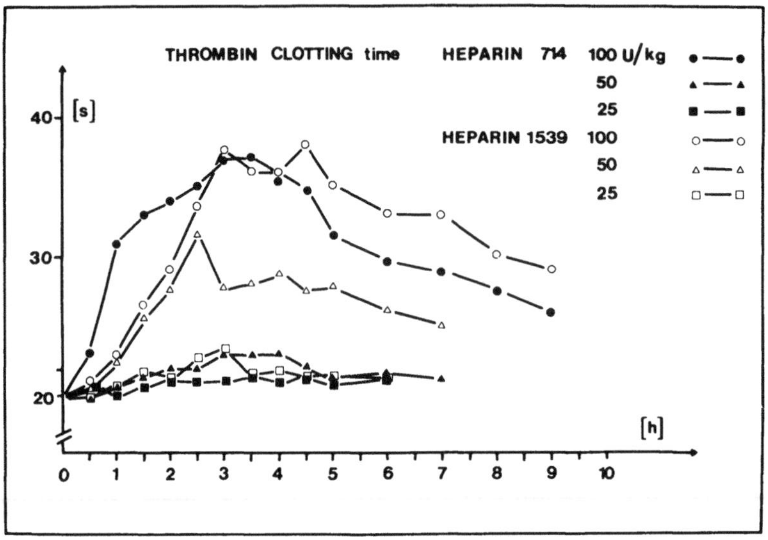

Fig. 2. The ex vivo effect of UF and LMW heparin on the thrombin clotting time is shown.

The ex vivo effect on the aPTT, thrombin clotting time and anti-Xa activity of 50 USP LMW heparin/kg body weight was significantly higher than that of UF heparin ($p < 0.05$, Fig. 1, 2, 3). The anti-Xa activity showed quite a different pattern than the other coagulation test systems. The effects of 50 USP LMW heparin and 100 USP UF heparin were found to be within the same range and did not differ significantly ($p > 0.05$). With regard to the ex vivo effect of these two doses on the aPTT and thrombin clotting time, the differences between 50 USP LMW heparin and 100 USP UF heparin were significant ($p < 0.05$).

No ex vivo effect of 25 USP LMW heparin/kg body weight subcutaneously was observed on the aPTT and thrombin clotting time. On the anti-Xa activity, however, a small but markedly higher effect was observed than after 25 USP UF heparin/kg body weight (Fig. 3).

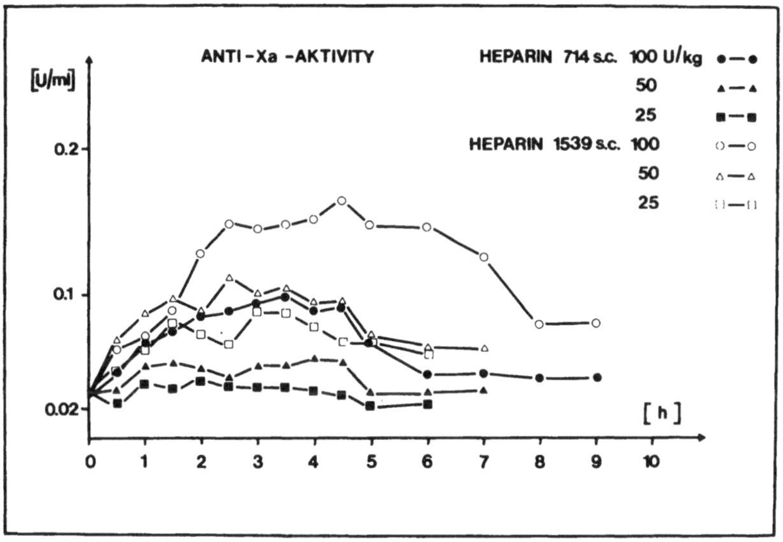

Fig. 3. The ex vivo effect of heparin (714) and LMW heparin (1539) on the anti-Xa activity (expressed in USP heparin/ml plasma, ordinate) is depicted (mean values) before and after application of 100, 50 and 25 USP heparin/kg body weight.

Discussion

Unfractionated heparin is known to have fractions with high and low affinities to antithrombin III in vitro (18). This has been demonstrated also for heparin preparations with low molecular weight (19).

In vitro, the different affinities of the heparins to antithrombin III were related to different binding constants of heparin (20). Furthermore, different binding sites were identified on the antithrombin III molecule for different heparin preparations (20).

Ex vivo, the effect of intravenously injected heparin prepared from pig intestinal mucosa and bovine lung supported the in vitro results in which the bovine lung heparin revealed lower anti-Xa activity (21). Different heparin preparations of the same molecular weight range of different origins revealed different effects on the aPTT and anti-Xa activity in vivo, whereas on anti-IIa activity they did not differ (21). Thus, different affinities to antithrombin III in vivo were assumed by these authors.

The present data provide some evidence that heparin preparations with different molecular weights have different affinities to antithrombin III in vivo. In vivo, heparin binds to several plasma proteins such as antithrombin III, lipases and platelet factor 4 (3-5). It can be assumed that heparins with different molecular weights have different physicochemical properties and thus different affinities to the various plasma proteins. This has been demonstrated especially for antithrombin III. The present data show that the LMW heparin has a higher ex vivo effect on the anti-Xa activity at all doses applied subcutaneously than the UF heparin. At lower doses (50 USP/kg body weight), however, also a higher anti-IIa and aPTT effect was observed ex vivo after the application of the LMW heparin. These differences can be explained by a higher affinity of the LMW heparin to antithrombin III in vivo (Fig. 4). The effect on the lipolytic activity and the platelet factor 4 activity, however, was not investigated in this study.

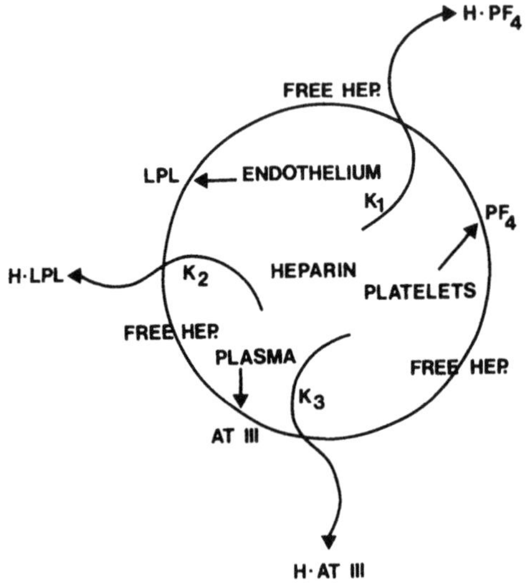

Fig. 4. The binding of heparin in vivo to the different plasma proteins is shown. The binding constants (K_1, K_2, K_3) are determined by the physicochemical properties of the heparin. Because the binding constants have not been determined in vivo or ex vivo, it is also called affinity of heparin.

The data further indicate that the heparin-antithrombin III complexes of the different heparin preparations exhibit different affinities and/or binding sites to the coagulation factors IIa and Xa (Fig. 5) in vivo. Thus, the UF heparin used here showed a marked ex vivo effect only at a dose of 100 USP/kg body weight, whereas at 50 USP/kg no differences were observed. Furthermore, no difference of these patterns were found between effects on the anti-Xa, anti-IIa and aPTT. The LMW heparin, however, exhibited about twice the ex vivo effect on the anti-Xa assay, compared to the UF heparin. This was not observed on the anti-IIa determination. These differences might be explained by a higher affinity of the LMW heparin-antithrombin III complex than the UF heparin-antithrombin III complex to factor Xa.

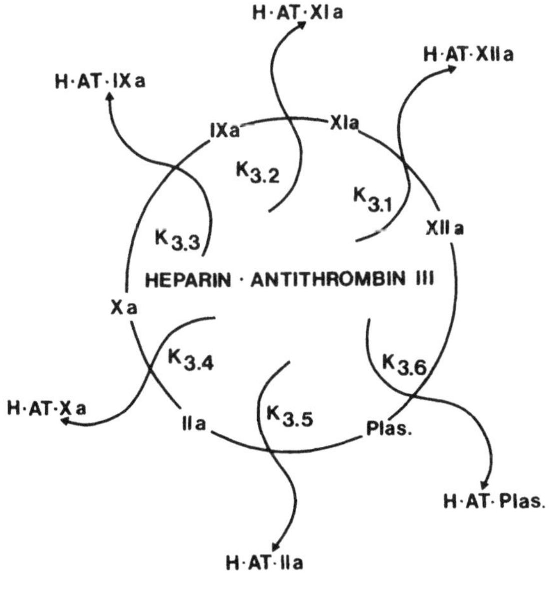

Fig. 5. The different proteases which are inhibited by the heparin-antithrombin III complexes are shown. From the present ex vivo results it is supposed that different binding constants ($K_{3.1 - 3.6}$) or affinities of the heparin-antithrombin III complexes of each heparin do exist in vivo.

Alternatively to this hypothesis and in agreement with the in vitro results of Rosenberg, the present data indicate that different binding sites on the antithrombin III molecule can be assumed for the UF and LMW heparin in vivo. Thus, the LMW heparin binding site of the antithrombin III molecule would have a higher affinity for the LMW heparin than the UF heparin binding site for the UF heparin. However, further in vivo studies with more highly purified heparin preparations are necessary to confirm this.

References

1. Zöllner, N., Kaiser, W.: Exp. Med. Zschr. ges. exp. Med. einschl. Chir. 158, 89-94 (1972).

2. Dawes, J., Pepper, D. S.: Thromb. Res. 14, 845-869 (1979).

3. Estes, J. W., Poulin, P. F.: Thromb. Diathes. Haemorrh. 33, 26-37 (1974).

4. Brown, W. V., Wang-Iverson, P., Paterniti, J.: Chemistry and Biology of Heparin, 175-185 (1981) Elsevier/North Holland.

5. Cella, G., Girolami, A.: Chemistry and Biology of Heparin. 403-406 (1981) Elsevier/North Holland.

6. Anderson, L. O., Barowcliffe, T. W., Holmer, E., Johnson, E. A., Sims, G. E. G.: Thromb. Res. 9, 574-583 (1976).

7. Laurent, T. C., Tengblad, A., Thunberg, L., Höök, M., Lindahl, U.: Biochem. J. 175, 691-701 (1978).

8. Thunberg, L., Lindahl, U., Tengblad, A., Laurent, T. C.: Biochem. J. 181, 241-243 (1979).

9. Lane, D. A., Michalski, R., v. Ross, M. E., Kakkar, V. V.: Brit. J. Haematol. 37, 239-245 (1975).

10. Thomas, D. P., Merton, R. E., Lewis, W. E., Barowcliffe, T. W.: Thrombos. Haemostas. 45, 214-218 (1981).

11. Teien, A. N., Lie, M.: Thromb. Res. 7, 777-788 (1975).

12. Vinazzer, H.: Anaesthesist 28, 299-303 (1979).

13. Harenberg, J., Fussi, F., Grün, M., Schlegel, A., Mattes, K., Zimmermann, R., Weber, E.: Mikrozirkulation und Prostaglandinstoffwechsel. 399-402 (1981). F. K. Schattauer Verlag, Stuttgart - New York.

14. Harenberg, J., Junker, W., Fussi, F., Mattes, K., Zimmermann, R., Weber, E.:Thrombos. Haemostas. 46, 235 (1981).

15. Harenberg, J., Fussi, F., Grün, M., Schlegel, A., Mattes, K., Zimmermann, R., Weber, E.: Thrombos. Haemostas. 46, 375 (1981).

16. Fussi, F.: US Pat. Appl. (January 28, 1980).

17. Fussi, F., Girolami, A., Cella, G.: Chemistry and Biology of Heparin. 535-546 (1981) Elsevier/North Holland.

18. Höök, M., Björk, J., Hopwood, J., Lindahl, U.: FEBS Letters 66, 90-93 (1976).

19. Rosenberg, R. D., Armand, G., Lam, L.: Proc. Natl. Acad. Sci. USA 75, 3065-3069 (1978).

20. Rosenberg, R. D., Jordan, R. E., Faureau, L. U., Lam, L. H.: Biochem. Biophys. Res. Comm. 86, 1319-1324 (1979).

21. Barowcliffe, T. W., Johnson, E. A., Eggelton, C. A., Thomas, D. P.: Thromb. Res. 12, 27-36 (1977).

Discussion

Witt asked if *Harenberg* had estimated the lipoprotein lipase activity after administration of the different types of heparin.

Harenberg had not measured it.

Wenzel asked if the different heparins were administered to the healthy volunteers one after the other.

Harenberg explained that they had performed two studies: in the first study they administered all types of heparin to each volunteer in weekly intervals. In the second, each volunteer received six administrations at different rates.

Bhargava asked for the activity of the low molecular weight heparin in anti-Xa units.

Harenberg explained that the low molecular weight heparin had an activity of 200 units/mg substance. This was a little bit higher than the activity of the 15000 molecular weight heparin. It was different from the heparin used by *Kakkar*. Standard curves were obtained according to the USP standard.

Zimmer pointed out that *Harenberg* had measured the Xa-activity with a chromogenic substrate and the thrombin activity with a clotting method. He thinks that it is not correct to compare these two methods because the thrombin time is influenced by several factors and does not depend only on the heparin activity.

Harenberg replied that he had found a good correlation between several methods for measuring thrombin activity and therefore chosen to measure the thrombin clotting time.

Determination of Heparin and Fractionated Heparin with Different Molecular Weights

Ulrich Schmitz-Huebner*
Medizinische Klinik und
Poliklinik der Universität Münster
D-4400 Münster

Summary

The anticoagulant activity of ordinary and fractionated heparin preparations with different molecular weight distributions has been studied in vitro and ex vivo after subcutaneous administration to healthy volunteers. Different clotting and chromogenic assays were used for the determinations of heparin activity. In vitro the differences between the specific activities of the preparations determined with different assays were relatively small, while ex vivo a large discrepancy between the levels of anti-Xa activity and the effects on the APTT and TCT induced by low molecular weight heparin was observed. Possible explanations for the different action of certain heparin preparations in vivo are still hypothetical.

Introduction

Heparin is a chemically and functionally heterogeneous polyanion. No precise and sensitive method for its direct chemical determination in blood has yet been devised. Clotting tests and more recently assays with synthetic substrates have been used to quantify the activity of heparin in terms of International or USP units. These methods in general only measure one aspect of the anticoagulant activity of the drug. Therefore determinations of

*Supported by Deutsche Forschungsgemeinschaft, grant Schm 345/3

Heparin · New Biochemical and Medical Aspects

heparin with several methods in parallel are needed to characterize the whole of its effect. Such experiments were performed in the present investigation designed to elucidate further the anticoagulant action of heparin preparations with different molecular weights both in vitro and in vivo.

Materials and Methods

Heparin preparations. 1. Unfractionated porcine sodium mucous heparin. Mean molecular weights: 9,600 (Lot no. 79093 DP) and 13,000 (Lot no. 02A). 2. Heparin fractions with high (HMW) and low (LMW) molecular weights prepared from Lot no. 02A by gel filtration chromatography (Schmitz-Huebner et al., submitted for publication).

Determination of heparin activity. Standard curves were made with each subject's pre-injection plasma and levels of heparin activity in the post-injection plasma were measured from single point estimates against a heparin standard curve prepared with a USP reference heparin. For the estimation of in vitro anticoagulant potencies, a calibration curve was established with the USP standard and a normal plasma pool. Each heparin preparation was diluted into the range of the calibration curve and assayed three times at different dilutions. The following assays and reagents were employed:

APTT (1): Pathrombin (Behringwerke AG, Marburg), Standardised APTT Reagent (Dr. L. Poller, Manchester, UK).
Anti-Xa Clotting Test (2): Plasma-CEF/Activated Factor X set (Sigma, Saint Louis, Missouri, USA).
Amidolytic Assays: Substrates S-2222 (3) and S-2238 (4) (Deutsche Kabi, München).
Thrombin Clotting Time = TCT (5):Test-Thrombin (Behringwerke AG, Marburg).

Plasma. Blood used for heparin estimations was centrifuged immediately after collection at 4 °C (2500 g for 40 min.) and the plasma was stored at -30 °C for not longer than 3 months, when not processed on the same occasion for the determinations of the APTT.

In vivo experiments. Unfractionated and fractionated heparin preparations were administered by subcutaneous injections of 5,000 U to six healthy human volunteers from whom informed consent had been obtained. This dosage was injected twice daily over a period of three days. Intervals of at least one week were observed between the treatments. Any other sort of therapy before and during the trials was refrained from.

Results

1. **In vitro activities.** Table 1 shows the mean molecular weights and the specific anticoagulant activities of the four heparin preparations used. As it was to be expected the potencies of the preparations vary considerably depending on the type of assay. Also the medium in which the assay is performed seems to have influence on the activity of heparin. Its anti-Xa activity in particular is higher when purified AT III preparations are employed than when heparin is determined in plasma.

2. **Ex vivo activities.** The kinetics of heparin activities after subcutaneous administration of 5,000 U of two ordinary heparin preparations are shwon in Fig. 1. While the effect of these preparations on the APTT is very similar, it differs when measured by anti-Xa assays. In fact, heparin lot no. 79093 having the lowest average molecular weight induces significantly higher anti-Xa activities than the other unfractionated preparation. Corresponding results were obtained when two heparin fractions separated during the same gel filtration chromatography were injected (Fig. 2). Again, the anti-Xa effect of the LMW preparations was considerably more pronounced than the same activity induced by the HMW fraction. No significant difference was observed between the APTT results. In order to facilitate comparisons, the APTT results obtained with the LMW fraction as well as its effects on the simultaneously performed TCT were read as levels of heparin in plasma (Fig. 3). Both heparin activities were in the same range and markedly lower than the corresponding anti-Xa activities.

3. **Correlations between different anti-Xa tests.** The effects of the LMW fraction on the two anti-Xa tests performed were studied comparing the

Table 1: Anticoagulant and molecular weight characteristics of the four heparin preparations studied. Anticoagulant potencies assayed as specific activities in vitro (U/mg)

Method	Source of AT III	7 9 0 9 3	0 2 A	Fraction 05	Fraction 04
USP	Sheep Plasma	128	152	194	105
APTT	Human Plasma	128	151	156	87
Anti-Xa Clotting	Human Plasma	172	136	136	105
S-2222	Human Plasma	192	148	145	104
S-2222	Purified AT III	220	161	186	109
S-2238	Human Plasma	156	170	171	108
S-2238	Purified AT III	151	153	169	106
Estimated Mean Molecular Weight		9,300	13,000	16,000	8,900

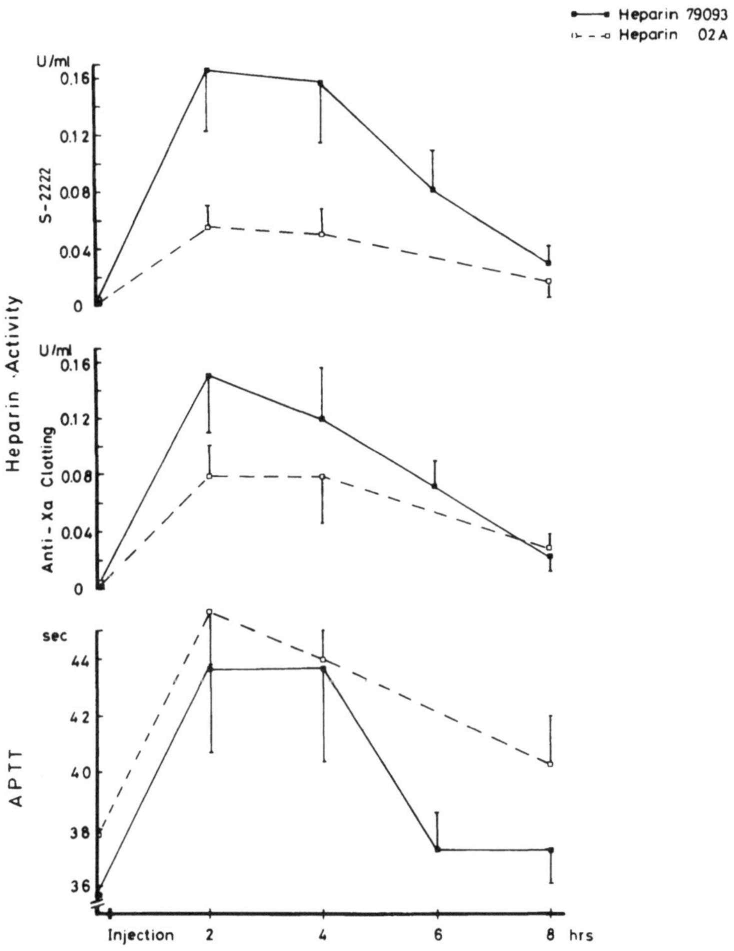

Fig. 1. Kinetics of heparin activities and APTT results after one subcutaneous injection of each heparin preparation. Mean values ± S. E. M.

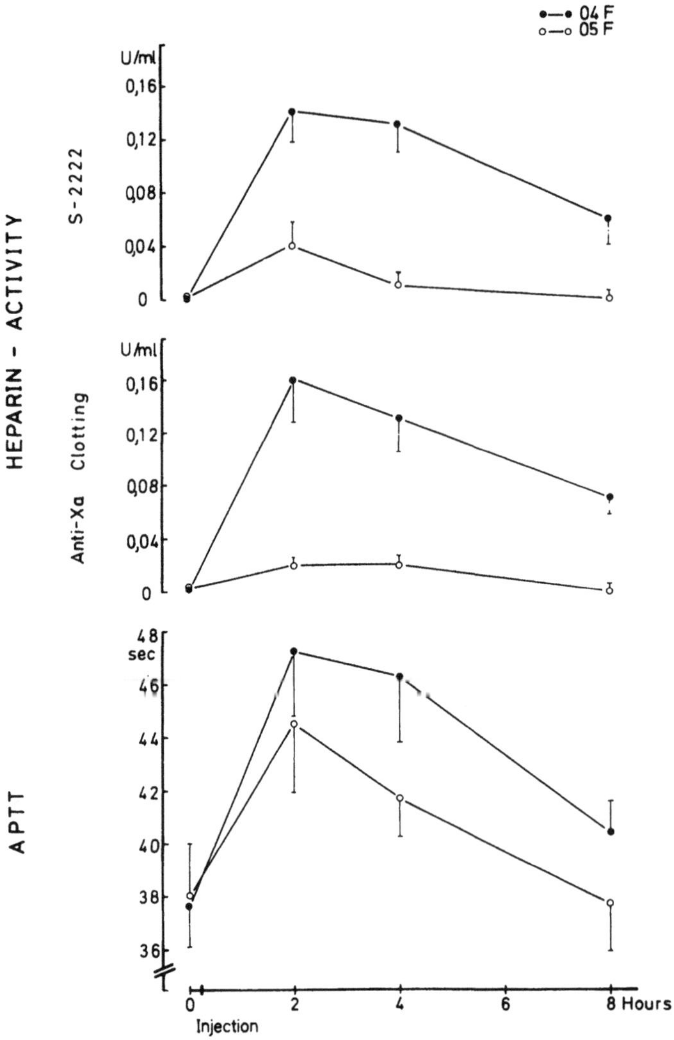

Fig. 2. Kinetics of heparin activities and APTT results after one subcutaneous injection of each heparin fraction. Mean values ± S. E. M.

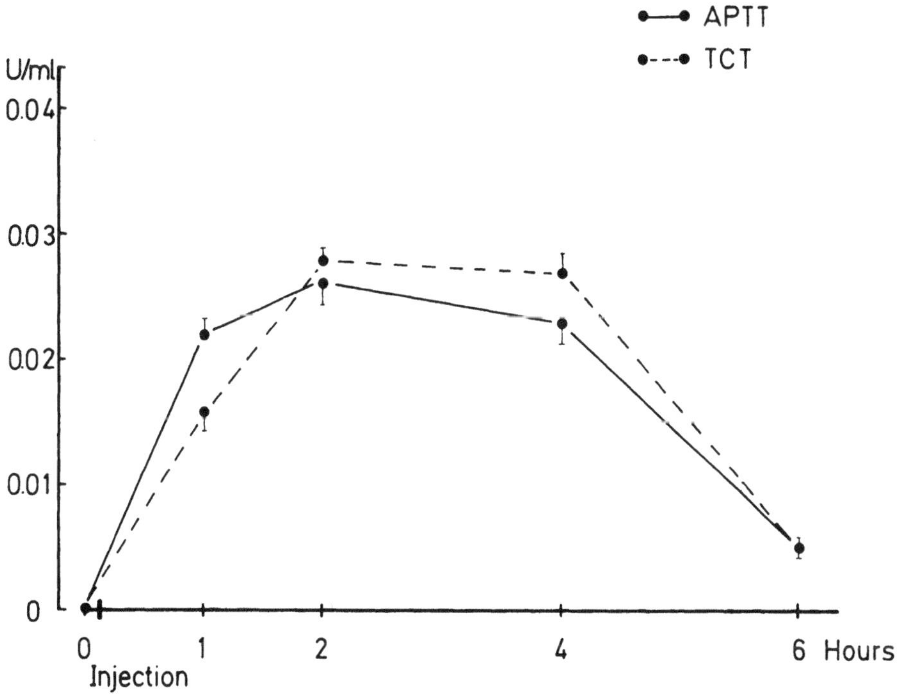

Fig. 3. Kinetics of heparin activities determined by the APTT and TCT after one subcutaneous injection of the LMW heparin fraction. Mean values ± S. E. M.

results of 78 parallel determinations. A significant positive correlation was found (Fig. 4). The corresponding activities obtained after injections of the other heparin preparations also correlated significantly.

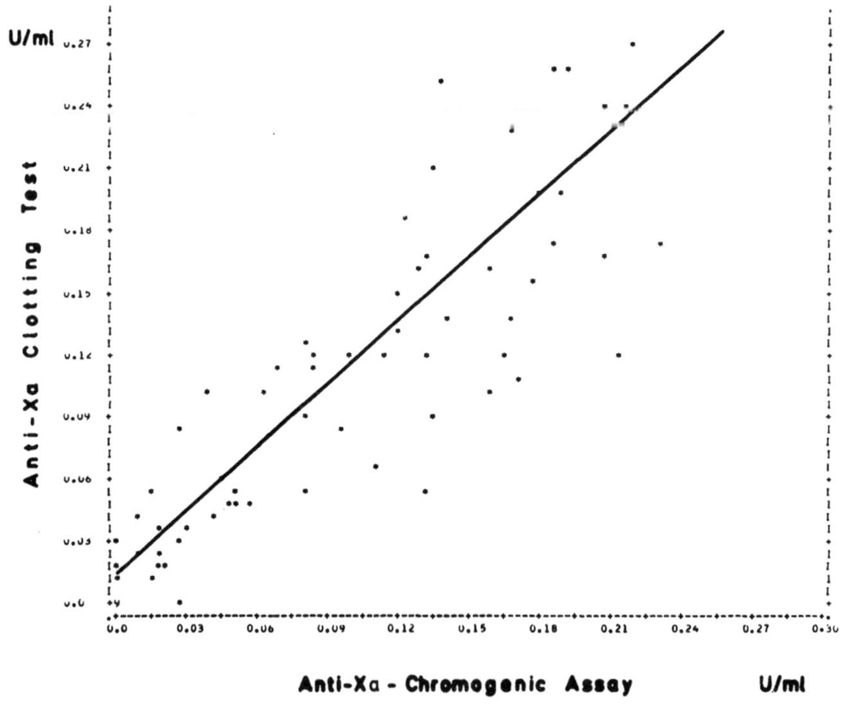

Fig. 4. Correlation analysis between the effects induced by the LMW heparin fraction on anti-Xa clotting respectively chromogenic assays. n = 78, r = 0.93, y = 0.96 + 0.01

Discussion

The anticoagulant activity of heparin preparations in vitro depends on several factors. It is generally accepted that affinity to antithrombin III is a prerequisite for the anticoagulant effect of a heparin molecule. Recent investigations (6,7) have provided evidence that the molecular weight plays an important role in determining the specific inhibitory effect of heparin on the clotting mechanism. In addition, plasma seems to contain one or more components able to inhibit certain heparin activities. To date, the way in which plasma exerts this modulating effect on heparin is controversial (8, 9). Obviously, these factors acting in vitro also have influence on the activitiy of heparin in vivo. However, as demonstrated by the present investigations, it is not possible to predict the in vivo effects of a preparation of heparin on the basis of in vitro assays. After subcutaneous administration the preparations chiefly containing low molecular weight species induced higher anti-Xa activities than was to be expected from the in vitro results. Although the reasons for this discrepancy are not yet clear, two mechanisms might be responsible:

1. HMW heparin chains are possibly neutralized and/or eliminated from circulation more rapidly than LMW molecules.
2. LMW heparin fractions might release endogenous polysaccharides exhibiting heparin-like properties.

Preliminary studies performed in our laboratory show that HMW heparin can indeed be neutralized to a greater extent by heparin antagonists than LMW preparations. The second possibility has also been discussed in connection with a heparin analogue which is practically inactive in vitro but which induces considerable anti-Xa activity in vivo (10).

The determination of heparin activities with different assays is indispensable when the effect of fractionated heparin is to be studied. It could be shown that under the conditons of the present investigations the results obtained with some of these tests correlated very well.

References

1. Proctor, R. R., Rapaport, S. I.: Amer. J. Clin. Pathol. 36, 212 (1961).

1. Yin, E. T., Wessler, S., Butler, J.: J. Lab. Clin. Med. 81, 298 (1973).

3. Teien, A. N., Lie, M., Abildgaard, U.: Thromb. Res. 8, 413 (1976).

4. Larsen, M. L., Abildgaard, U., Teien, A. N., Gjesdal, K.: Thromb. Res. 13, 285 (1978).

5. Godal, H. C.: Scand. J. Clin. Lab. Invest. 13, 153 (1961).

6. Oosta, G. M., Gardner, W. T., Beeler, D. L., Rosenberg, R. D.: Proc. Natl. Acad. Sci. 78, 829 (1981).

7. Holmer, E., Kurachi, K., Söderström, G.: Biochem. J. 193, 395 (1981).

8. Holmer, E., Lindahl, U., Bäckström, G., Thunberg, L., Sandberg, H., Söderström, G., Andersson, L.-O.: Thromb. Res. 18, 861 (1980).

9. Mac Gregor, I., Lane, D. A., Kakkar, V. V.: Biochim. Biophys. Acta 617, 472 (1980).

10. Thomas, D. P., Lane, D. A., Michalski, R., Johnson, E. A., Kakkar, V. V.: Lancet 1, 120 (1977).

Discussion

In answer to *Spaethe's* question concerning the regression line *Schmitz-Hübner* stated that it did not go through the zero point. The low activities gave higher values with the Yin and Wessler test and the higher activities produced higher values with the chromogenic substrate method.

Róka asked *Aronson*, if he had any evidence that the uptake of heparin by macrophages depends on the molecular weight of the heparin. The different activities of high and low molecular weight heparin after subcutaneous injection might depend on the different uptake by macrophages.

Aronson answered that this question is under investigation but that he cannot report on any results yet.

Spaethe wondered if *Schmitz-Hübner* had measured both the anti-Xa and the anti-thrombin activity of the different heparins with chromogenic substrates. This would be a good comparison because as *Rosenberg* reported there are different binding capacities of different heparins towards factor Xa and thrombin.

Schmitz-Hübner reported that he had made some heparin measurements with the low molecular weight heparin fraction with S-2238. It was seen that the low molecular weight heparin had higher activity than the high molecular weight heparin, but it was not so high as with the substrate S-2222.

Rosenberg stated that the anti-Xa activity is sometimes said to be higher with low molecular weight fractions compared to anti-thrombin activity, which is low.
It is thought that a high anti-Xa activity is desirable, but it may be that a low anti-thrombin activity is undesirable.
Part of the problem is that heterogenous all-molecular weight fractions are used as a titrant for standard curves. These fractions contain heparins with multiple binding sites for antithrombin which results in a high anti-thrombin activity relativ to the anti-Xa activity. The low molecular weight heparin fractions may perhaps have the more undesirable characteristics.

Schmitz-Hübner admitted that it is not certain what the desirable characteristics of heparin should be for the in vivo model.

III. Clinical Usage of Heparin

Low Molecular Weight Heparin and the Prevention of Postoperative Deep Vein Thrombosis

V. V. Kakkar, B. Djazaeri, J. Fok, M. Scully, J. Westwick
Thrombosis Research Unit
King's College Hospital Medical School
Denmark Hill
London SE5 8RX

Summary

Equal amounts of the LMW and UF heparin injected intravenously and subcutaneously in healthy volunteers produced different responses in anti factor Xa and APTT assays. Significant difference in prolongation of APTT was observed following intravenous injection while the LMW heparin produced nearly 4 times greater anti-factor Xa activity following sucutaneous injection. Both preparations of heparin affected the coagulation mechanism and in-vivo platelet function to the same extent when administered subcutaneously for 7 postoperative days in 30 patients undergoing major abdominal surgery.

The efficacy of LMW heparin as a prophylactic agent was assessed in 150 consecutive patients over the age of 40 undergoing major abdominal surgery. 50 of these received 1250 APTT units of the LMW heparin every 12 hourly i. e. 2 injections per day; isotopic DVT was diagnosed in only 1 (2 %) patient during prophylaxis. 100 patients received a single injection of 1850 APTT units of LMW heparin; 3 developed isotopic DVT, venography failed to confirm the presence of thrombi in each case. None of the 150 patients investigated died due to fatal or contributory pulmonary emboli. LMW heparin was not associated with any increase in peroperative or postoperative bleeding.

Heparin · New Biochemical and Medical Aspects

Introduction

Several clinical trials have established that low dose heparin provides effective prophylaxis not only against deep vein thrombosis but also against death from pulmonary embolism in the post operative patient (1-5). However, in two reported studies investigating large numbers of patients, a significant difference was observed between those receiving heparin who developed wound heamatoma and their control counter parts (1, 2).

Commercially available heparin represents a heterogenous mass which is the result of a degree of randomness in the biosynthetic process (6). Therefore, it is considered to be a family of straight chain anionic polysaccharides of highly variable molecular weight extending from perhaps 3000 to 40,000 Daltons (6,7). Fractionation of heparin using gel filtration yields fractions of different molecular weights (7, 8, 9).

Antithrombin III inhibits a number of activated coagulation factors in addition to thrombin, including Factor IXa, Xa, XIa, and XIIa; all these inhibition reactions are markedly accelerated in the presence of heparin (10-15). Recent studies have demonstrated that heparin activity is modulated by its molecular weight. The potentiation of the inhibition of Factor Xa in plasma system is strongly dependent on the molecular size of heparin, this specific activity per unit weight increasing with decreasing molecular weight (16-20). In contrast, measurements on the effect on activated partial thromboplastin time (APTT) which reflects a change in overall clotting mechanism, showed that this activity of heparin increased with increasing molecular weight (18-20).

The investigations described in this paper were aimed at answering three questions: what is the response when the LMW and the UF heparin is administered intravenously and subcutaneously; whether the LMW and the UF heparin effect the coagulation mechanism and in-vivo platelet function to the same extent in patients undergoing major abdominal surgery, and whether a low or moderate dose of LMW heparin is effective in preventing postoperative deep vein thrombosis without producing excessive bleeding.

Patients and Methods

Studies were performed in healthy volunteers and in patients undergoing major abdominal surgery. All received a written and oral description of the study protocol, and gave their consent to participate.

LMW and UF heparin. Both preparations of heparin were supplied by Laboratoire Choay, Paris (France). The UF heparin was commercial calcium heparin (Calciparine®). For preparing LMW fraction, is was extracted with a mixture of ethanol and water (21) and purified. This fraction was studied by physical (^{13}C-n.m.r. spectroscopy) and chemical techniques. Compared with the UF heparin, it contained a higher percentage of non sulfated uronic acid and particularly glucuronic acid (about 30 % of total uronic acids) as well as a higher percentage of N-acetyl-glucosamine, whereas the content in sulfate groups was lower (22). The molecular weights of the UF heparin and the LMW fractions were estimated by comparing their elution positions from a column of Ultrogel with the fractions whose molecular weights had been determined by a sedimentation diffusion equilibrium method. The mean molecular weight of the UF heparin and the LMW fraction was 18.000 and 6,000 Daltons respectively. The anticoagulant activities of the two heparin preparations were assessed using APTT (23) and anti-Xa clotting assays (24). The LMW fraction had a specific activity of 200 iu/ml in anti-factor Xa assay and 50 iu/ml in APTT assay. The ratio between both types of activities in tests using human plasma was thus 4. The UF heparin had a specific activity of 150 iu/ml on both assays. The LMW fraction was supplied in a single dose vial prepared under approved pharmaceutical conditions and containing either 1250 APTT units (5000 anti-Xa units) in 0.2 ml or 1850 APTT units (7500 anti-Xa units) in 0.3 ml. Tests for sterility and pyrogens were satisfactory.

Studies in healthy volunteers. Six healthy volunteers (4 males and 2 females), mean age 28 years (range 25-34), consented to receive subcutaneous and intravenous injections of the LMW and the UF heparin. The injections were given on a randomised basis at weekly intervals and the amount of heparin given was based on APTT assay. Venous blood samples were obtained before and at 5, 15, 30 and 60 mins after intravenous injection and 1, 3 and 5 hr following subcutaneous administration. In another 5 healthy volunteers aged 24-38 years, (4 male and 1 female) who received the LMW heparin only, blood samples were withdrawn up to 24 hours after subcutaneous injection.

Studies in Patients

Effect on coagulation and platelet function

Thirty patients who were admitted for major abdominal surgery were randomly allocated to receive either 1250 APTT units of the LMW or 5000 APTT units of the UF heparin subcutaneously, starting 2 hours before surgery and then every 12 hours for 7 postoperative days. Blood samples were obtained before administration of heparin, before surgery in the anaesthetic room, midway during operation, in the recovery room and on the first and seventh postoperative days. They were analysed for heparin levels measured by anti-factor Xa assay, antithrombin III concentration, lipoprotein lipase release, activated partial thromboplastin time (APTT), plasma fibrinopeptide A (FPA) and pre-kallikrein levels, and tests of in-vivo platelet function measured by estimating the level of β-thromboglobulin (βTG), platelet factor 4 (PF4) and thromboxane B_2 (TxB_2) formation.

Prevention of Deep Vein Thrombosis

The efficacy of the LMW heparin in preventing postoperative DVT was assessed in 150 consecutive patients aged over 40 years undergoing major elective abdominal surgery. The details of age, sex, type of operation performed and other risk factors likely to influence the incidence of DVT are shown in Table I and II. The first 50 of these received 1250 units of the LMW heparin subcutaneously starting 2 hours prior to surgery and 12 hourly thereafter for seven days. The other 100 patients received a single daily injection of 1850 APTT units of LMW heparin again starting 2 hours before surgery, and continuing for seven postoperative days. In 25 of these, simplate bleeding time was measured before, during and 24 hours after surgery.

Table I. Details of Patients Investigated

Patients Studied	Two injections per day	One injection per day
No.	50	100
Sex	23 m, 27 f	39 m, 61 f
Age (yrs) Mean	61.4 ± 11.7	60.3 ± 13.2
<40	4 (4 %)	2 (4 %)
40-49	19 (19 %)	9 (18 %)
50-59	23 (23 %)	11 (22 %)
60-69	30 (30 %)	18 (36 %)
>70	24 (24 %)	10 (20 %)
Predisposing risk factors		
Varicose veins	6 (12 %)	11 (11 %)
Varicose ulcer	1 (2 %)	7 (7 %)
Malignancy	12 (24 %)	30 (30 %)
Previous DVT #PE	2 (4 %)	3 (3 %)
Previous myocardial infarction	2 (4 %)	5 (5 %)
Chronic bronchitis	3 (6 %)	4 (4 %)
Oestrogen therapy	0	5 (5 %)

Assessment

Diagnosis of DVT

DVT was detected by the radioactive fibrinogen uptake test using the technique previously described (25). Patients were scanned for at least 10 days. DVT was diagnosed if the counts at any site differed by 20 % or more from those at the adjacent points on the same leg or at the same position in the opposite limb, and if this difference persisted or increased in the subsequent 24 hours (25). In patients, who had raised counts, ascending venograms were performed to determine the exact site and extent of the thrombus (26).

Table II. Operations performed

	Two injections per day	One injection per day
No. of patients	50	100
Gastric	15 (30.0 %)	21 (21.0 %)
Oesophagectomy	1	3
Total and partial Gastrectomy	4	10
Vagotomy and Pyloroplasty	6	6
Gastroenterostomy	4	2
Biliary	16 (32.0 %)	31 (31.0 %)
Cholecystectomy alone	12	23
Cholecystectomy and Exploration of CBD	3	5
Cholecystoenterostomy	1	2
Partial Pancreatectomy or Drainage	0	3
Large Bowel	16 (32.0 %)	27 (27.0 %)
Total and Partial Colectomy	7	9
Anterior Resection	4	6
A-P Resection	3	4
Closure of Colostomy	2	8
Miscellaneous	3 (6.0 %)	21 (21.0 %)
Hysterectomy	0	7
Laparotomy and Biopsy	1	6
Mastectomy	2	5
Nephrectomy	0	3

Operative and Postoperative Blood Loss

Operative blood loss was recorded as being excessive or not on the assessment of the surgeon. Surgical wounds and heparin injection sites were examined every day for haematoma formation. In addition, the preoperative haemoglobin and the haemoglobin value a week after surger, together with blood transfusion requirements were also noted.

Laboratory Tests

Venous blood for haematological tests were collected in trisodium citrate (3.8 %) solution at a ratio of one part citrate to nine parts blood. Blood for fibrinopeptide A (FpA) was collected on o.5 ml of an anticoagulant mixture containing 500 U of heparin and 500 U of Aprotinin (Trasylol®), 0.5 mmol epsilon aminocaproic acid (EACA). The first 2 ml of blood after a venepuncture was discarded and the following 4.5 ml was collected into 0.5 ml of the anticoagulant mixture. Platelet poor plasma was prepared by centrifugation at 3000 g for 30 minutes at 4 °C and stored at -20 °C until assayed. Chromogenic assays were used for measuring heparin levels using substrate S-2222, and for determining antithrombin III concentrations using substrate S-2238. The details of the techniques of those assays have already been described (27). The standard curves were prepared using a normal pool of plasma with the Third International Heparin Standard (NIBSC, Holly Hill, London). APTT was measured on platelet poor plasma samples within one hour of blood collection using techniques described by Hardisty et al. (28). The cephalin used for these measurements was kindly provided by Dr. Leon Poller, National Reference Laboratory for Anticoagulant Control Reagents, Manchester, (UK). Assays of lipoprotein lipase activity were carried out by the method of Nilsson-Ehle and Schotz (29). Plasma pre-kallikrein and fpA levels were measured using the method of Kluft et al. (30) and Kockum et al. (31), respectively.

Platelet Function Tests

5 ml of blood was collected via 19 G base needle using clean venepuncture without stasis, and one half volume aliquots were placed in ice tubes containing EDT and theophylline and the other half in similar tubes containing in addition freshly prepared 180 M indomethacin to reduce artefactual production of TxB_2. These tubes were kept in ice and were centrifuged within 30 minutes at 2300 g for 30 minutes at 4 °C, to produce platelet poor plasma. Plasma was removed and stored frozen at -20 °C. The plasma concentration of βTG and PF4 were measured by using a radioimmunoassay kit (Radiochemical Centre, Amersham, UK, and Abbott Laboratories, Queen-

borough, Kent, UK). Concentration of TxB_2 was measured by using techniques described by Levy et al. (32). the antisera was generously donated by Dr. J. B. Smith of Philadelphia, USA.

The Simplate Bleeding Time (SBT)

The SBT was determined using the method as described by Mielke et al. (33). The Simplate is a springloaded device which produces a guillotine-like incision of constant length and depth. A blood pressure cuff was applied to the upper arm and then inflated to 40 mm Hg and after waiting 30 seconds to permit uniform capillary filling, the Simplate was placed on the skin with the slot running parallel to the elbow crease. A stop watch was started and a circular filter paper was used to blot the drops of blood at 30 second intervals. The end point was reached when the blood no longer stained the filter paper.

Statistical Analysis

An analysis of variance was performed on the data obtained following subcutaneous and intravenous injection of the LMW and the UF heparin using a Commodore S61 preprogrammed statistical calculator. A significant difference was determined by the student t test for paired values. Whenever the variables were not normally distributed, the non-parametric statistics in the form of Mann Whitney two tail test was used to analyse the data.

Results

Studies in Healthy Volunteers

The results of intravenous and subcutaneous administration of the LMW and the UF heparin are shown in Fig. 1 and 2. When 5000 anti-Xa units of both heparins were given intravenously, the LMW fraction produced higher levels of anti-Xa activity measured as heparin units (Fig. 1 a) compared to that

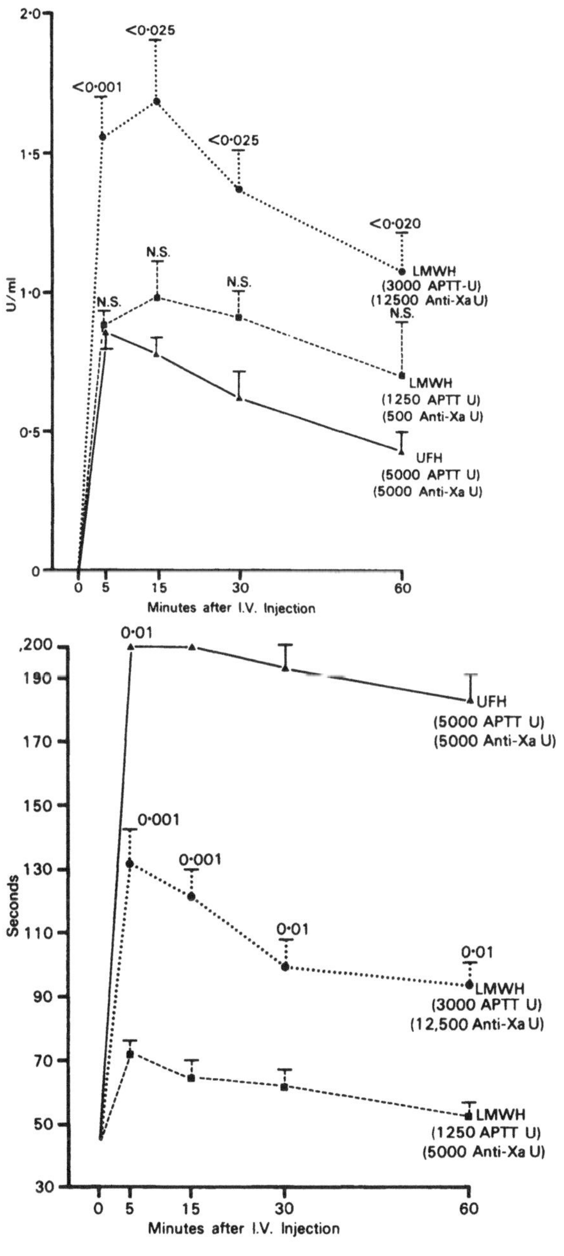

Fig. 1. The response following intravenous administration of equal amount of the LMW and UF heparin assessed in anti-factor Xa assay (Fig. 1 a) and APTT assay (Fig. 1 b).

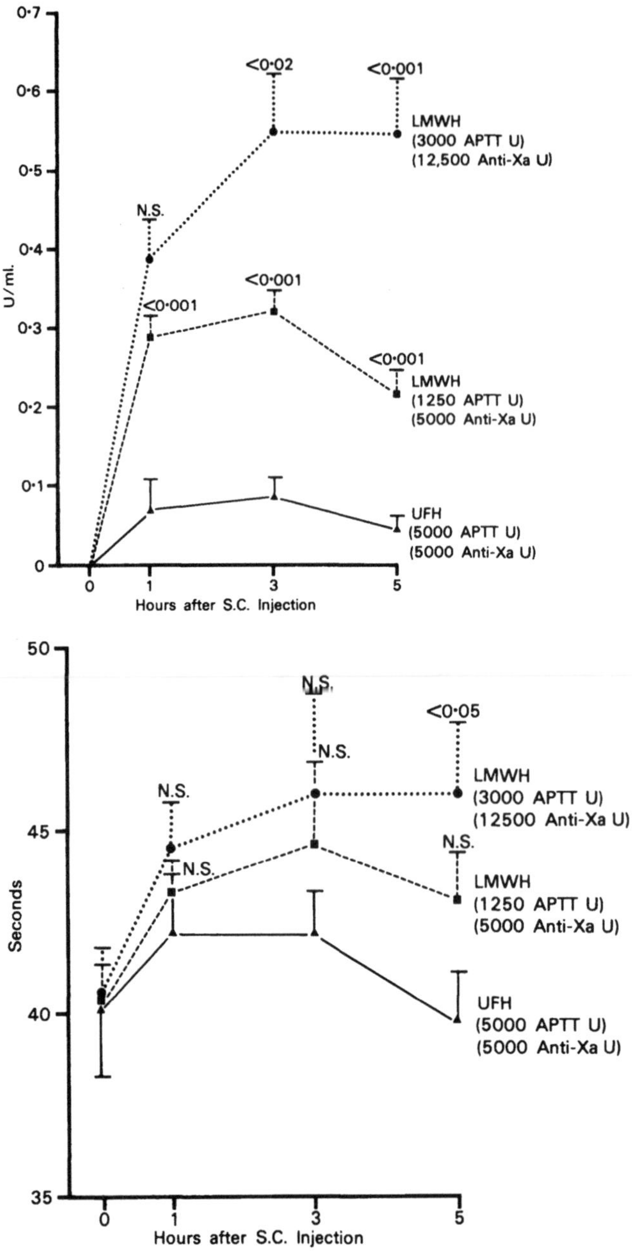

Fig. 2. The response following subcutaneous administration of equal amount of the LMW and UF heparin assessed in anti-factor Xa assay (Fig. 2 a) and APTT assay (Fig. 2 b).

produced by the UF heparin, but the difference was not statistically significant (p = 0.20). However, there was a highly significant difference in the APTT response, the UF heparin giving a prolongation in excess of 200 seconds compared to 132 seconds above the normal control value following administration of LMW heparin (Fig. 1 b). Different response was obtained when the same amount of both preparations of heparin were administered subcutaneously. The LMW heparin produced nearly 4 times greater anti-factor Xa activity compared to the UF heparin (Fig. 2 a) and yet there was no significant difference in the APTT response (Fig. 2 b). Similar changes were observed when a larger amount (12,500 anti-Xa units) of the LMW heparin was administered subcutaneously and intravenously.

When blood samples were withdrawn up to 24 hours following a single subcutaneous injection of 1250 APTT units (5000 anti-Xa units) of LMW heparin, the anti-Xa activity measured as heparin units persisted up to 18 hours (Fig. 3).

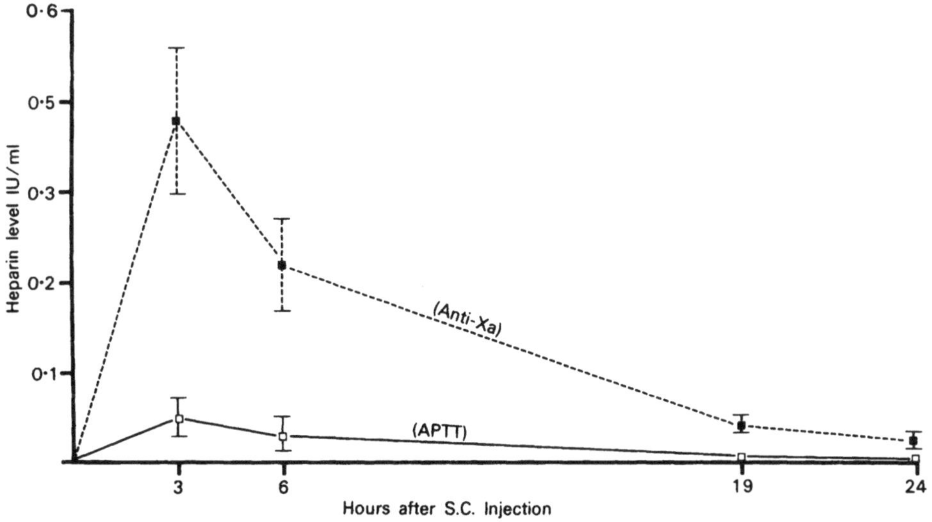

Fig. 3. The mean heparin levels and APTT in 5 healthy volunteers who received 1250 APTT units subcutaneously.

Studies in Patients

Effect of coagulation and platelet function

The results of clotting assays and platelet function tests following subcutaneous administration of the LMW and the UF heparin in patients undergoing major abdominal surgery are shown in Tables III, IV and V.

APTT, Heparin levels and ATIII Concentration (Table III)

There was no significant difference in the mean APTT value following administration of two preparations of heparin in the samples withdrawn in the anaesthetic room, during surgery, in the recovery room, on 1st and 7th postoperative day. Heparin levels measured by an anti-factor Xa assay, showed a different response in the two groups; the mean level in the sample withdrawn during surgery was 0.175 ± 0.02 units/ml in the group who received the LMW heparin and 0.090 ± 0.03 units/ml in the group receiving the UF heparin; this difference is statistically significant ($p < 0.05$). The mean ATIII concentration before surgery was 99.5 % of the normal in the patients who received the LMW heparin and a significant fall was observed during and after surgery. Similar changes were also seen in patients who received the UF heparin.

Pre-kallikrein, lipoprotein lipase and FPA (Table IV)

A significant difference in plasma pre-kallikrein level was observed on 1st and 7th postoperative day compared to the preoperative value in the patients who received the UF heparin; the preoperative value was 64.4 ± 6.2 % of the normal and this fell to 37.4 ± 8.3 % on the 1st and 32.0 ± 4.6 % on the 7th postoperative day ($p < 0.01$). The plasma pre-kallikrein did not fall throughout the observation period in the group receiving the LMW heparin (Table IV).

Table III. Effect of the LMW and UF Heparin on Clotting Assays

Test	Type of Heparin	Mean ± S.E.M.	Pre-op	Anaesthetic Room	Mid-op	Recovery Room	Postop Day 1	Postop Day 7
Heparin levels Anti Xa u/ml	LMWH	Mean ± SE	0	0.124±.02	0.175±.33	0.129±.33	0.-208±.06	0.151±.03
	UFH	Mean ±SE	0	0.125±.43	0.090±.03°	0.090±.02°	0.200±.06	0.109±.02
APTT ratio patients/ control	LMWH	X ± SE	1.36±0.13	1.47 ±0.12	1.51 ±0.12	1.31 ±.133	1.64 ±.22	1.03 ±.06
	UFH	X ± SE	1.4 ±0.25	1.33 ±0.13	1.37 ±0.13	1.24 ±.20	1.62 ±.27	1.26 ±.09
ATIII Concentration % normal	LMWH	X ± SE	99.5 ±2.49	84.0 ±4.31**	89.5 ±3.41**	75.3 ±5.61**	82.3 ±4.7**	89.2 ±3.75**
	UFH	X ± SE	101.5 ±4.3	94.5 ±4.8	82.6 ±3.5**	85.3 ±4.8**	85.3 ±4.5**	87.6 ±8.8*

° $p < .05$ LMW v UF heparin

** $p < .01$) compared to preop value

* $p < .05$)

Table IV. Effect of the LMW and UF Heparin on Coagulation Assays

Test	Type of Heparin	Mean ± S.E.M.	Preop	Anaesthetic Room	Mid-op	Recovery Room	Postop Day 1	Postop Day 7
Prekallikrein % normal	LMWH	X ± SE	67.8 ±8.9	71.8 ±8.9	66.6 ± 8.2	64.9 ±12.2	62.1 ±12.2	48.6 ± 9.0
	UFH	X ± SE	64.3 ±6.2	60.5 ±5.6	61.5 ± 5.7	64.8 ± 6.8	37.4 ± 8.3**	32.0 ± 4.6***
Lipoprotein lipase release IU/ML	LMWH	X ± SE	12.9 ±3.6	25.7 ±3.9***	21.1± 4.0***	26.14 ± 5.0***	24.8 ± 6.5***	16.5 ± 7.5***
	UFH	X ± SE	9.1 ±3.0	45.0 ±9.4°***	33.3±10.2***	35.2 ± 7.1***	22.5 ± 5.3***	20.5 ± 7.5***
Fibrinopeptide A ng/ml	LMWH	X ± SE	1.5 ±.42	1.8 ±.46	3.55±.55***	2.9 ± .64**	2.55 ± .63*	2.2 ± .44
	UFH	X ± SE	1.48 ±.29	2.56 ±.45	3.7 ±.39***	3.09 ± .47***	2.16 ± .62	2.5 ± .53

*** p <.001)
** p <.01) compared to preop value
* p <.05)
° p <.05 LMW v UF heparin

Both the LMW and the UF heparin caused a significant increase in lipoprotein lipase compared with pre heparin values, and the raised levels subsequently persisted throughout the period of observation (Table IV). The increase was even greater in those who received the UF heparin. The difference in the lipoprotein lipase release in the two groups following the LMW and the UF heparin administration was statistically significant ($p < 0.05$). A significant increase in the levels of fpA was also observed during and after surgery following administration of both heparins but the difference between the two groups was not significant (Table IV).

βTG, PF4, TxB_2 and Bleeding Time (Table V)

Analysis of the results of platelet function tests showed them not to be normally distributed in both groups. Therefore, non-parametric statistics in the form of Mann Whitney two tail test was used to analyse the data obtained. In the group who received the LMW heparin, the median βTG levels increased from 63 ng/ml before surgery to 72 ng/ml during operation, the difference is not statistically significant. A similar increase was also observed in the group receiving UF heparin (Table V). The median PF4 levels in the patients receiving the LMW heparin was 18 ng/ml before and 19 ng/ml during surgery. The group who received the UF heparin, median PF4 level increased from 26 ng/ml before surgery to 36 ng/ml during operation, the difference is not statistically significant (Table V). The median levels of TxB_2 increased from 110 pg/ml before surgery to 300 pg/ml during operation, this difference being statistically significant ($p < 0.02$). Raised levels were also observed in the samples withdrawn in the recovery room (Table V). Similar significant difference in the median TxB_2 level was also observed in the patient receiving the UF heparin (Table V).

The results of SBT in 25 patients who received a single injection of 1850 APTT units of the LMW heparin are shown in Fig. 4. The difference between the mean SBT before, during and 24 hours after surgery is not statistically significant though a rise greater than 1 SD was observed in 6 patients. In 7 patients, the bleeding time was reduced to below 1 SD, 5 of these were being operated upon for malignant disease. Blood samples were

Table V. Effect of the LMW and UF Heparin on in-vivo Platelet Function

Test	Type of Heparin	Median UQ-LQ	Preop	Anaesthetic Room	Mid-Op	Recovery Room	Postop Day 1	Postop Day 7
	LMWH	Median	63	53	72	50.5	51	43
BTG ng/ml		UQ-LQ	42-80	38-69	29-182	36-129	30-74	34-48
	UFH	Median	57	52	74	80	35	40
		UQ-LQ	28-84	27-56	49-148	39-122	26-54	32-57
	LMWH	Median	18	17	16	20	18	22
PF4 ng/ml		UQ-LQ	12-32	13.32	8-20	18-28	16-20	12-21
	UFH	Median	26	29	36	40	20	21
		UQ-LQ	13-32	23-31	20-39	13-53	16-23	14-31
	LMWH	Median	90	140	190*	160*	130	80
TXB2 pg/ml		UQ-LQ	40-120	120-160	130-280	110-260	60-180	50-200
	UFH	Median	110	150	300**	250**	200	180
		UQ-LQ	30-160	80-350	180-790	160-600	100-390	90-400

* p < .05 Compared to preop value

** p < .02

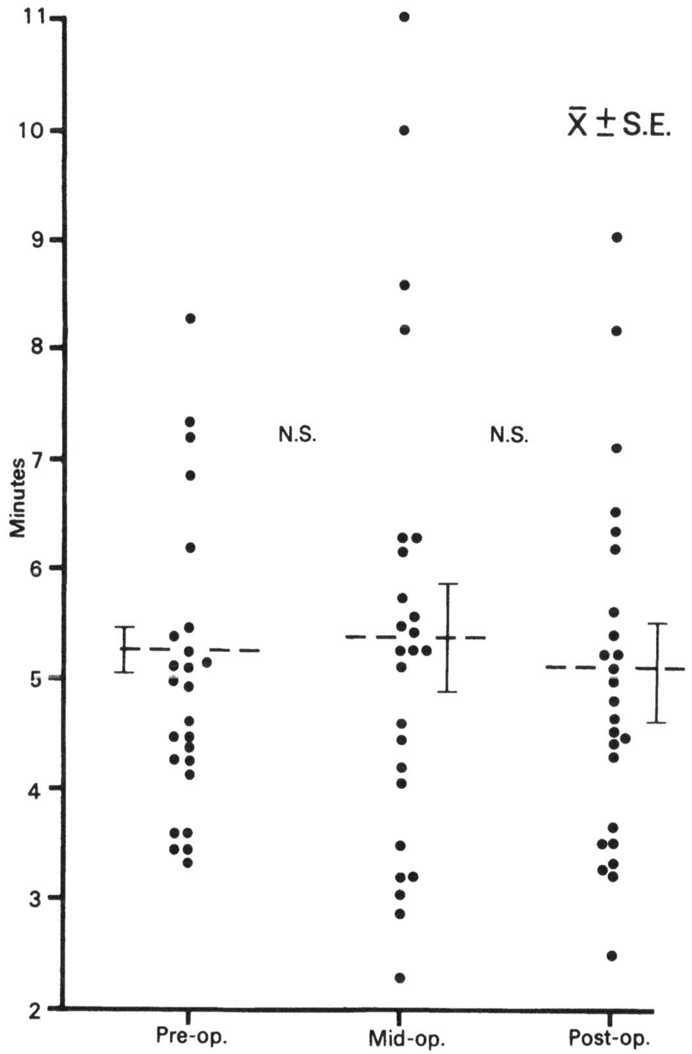

Fig. 4. Simplate Bleeding Time in 25 patients who received a single injection of 1850 APTT units of LMW heparin 2 hours before surgery.

also obtained at the time when SBT was measured and these were analysed for the plasma heparin level. The mean plasma heparin level during surgery was 0.28 u/ml, the range being 0.08 to 0.6 u/ml. Increases in the SBT were unrelated to changes in the plasma heparin concentration. In 9 of 25 patients, circulating heparin could still be detected after 24 hours of a single subcutaneous injection (Fig. 5).

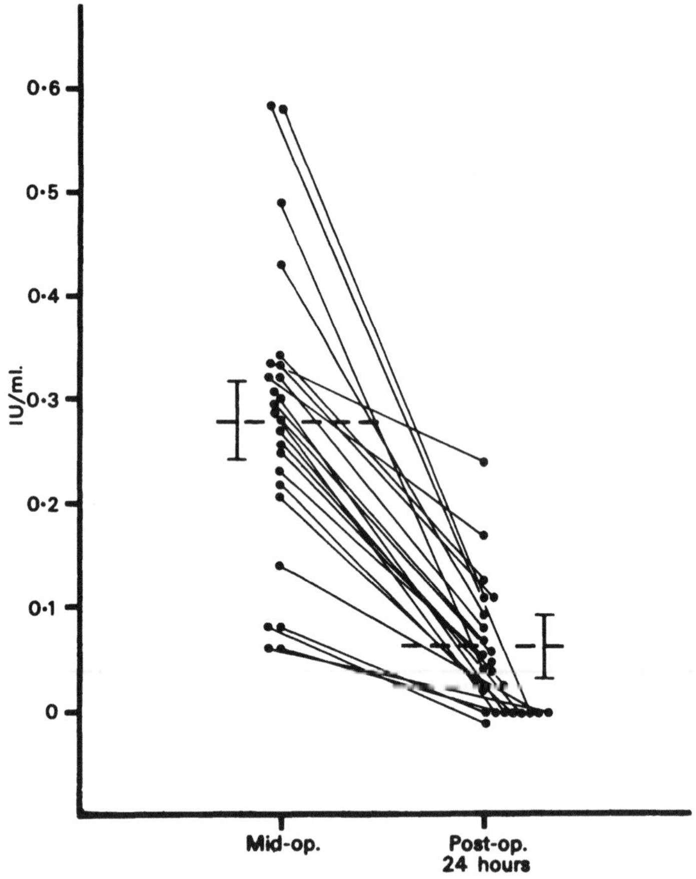

Fig. 5. Plasma heparin level in 25 patients who received a single injection of 1850 APTT units of LMW heparin two hours before surgery.

Prevention of DVT

150 consecutive patients over the age of 40 undergoing major abdominal surgery were investigated in this study; the first 50 of these received 1250 APTT units of the LMW heparin every 12 hourly i. e. 2 injections per day while the other 100 patients received a single injection of 1850 APTT units of LMW heparin per day during the first 7 postoperative days. There were no significant differences between these two groups as far as their age, sex, type or duration of operation, presence of malignancy and other risk factors known to predispose to occurrence of DVT (Table I and II).

Group receiving TWO injections per day

Isotopic DVT was diagnosed in 3 of 50 patients (Table VI); venography confirmed the presence of thrombi in only 2 cases. In each instance, thrombi were confined to calf veins only. Thrombi were detected on 7th, 11th and 15th postoperative days. The prophylaxis was given for the 7 postoperative days. Therefore the incidence of isotopic DVT during prophylaxis was 2 % (1 out of 50). 12 (24 %) of 50 patients were operated for malignant disease, and none of these developed DVT. None of these patients developed symptoms or signs of minor pulmonary embolism. There were no fatalities during the postoperative period.

Group receiving ONE injection per day

Isotopic DVT was detected in 3 of 100 patients receiving one injection of LMW heparin per day (Table VI). Thrombi were detected on 2nd, 4th and 6th postoperative days and the raised counts persisted for 48 to 72 hours only. Venography performed failed to confirm the presence of thrombi in each instance. Three patients died during the postoperative period and autopsy was performed in each case. The cause of death was as follows: one patient died on the 9th postoperative day due to Gram negative septicemia following the resection of carcinoma of the sigmoid colon; the second and third patients died on the 14th and the 19th postoperative days due to advanced carcinomatosis secondary to carcinoma of stomach. Both patients has palliative gastro-jejunostomy. In none of the patients pulmonary emboli or thrombi in the deep veins could be demonstrated at autopsy.

Operative and Postoperative Bleeding

Prophylaxis was discontinued in 2 patients who received LMW heparin every 12 hourly; one developed extensive bruising at the site of injection and in the other blood loss at the time of surgery was considered to be excessive. Two of 100 patients who received a single injection per day developed wound haematoma; one following an anterior resection and the other following abdomino-perineal resection of rectum. An objective assessment of operative and postoperative bleeding showed that there was no statistically significant difference in the amount of blood transfused in both groups; the mean transfusion requirement of each patient is shown in Table VII. There was no statistically significant difference in the fall in the postoperative haemoglobin in the two groups when analysed on the basis of different operations or in the groups as a whole.

Table VI. DVT diagnosed by the radioactive Fibrinogen test and confirmed by Venography

	Two injections per day	One injection per day
Patients studied	50	100
DVT diagnosed	3 (6 %)	3 (3 %)
Bilateral DVT	1 (2 %)	0
Confirmed by venography	2 (4 %)	0
Day of onset	7th, 11th, 15th	2nd, 4th, 6th
During prophylaxis	1 (2 %)	3 (3 %)

Table VII. Blood Transfusion Requirements (Mean) and Postoperative Fall in Haemoglobin (Mean)

	Two injections per day	One injection per day
Patients no.	50	100
No. requiring transfusion	8 (16 %)	17 (17.0 %)
Transfusion requirements (mean ml)	1312 ± 393.9	1035.2 ± 407.1
Mean preop Hb (g/dl)	14.2 ± 1.3	14.9 ± 1.8
Mean postop Hb (g/dl)	12.4 ± 1.38	13.6 ± 1.6

Discussion

Presently available information strongly indicates that the anticoagulant action of heparin is mediated mainly or completely through antithrombin III (10-12). Only a portion of the heparin in commercially available preparation has affinity for At III and displays anticoagulant activity. Thus, by using affinity chromatography on matrix-bound At III, heparin can be divided into one fraction (about one third of the total amount) with high anticoagulant activity (high activity heparin) and other almost inactive fraction (low activity heparin) (8-9). The difference in biological activity between the two fractions has been shown to be related to the molecular size (16-20). In the present study, we have compared in vivo the anti-factor Xa and the APTT response following intravenous and subcutaneous administration of two different doses of the LMW fraction with a standard dose of the UF heparin in the same healthy volunteers. The results indicate that equivalent amounts of the two preparations of heparin produced different. responses. When 5000 anti-Xa units of both heparins were administered intravenously, there was a highly sifnificant difference in the prolongation of the APTT following injection of the UF compared to LMW heparin yet the difference in the anti-factor response was not statistitcally significant. In contrast, when equivalent amounts of both heparins were administered subcutaneously, a highly significant difference was observed in the anti-factor Xa response following injection of the LMW fraction while the differences in the APTT response were not significant. The other interesting finding was the duration of the anti-factor Xa response which persisted for nearly 18 hours following a single subcutaneous injection of the LMW fraction. It is not clear why the same amount of the LMW heparin should have less anticoagulant activity in the multiple-role clotting assays such as the APTT assay than the UF heparin when administered intravenously. The most plausible explanation for this discrepancy is as follows. We have previously reported that a plasma inhibitor, low density lipoprotein (LDL), modifies the heparin accelerated neutralization of activated factor X (Xa) by At III in vivo as well as in vitro, and that this is dependent upon the molecular weight of the injected heparin (34).

The reduction in heparin activity by this inhibitor is related to its molecular weight such that high molecular weight heparin is more greatly inhibited, the standard commercially available heparin less so and the LMW least of all (35). The response after subcutaneous injection of the LMW and the UF heparin can be more easily explained since the concentration of heparin which reaches the circulation is inversely related to its molecular weight. Thus a greater percentage of the LMW than the UF heparin reaches its site of pharmacological action, and that the heparin once it reaches circulation, behaves as it would when an intravenous injection is given. Therefore, when the UF heparin was given by subcutaneous injection, the probability is that only the heparin species of LMW reaches the circulation in significant concentration.

The second aim of our studies was to find out whether the two preparations of heparin effect the coagulation mechanism and in vivo platelet function to the same extent. The clotting assays and platelet function tests indicated that both the LMW and UF heparin in general produced similar effect. However, intra-group comparison showed a significant difference in the anti-Xa activity, lipoprotein lipase, and plasma pre-kallikrein and TXB_2 levels. Both heparins caused a significant increase in lipoprotein lipase compared with preheparin values but the increase was even greater in those who received the UF heparin. The ability of heparin to interact with lipoprotein lipase increases with the molecular weight, suggesting that the LMW fragment may cause less release of free fatty acids on administration in vivo than does the UF heparin (36). Endothelial cells have been demonstrated to contain heparin sulphate, platelet factor 4 (PF4) and lipoprotein lipase in a complex bound to their cell surface (37). The UF heparin being a highly charged molecule, probably displaces this complex from the endothelial cell surface to a greater extent than the LMW fraction and thus causing a greater release of lipoprotein lipase. Platelets produce prostaglandins, prostaglandin endoperoxide and thromboxanes during aggregation and blood clotting. Therefore, the high levels of plasma TXB_2 observed in patients receiving UF heparin may reflect greater activation of platelets. Such observation is supported by the previously reported findings that the LMW heparin fraction also showed very low platelet aggregation enhancing activity while the heparin fractions with molecular weights of 17,000 had a higher aggregation enhancing activity (38). These results suggest that the molecular weight of heparin is a major factor with regard to the effect on platelets (39). However, in our studies, the difference in the BTG levels was not statistically significant. A significant fall in the plasma pre-kallikrein level was only observed on 1st and 7th postoperative day in the patients who received the UF heparin. Plasma pre-kallikrein levels are directly related to the degree of activation of factor XII. Recent studies have also demonstrated that heparin fractions of different molecular weight and with affinity for antithrombin differ in their ability to potentiate the inhibition of clotting factors by At III (39), inhibitor of thrombin. Factor IXa, and Factor XIa were found to decrease with decreasing molecular weight. Inactivation of Factor Xa, Factor XIIa and Kallikrein was potentiated by LMW heparin fractions that had virtually no effect on the inhibition of thrombin, Factor IXa and XIa. This suggests the possibility that the anti-thrombotic properties of LMW heparin may be related to its ability to potentiate inactivation of serine proteinases in the initial stages of the coagulation cascade (39). According to this hypothesis, the LMW heparin would possess anti-thrombotic properties with little effect on the clotting time, and possibly, without causing bleeding.

The third aim of this study was to determine the efficacy of LMW heparin as a prophylactic agent against venous thromboembolism. The results indicate that the LMW heparin almost abolished the occurrence of postoperative DVT. During prophylaxis, isotopic DVT was diagnosed in only one of 50 patients who received 2 injections of 1250 units of LMW heparin per day. In 3 out of 100 patients who received a single daily injection of 1850 units of the LMW fraction, the raised counts were detected by the venography performed failed to confirm the presence of thrombi in each instance. The most likely explanation for this discrepancy is the small thrombi detected by the ^{125}I-fibrinogen uptake test in the muscular veins of the calf may not be demonstrated by venography which often fails to visualize such veins.

None of the 150 patients who received LMW heparin died due to fatal or contributory pulmonary emboli. These results compare favourably with the data reported in the studies using UF heparin (1-5). The other advantage of using the LMW fraction for prophylaxis would seem to be the reduced frequency of bleeding complications during postoperative period. Prophylaxis was discontinued due to bleeding complications in 2 of 50 patients who received injections every 12 hourly and in none of 100 patients receiving one injection per day. Three patients developed wound haematoma; 2 had received LMW heparin everly 12 hourly while the 3rd belonged to the group who received one injection per day. In contrast, in the MCT, heparin administration was discontinued in 53 (2.59 %) of 2045 patients of excessive bleeding and 158 (7.77 %) developed minor or major wound haematoma (1). In the MCT, each patient received 15,000 APTT units of the UF heparin (5000 units x 8 hourly) per day. In the present study, the patients received either 2500 APTT units (1250 units x 12 hourly) or 1850 APTT units (one injection per day). Therefore the reduced frequency of bleeding complications in patients receiving the LMW fraction is not surprising.

One of the disadvantages of the low dose heparin prophylaxis is that the drug has to be administered every 8 or 12 hourly. Adoption of such a regimen to protect a large number of high risk patients requires considerable nursing time. Thus a single injection of the LMW heparin per day will not only reduce the frequency of haemorrhagic side effects but would also overcome the need for frequent drug administration.

The results of this study indicate that a single injection of the LMW heparin represents a convenient method of preventing deep vein thrombosis in the high risk patients undergoing major abdominal surgery. It avoids the complication of haemorrhage - one of the major drawbacks when UF heparin is used.

Acknowledgements

We thank the Consultant Surgeons of King's College Hospital for allowing us to study their patients; Choay Pharmaceuticals Ltd (Paris) for supply of the LMW and UF heparin. We also acknowledge the help of Mr. J. Choay and Dr. F. Toulemonde in designing the studies reported in this paper.

We are grateful to Miss C. Privett and MIss M. Fry for excellent technical assistance and Miss M. Johnson for secreterial help. The study was supported by the MRC Programme Grant No 973/756 and a grant from the Sir Jules Thorn Charitable Trust.

References

1. An International Multicentre Trial. Prevention of Fatal Postoperative Pulmonary Embolism by Low Doses of Heparin. Lancet 1975, II, 45-51

2. Gallus, A. S., Hirsh, J., Tuttle, R. J., Trebilcock, R., O'Brien, S. E., Carroll, J. J., Minden, J. H., Hudecki, S. M. Small subcutaneous doses of heparin in prevention of venous thrombosis. N. Engl. J. Med. 1963, 288, 545-549.

3. Kakkar, V. V., Spinder, J., Flute, P. T., Corrigan, T., Fossard, D. P., Crellin, R. Q., Wessler, S., Yin, E. T.: Efficacy of low doses of heparin in prevention of deep vein thrombosis after major surgery; a double blind trial. Lancet 1972, II, 101-106.

4. Nicolaides, A. N., Desai, S., Douglas, J. N., Fourides, G., Dupont, P. A., Lewis, J. D., Dodsworth, H., Luck, K. J., Jamieson, C. W. Small doses of sodium heparin in preventing deep venous thrombosis after surgery. Lancet 1972, II, 890-893.

5. Kill, J., Axelsen, F., Andersen, D. Prophylaxis against postoperative pulmonary embolism and deep vein thrombosis by low dose heparin. Lancet 1978, I, 1115-1116.

6. Cifonelli, J. A. The relationship of molecular weight, and sulfate content and distribution to anticoagulant activity of heparin preparations. Carbohydrate Research 1974, 37, 145-154.

7. Johnson, E. A., Malloy, B. The molecular weight range of mucosal heparin preparations. Carbohydrate Research 1976, 51, 119-123.

8. Andersson, L. O., Barrowcliffe, T. W., Holmer, E., Johnson, E. A., Sims, G. E. C. Anticoagulant properties of heparin fractionated by affinity chromatography on matrix bound antithrombin III and by gel filtration. Thromb. Res. 1976, 9, 575-583.

9. Lam, L. H., Silbert, J. E., Rosenberg, R. D., The separation of active and inactive form of heparin. Biochem. Biophys. Res. Commun. 1976, 69, 570-576.

10. Rosenberg, R. D. Actions and interactions of antithrombin and heparin. N. Engl. J. Med. 1975, 292, 146-148.

11. Abildgaard, U. Inhibition of the thrombin-fibrinogen reaction by heparin and purified cofactor. Scand. J. Haematol. 1968, 5, 440-445.

12. Rosenberg, J. S., McKenna, P. W., Rosenberg, R. D. Inhibition of human factor IXa by human anti-thrombin. J. Biol. Chem. 1975, 250, 8883-8888.

13. Østerud, B., Miller-Andersson, M., Abildgaard, U., Prydz, H. The effect of antithrombin III on the activity of the coagulation factor VII, IX and X. Thromb. Haemostas. 1976, 35, 295-301.

14. Johnson, E. A., Kirkwood, T. B. L., Stirling, Y., Perez-Requejo, L. J., Ingram, G. I. C., Bangham, D. R., Brozovic, M. Four heparin preparations. Anti-Xa Potentiating Effect of Heparin after Subcutaneous Injection. Thromb. Haemostas. 1976, 35, 586-591.

15. Damus, P. S., Hick, S., Rosenberg, R. W. Anticoagulant action of heparin. Nature (Lond) 1973, 246, 355.

16. Anderssson, L. O., Barrowcliffe, T. W., Holmer, E., Johnson, E. A., Söderström, G. Molecular weight dependency of the heparin potential inhibition of thrombin and activated factor X. Effect of heparin neutralisation in plasma. Thromb. Res. 1979, 15, 531-541.

17. Laurent, T. C., Tengblad, A., Thunberg, L., Höök, M., Lindahl, U. The Molecular weight dependence of the anticoagulant activity of heparin. Biochem. J. 1978, 175, 691-701.

18. Lane, D. A., MacGregor, I. R., Michalski, R., Kakkar, V. V. Anticoagulant activities of four unfractionated and fractionated heparins. Thromb. Res. 1978, 12, 257-271.

19. Barrowcliffe, T. W., Johnson, E. A., Eggleton, C. H., Thomas, D. P. Anticoagulant activities of lung and mucous heparins. Thromb. Res. 1978, 12, 27-36.

20. Barrowcliffe, T. W., Johnson, E. A., Eggleton, C. A., Kemball-Cook, G., Thomas, D. P. Anticoagulant activities of high and low molecular weight heparin fractions. Brit. J. Haematol. 1979, 41, 583.

21. Choay, J., Lormeau, J. C., Petitou, M., Sinay, P., Casu, B., Oreste, P., Torri, G., Gatti, G. Anti-Xa active heparin oligosaccharides. Thromb. Res. 1980, 18, 573-578.

22. Choay, J. Personal communication.

23. Caen, J., Larrieu, M. J., Samama, M. In: L'hemostase. Paris. Expansion Scientifique Francaise, 1968, pp. 133-135.

24. Yin, E. T., Wessler, S., Butler, J. V. Plasma heparin: a unique practical, submicrogram-sensitive assay. J. Lab. Clin. Med. 1973, 81, 298-310.

25. Kakkar, V. V., Nicolaides, A. N., Renney, J. T. G., Friend, J. R., Clarke, M. D. ^{125}I-fibrinogen test adapted for routine screening. Lancet 1970, I, 540-542.

26. Kakkar, V. V. The problems of thrombosis in the deep veins of the legs. Ann. Roy. Coll. Surg. Engl. 1969, 45, 257-276.

27. Scully, M. F., Kakkar, V. V. Methods for semimicro or automated determination of thrombin, antithrombin, and heparin co-factor, using the substrate H-D-Phe-Pip-Arg-p-Nitroanalide 2-HCl. Clin. Chim. Acta 1977, 79, 595-602.

28. Hardisty, R. M., Ingram, G. I. C. In Bleeding disorders. Oxford, 1965.

29. Nilsson-Ehle, P., Schotz, N. C. A stable radioactive substrate emulsion for assay of lipoprotein lipase. Journal of Lipid Research. 1976, 17, 536-541.

30. Kluft, C. Determination of pre-kallikrein in human plasma. Optimal conditions of activating pre-kallikrein. J. Lab. Clin. Med. 1978, 91, 83-95.

31. Kockum, C., Frebeluis, S. Rapid radio immunoassay of human fibrinopeptide A. Removal of cross reacting fibrinogen with Bentonite. Thromb. Res. 1980, 18, 589-596.

32. Lewy, R. C., Smith, J. B., Silver, M. T., Saia, J., Walnski, P., Weiner, L. Detection of thromboxane B_2 in variant angina. Prostaglandin Med. 1979, 2, 243-249.

33. Mielke, C. H. Jr., Kaneshiro, M. M., Maher, I. A. The standardised normal Ivy bleeding time and it's prolongation by aspirin. Blood 1969, 34, 204-210.

34. MacGregor, I. R., Lane, D. A., Kakkar, V. V. Evidence for a plasma inhibitor of the heparin accelerated inhibition of factor Xa by Antithrombin III. Biochim. Biophys. Acta. 1979, 586, 584-593.

35. MacGregor, I. R., Lane, D. A., Kakkar, V. V. The antiheparin properties of human low density lipoprotein. Biochim. Biophys. Acta 1981 (in press).

36. Bengtsson, G., Olivecroma, T., Höök, M., Riesenfeld, J., Lindahl, U. Interaction of lipoprotein lipase with native and modified heparin-like polysaccharides. Biochem. J. 1981 (in press).

37. Buonassisi, V. Sulphated mucopolysaccharide synthesis and secretion in endothelial cell culture. Exp. Cell. Res. 1973, 76, 363-378.

38. Holmer, E., Lindahl, U., Bäckström, G., Thunberg, L., Sandberg, H., Söderström, G., Anderson, L. O. Anticoagulant activities and effects on platelets of a heparin fragment with high affinity for antithrombin. Thromb. Res. 1980, 18, 861-869.

39. Holmer, E., Kirchi, K., Söderström, G. The molecular weight dependence of the rate enhancing effect of heparin on the inhibition of thrombin, Factor Xa, Factor IXa, Factor XIIa and kallikrein by antithrombin. Biochem. J. 1981 193, 395-400.

Discussion

Rosenberg asked if there were significant differences between low molecular weight heparin and unfractionated heparin in respect to fibrinogen scan or phlebography in the small number of patients in *Kakkar's* study.

Kakkar replied that the data in his 150 patients show a total incidence of thrombosis during prophylaxis of 2 % to 7 %, which is significant. The rate of extention was more significant.
Kakkar has a study in progress of 500 patients with single injections and control of ventilation perfusion scan. Heparin prophylaxis is given for 14 days and also the perfusion scanning is done for 14 days.

Rosenberg stated that *Kakkar's* results seem to be similar to model experiments with rabbits where low molecular weight heparin is able at times to prevent fibrinogen accretion and larger molecular weight sizes are not.

Kakkar feels that his study offers a clear demonstration. With 1850 APTT units he saw thrombi, but they were very transitent.

Bhargava asked for the amounts of fractionated and unfractionated heparin given to the patients.

Kakkar explained that their aim was to give equivalent amounts of APTT units of unfractionated and of low molecular weight heparin.

Schmitz-Hübner wondered if it is possible to conclude from the last studies of *Kakkar* with patients that anti-Xa levels in circulation do not necessarily correspond to the preventing effect against thrombosis.

Kakkar explained that the difference between 1850 units of anti-Xa and 2500 units is still unknown. One would have to reduce the amount of low molecular weight heparin to 1250 anti-Xa units per day in order to answer this question.

Schmitz-Hübner reported that *Hirsh* had found no correlation between the anti-Xa level in plasma and the antithrombotic effect of heparin.

Kakkar replied that these results are difficult to explain. Many other things are happening, for instance lipoprotein lipase release or plasma prekallikrein activation.

Kakkar said that the differences observed in his patients could be quite significant if a larger number of patients had been studied.

Fussi wanted to know if the low molecular weight heparin used had 200 anti-Xa units per mg.

Kakkar replied that his normal (unfractionated) heparin had 150 anti-Xa units per mg.

Fussi asked for the administered doses of unfractionated and low molecular weight heparin in terms of weight.

Kakkar explained that one first has to look at the APTT units: 50 APTT units/mg of low molecular weight heparin and 150 APTT units/mg of unfractionated heparin. The dosage was based on APTT units, 1/3 of unfractionated heparin compared to low molecular weight heparin.

Fussi argued that if *Kakkar* had given three times as much low molecular weight heparin in terms of weight compared to unfractionated heparin, he must have given the same amount of both in terms of moles, assuming that unfractionated heparin has a molecular weight three times higher than low molecular weight heparin.

Kakkar stressed that one has to consider how much is absorbed if one gives the heparin subcutaneously. In giving unfractionated heparin one is fractionating it. Only that fraction is absorbed which has anti-Xa activity. Therefore one can show a difference in subcutaneous administration, and yet there is no difference in APTT assay.

Aronson asked if *Kakkar* could explain the way in which the material injected subcutaneously reaches the blood stream.

Kakkar wishes he knew that!

Bhargava wanted to know the difference in the cost and effect between application of unfractionated and low molecular weight heparin.

Kakkar said that this cannot be answered yet because the low molecular weight heparin is still under investigation. Moreover it is not produced in large amounts. The cost/effect ratio cannot be discussed yet. *Kakkar* had intended to show results supporting the hypothesis that the molecular weight of heparin is an important feature in determining its in vivo anti-Xa activity.

Wenzel asked if there were significant differences in the body weight of the patients studied.

Kakkar replied that the data will be published in detail in Lancet.

They have carefully taken into account the body weight.

Duckert pointed out that *Kakkar* had shown significant differences for the under operation and recovery state and wanted to know how this could be explained.

Kakkar replied that there were significantly higher levels of circulating heparin following administration of low molecular weight heparin compared to unfractionated heparin. For the release of lipoprotein lipase it was the contrary. But this has to be confirmed in larger numbers of patients for all the parameters. There were some significant trends, for instance, lower levels of plasma prekallikrein were observed on the postoperative day in the group of patients who had received unfractionated heparin. The level of circulating heparin and the release of lipoprotein lipase were also different. No other differences were found.

Rosenberg raised the question, if there is a real benefit of giving low molecular weight heparin or rather if it does not come back perhaps to the observation of *Hirsh* in the fibrin accretion model.

Kakkar said that it does come to the model of *Hirsh*. But he stressed that he was talking about anti-Xa activity.

Rosenberg wondered why *Kakkar* was emphasizing the anti-Xa activity. The problem is that the inactive fractions also have anti-Xa activity and they have clearly little antithrombotic activity in the fibrin accretion model. He suggested that the molecular explanation might not be so much the anti-Xa activity, but simply that the size of the heparins really determines the excess of the heparin-antithrombin complex in areas of the vascular circulation where perhaps clots are just beginning to form.
Large heparins basically electrostatically spoon them from certain areas in circulation, and in contrast small heparins induce the heparin-antithrombin complex formation and concentration in those areas. These considerations would fit with the data of *Hirsh's* fibrin accretion model.
Rosenberg feels that *Kakkar's* observations after surgery might be interesting but irrelevant.

Schöndorf asked for the kind of anesthesia because it might influence the results.

Kakkar replied that all patients had received the same kind of premedication, anesthesia etc.

Schöndorf wanted to know how much blood volume replacement the patients had received.

Kakkar said that they received 1325 and 1270 ml as a normal saline infusion.

Verstraete wondered about *Kakkar's* conclusion on haemostasis that there were no differences between unfractionated and low molecular weight heparin. He wanted to know what he had measured.

Kakkar explained that his conclusion was based on APTT ratio and also on bleeding time.

The Effect of Heparins on Platelet Release Reaction*

F. Fabris, G. Cella, M. Randi, A Casonato,
F. Fussi, A. Girolami
University of Padua
Medical School
Institute of Semeiotica Medica
Padua, Italy

Important physiopathological inferences can be drawn from the interrelationships between heparin and platelets. The influence of heparin on platelet function (30) and the ability of the platelet specific proteins to neutralize the heparin itself (24) are well known. Moreover, frequent clinical observations have dealt with heparin induced thrombocytopenia (15). In most cases the phenomenon was transient, but in a few instances, a severe clinical picture with recurrent arterial thrombosis was induced (1, 27).

Conflicting results have been reported on the effect of heparin on platelet aggregation depending on the experimental model used (30) and the source of heparin employed (10). A number of workers have found inhibition of platelet aggregation and release by heparin in vitro (16, 15); others have found potentiation both in vitro and in vivo (17, 29) or no detectable effect (21).

Using the common inductors, normal platelet aggregation was obtained in control subjects using citrated or heparinized plasma. In contrast, ristocetin induced platelet agglutination is completely absent in heparinized plasma (50 I.U/ml of blood) (13) (Table 1). Inhibition of ristocetin induced

*This study was supported by grants from the M. P. I., Rome (grant 1592-1979) and from the Venetian Regional Government, Venice.

Heparin · New Biochemical and Medical Aspects

platelet agglutination is also obtained adding increasing amounts of heparin in citrated platelet rich plasma (PRP), and washed or formalin fixes platelets (8). This inhibition is probably due to the highly ionized molecule of heparin that, affecting the surface charge of the platelets, hampers the electrostatic interaction between factor VIII and platelets (8, 19). The same mechanism may justify the inhibition by heparin on collagen induced release (11, 25). The assumption that heparin potentiates the first wave of aggregation (29) by common inductors may be supported by the results obtained in patients with congenital afibrinogenemia (14). The abnormal aggregation pattern found in congenital afibrinogenemia seems to be improved using heparin as an anticoagulant while the release of serotonin (^{3}H-5HT) is not improved (Fig. 1, 2, 3).

Table 1. Platelet aggregation by Ristocetin, ADP, adrenalin and collagen in citrated and heparinized blood in normal subjects. (M. A. = maximal amplitude; Time = seconds to reach M. A.)

			Normal Subjects*	
			Heparinized Blood 50 IU/ml	Citrated Blood 1 : 10
Ristocetin	15mg/ml	Time (sec.)	0	240 ± 15.3
		M. A. %	0	74 ± 12.5
ADP	2 μM	Time (sec.)	210 ± 32	120 ± 28
		M. A. %	55 ± 8	55 ± 18.2
Adrenalin	10 μM	Time (sec.)	295 ± 35	300 ± 31
		M. A. %	69 ± 11	60 ± 12
Collagen	2 μg	Time (sec.)	257 ± 89	300 ± 67
		M. A. %	45 ± 17	70 ± 17
		Lag Phase	47 ± 16	90 ± 38

*M ± SD of 10 subjects

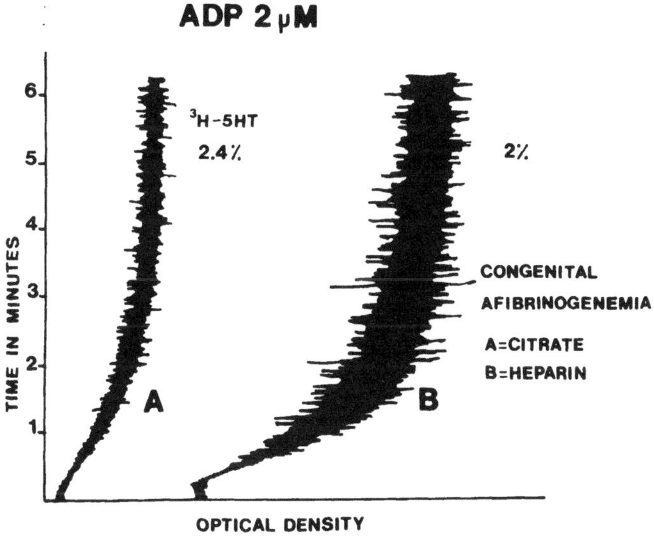

Fig. 1. Platelet aggregation by ADP (Fig. 1), adrenalin (Fig. 2) and collagen (Fig. 3) on citrated (curve A) and heparinized (curve B) plasma of a patient with congenital afibrinogenemia. (^{3}H-5HT = serotonin induced release after 4 min of aggregation).

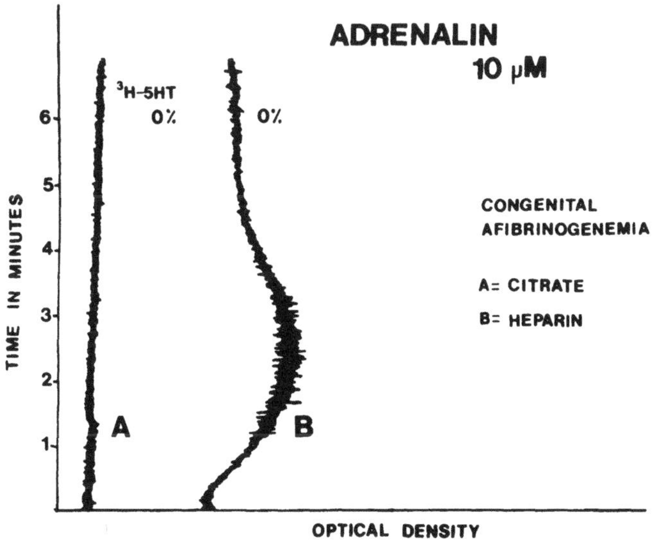

Fig. 2. Text see Fig. 1

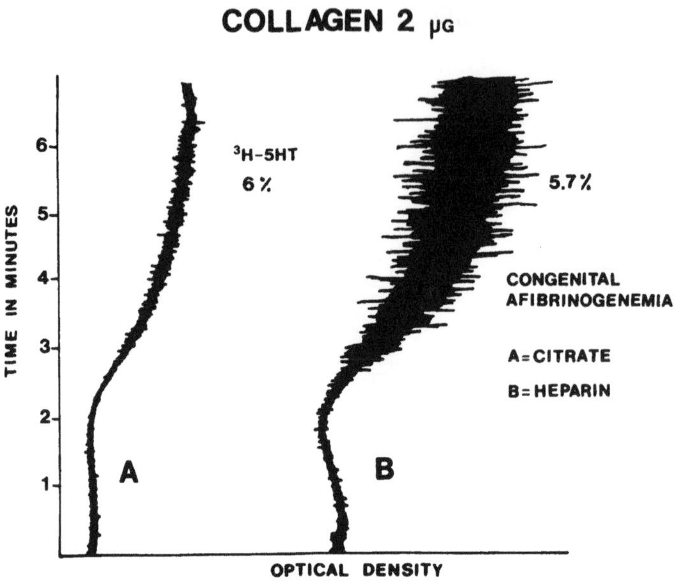

Fig. 3. Text see Fig. 1

Furthermore, aspirin which blocks the platelet release reaction, did not prevent the enhancement of primary aggregation induced by infusion of 5,000 I.U of heparin (5). Some relationship between platelet function and molecular size of heparin have been found in experimental models for heparins obtained by gel filtration and affinity chromatography (20). Some correlation between chemical structure, anticlotting activity and platelet aggregation has been also demonstrated (9).

We have taken into consideration different lots of normal heparins, chemically depolymerized heparin with different molecular weights kindly supplyed by Prof. F. Fussi (Hepar Ind. Ohio U. S. A) and other glycosaminoglycan sulphates chemically related to the heparin structure (HS + DS) in different systems for platelet aggregation (11) (Table 2). ^{3}H-serotonin (^{3}H-5HT) release in washed platelets (WP) was carried out in gel filtered platelets: 200 μl of WP were incubated with different heparin solutions for 1 h at 22 °C, centrifuged and the radioactivity measured in the supernatant. ADP

Table 2. Anticlotting activities of heparins and heparin-related substances

Compound	REL $\overline{MW}$	$(\alpha)^{20}_{D}$	APTT Specific activity	Anti Xa Specific activity	Anti Xa/APTT
Liquemin Roche	ND	+	444 ± 22.8*	1206 ± 90	2.7
Heparin SQUIBB	ND	+	568 ± 31.1	1645 ± 48	2.89
**Normal Heparin	1	+	353 ± 45	998 ±114	2.82
**LMW Heparin 1	0.85	+	204 ± 49	755 ±150	3.7
**LMW Heparin 2	0.5	+	38 ± 7.5	189 ± 18.5	4.97
**DS + HS	ND	-	397 ± 30	2110 ±300	5.3

*Mean ± 1 SD of three different experiments

**Hepar Industries U. S. A.

induced platelet ^{3}H-5HT release was performed in PRP : 500 µl of PRP were incubated with heparin solution for 2 min at 37 °C prior to ADP (2 µM) addition. No significant modifications in release from WP were observed for all tested heparins. It was observed that after very large additions (from 330 to 660 µg), Liquemin induces a significant ^{3}H-5HT release from WP in agreement with Eika (10).

In PRP, heparin increases the release of serotonin induced by ADP (Table 3). The potentiation of the release is related to the molecular weight for the depolymerized heparins, but is not significant. No release was noted using heparin alone.

Our results confirm the enhancement of platelet release induced by normal heparins (17, 28, 29). The mild effect shown by heparins with lower MW and by HS + SD could be related to a different affinity of different molecules for AT III (28) in comparison to normal heparin. In fact, we observed that the PRP of a patient suffering from an abnormal antithrombin III (AT III Padua) with an altered affinity for heparin showed an enhanced ADP induced release in presence of heparin (12) (Fig. 4).

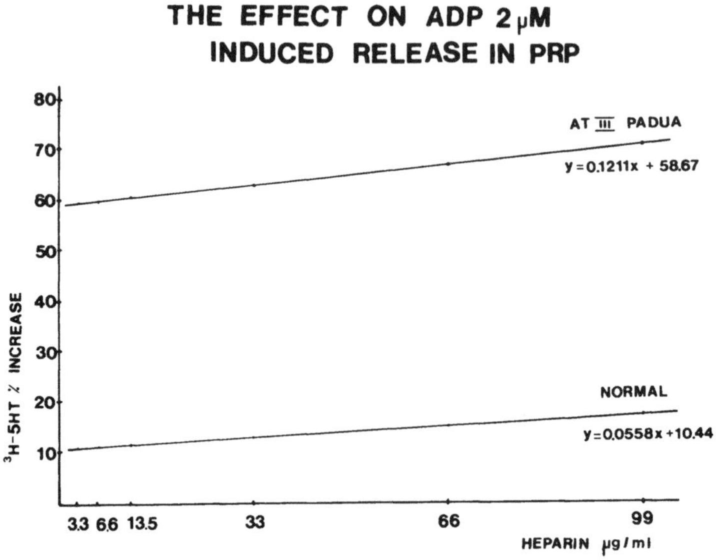

Fig. 4. The effect of heparin (Liquemin, Roche) on platelet release induced by ADP 2 µM in PRP of normal subjects and of a patient with AT III Padua

Table 3. The influence of heparins on platelet 3H-5HT release induced by ADP (2 μM) in PRP

Compound	Range of Additions	Rel. $\overline{MW}$	% Release*	F Ratio**	Q(U)**
Basal	-	-	40.4 ± 1.8	-	-
Liquemin Roche	0.5 - 15 IU (3.3-99UG)	ND	46.9 ± 21	5.6	0.043
Heparin SQUIBB	0.5 - 15 IU	ND	47.6 ± 2.8	411.9	0.000008
Normal Heparin	3.3 - 99 UG	1	47.9 ± 3.2	10.3	0.012
LMW Heparin 1	3.3 - 99 UG	0.85	42.9 ± 2	4.4	NS
LMW Heparin 2	3.3 - 99 UG	0.5	41.9 ± 1.1	0.2	NS
DS + SD	3.3 - 99 UG	ND	41.1 ± 1.4	0.15	NS

* Mean ISD of the values obtained by different Heparin additions

** Comparison of the single regression lines

We do not know yet if this is due to more heparin which has been left unbound or to an abnormal complex between heparin and the altered AT III.

Within the last few years a new approach for studying platelet function in vivo and in vitro has been developed which is the determination of two platelet specific proteins ß-thromboglobulin (ßtg) and platelet factor 4 (PF 4) (22, 24). ßtg and PF 4 are probably localized in alfa-granules and released during platelet release reaction (18). The two proteins are markedly similar in structure (23) but have different physical and biological properties. PF 4 binds strongly to heparin, neutralizing the anticoagulant activity, but ßtg has only a low anti-heparin action and its biological function has yet to be determined.

Recently, it has been shown that if heparin is given intravenously it causes an increase of PF 4; in contrast, ßtg does not seem to be affected by heparin itself (7). These features may open new approaches in the investigation of the interaction between heparin and platelets in vivo. Therefore, we studied the heparin induced release of ßtg, PF 4 and serotonin, a marker of platelet dense bodies content, both in vitro and in vivo.

Volunteer medical students were used as controls in addition to the four patients studied. Two patients presented with polycythemia vera and high platelet counts, and the other two presented with idiopathic thrombocytopenia. ßtg and PF 4 were determined in plasma and in platelets (PRP lysed by Triton) using commercially available radio-immunoassays (ßtg: Amersham Labs., England; PF 4: Abbott Labs. U. S. A.). Serotonin (5HT) assay was performed in platelet pellets according to a modification of the method of Crosti and Lucchelli (6). Sodium mucosal heparin (Liquemin Roche), calcium mucosal heparin (Calciparine Choay) and sodium beef lung heparin (Upjon) were used.

After hearpin injection (Liquemin) a great increase of approximately 20 fold of PF 4 levels was obtained in normal subjects with maximum peaks after 5 minutes and subsequently rapid clearance from the circulation (Fig. 5).

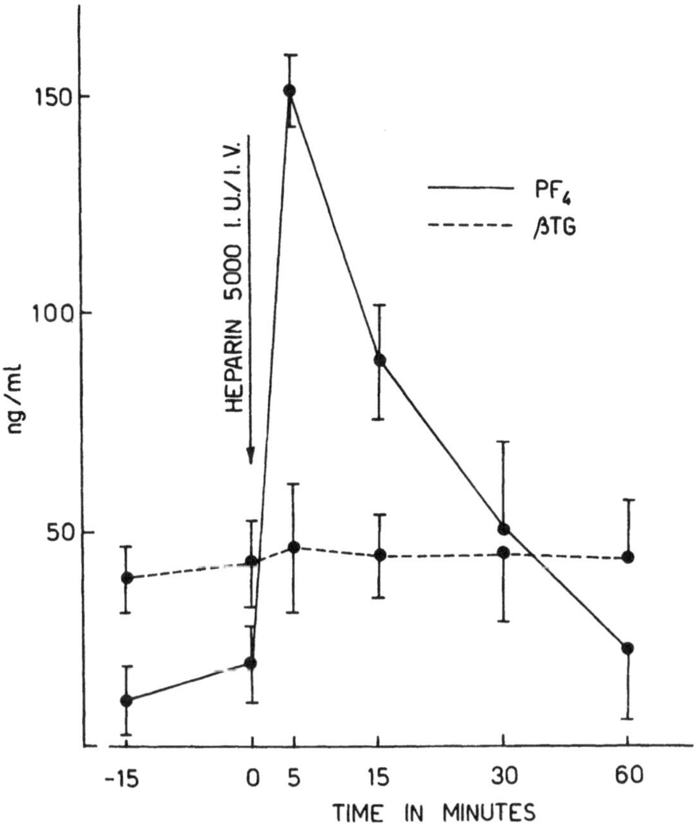

Fig. 5. Behaviour of PF 4 and ßtg in normal subjects after heparin (Liquemin, Roche) administration

In contrast, ßtg, the other specific protein which is supposed to be stored in the same granules of the platelet, seems not to be affected by heparin injection. A small and perhaps unspecific peak is present in ßtg levels immediately after heparin administration

Heparins from different sources seem to show different behaviour on platelet function (10), and beef lung preparations associated more frequently with thrombocytopenia (2).

Table 4. PF 4 and ßtg release induced in vivo by different heparins

Type of heparin		Platelet basal	Factor 4 ng/ml 5 min	60 min	β-Thromboglobulin ng/ml basal	5 min	60 min	Platelets mm³ basal
Mucosal Na salt	A	13.2	144	15.0	34	41	47	237000
	B	7.2	500	25.2	46	51	41	198000
	C	8.6	101	14.5	44	31	34	182000
Mucosal Ca salt	A	11.5	115	11.0	34	45	22	279000
	B	8.5	500	16.2	46	50	46	206000
	C	10.0	120	15.0	38	35	34	237000
Beef lung Na salt	A	20.7	84	17.3	28	33	33	253000
	B	11.7	259	14.0	54	50	30	210000
	C	14.3	83	21.5	34	33	31	216000

Five minutes after injection of two mucosal heparins a similar release of PF 4 was observed (Table 4) in three normal subjects although in two subjects the release was only 10 fold.

After beef lung heparin injection, the release was less evident and reduced by about 50 % as compared with the two intestinal mucosal heparins. No variations in platelet count were observed during the study with all three heparin preparations. The discrepancy in PF 4 release obtained with beef lung heparin is not clear (4). The increase of PF 4 was marked in two patients with thrombocythemia (100 and 50 fold respectively) and mild in the thrombocytopenic subjects (Fig. 6). The good correlation between platelet count and the increase of PF 4 may support the assumption of an activation of platelet specific release induced in vivo by heparin.

Platelet contents of ßtg, PF 4 and serotonin remained unchanged after heparin administration (Fig. 7) while PF 4 in blood increased (Table 5).

Furthermore, if platelet release reaction was blocked by Aspirin administration, the heparin injection was still able to induce release of PF 4 (Fig. 8).

Finally we then incubated in vitro (2 min, 37 °C) PRP with increasing amounts of heparin. After 4 min of stirring, ßtg and PF 4 were measured in the supernatent. Heparin was unable, in this model, to induce the release of ßtg and PF 4 (Fig. 9).

All these features seem to exclude that in vivo PF 4 increase after heparin administration was due to a release from blood platelets and suggest that the increase was due to the PF 4 bound to vascular endothelial cells (26). The clearance of PF 4 in vivo is extremely rapid and the T1/2 could not be determined, probably because of this binding to endothelial cells (7). Such interaction, demonstrated in vitro with cultured human endothelial cells (3), seems to be due to a specific and saturable binding with surface heparan sulphates of the endothelial cells (3).

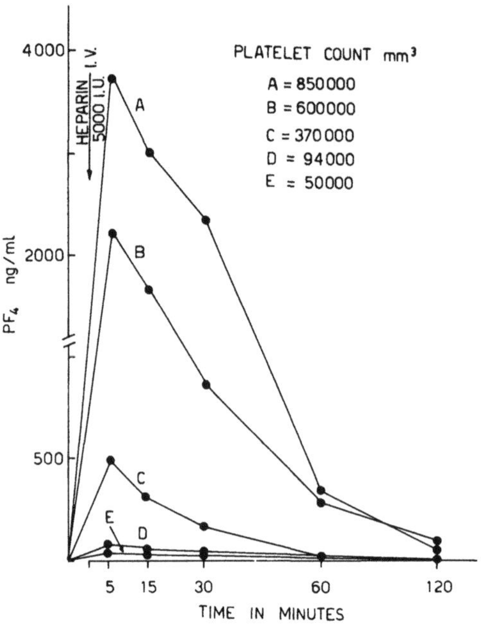

Fig. 6. PF 4 curves in patients with thrombocytosis (curves A-B) and thrombocytopenia (curves D-E). Curve C represents a normal subject. The numerical values of pre-injection PF 4 were: A = 45 ng/ml; B = 48 ng/ml; C = 9.5 ng/ml; D = 2.5 ng/ml; E = 1.5 ng/ml

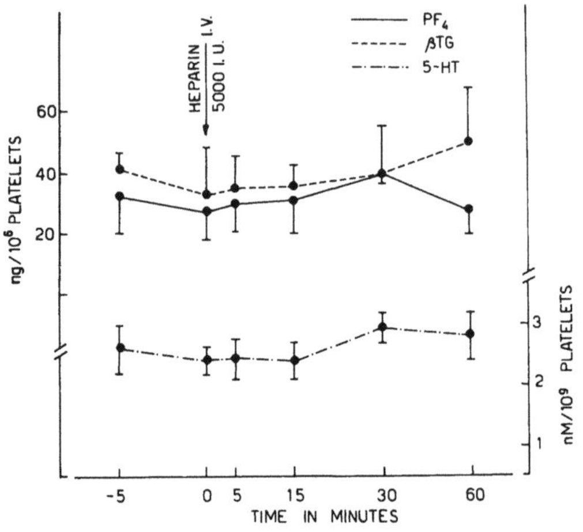

Fig. 7. Behaviour of platelet content of ßtg, PF 4 and serotonin after heparin injection (Liquemin, Roche)

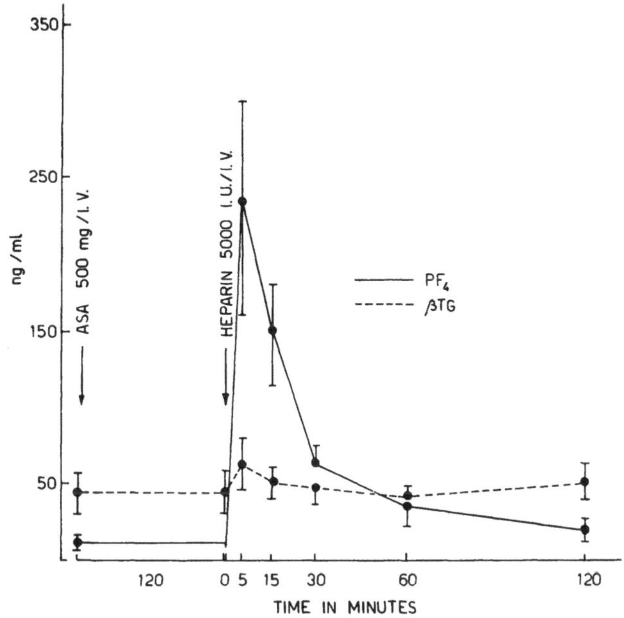

Fig. 8. Behaviour of PF 4 and ßtg in normal subjects after ASA and heparin (Liquemin, Roche) administration. Standard deviations are indicated by vertical bars.

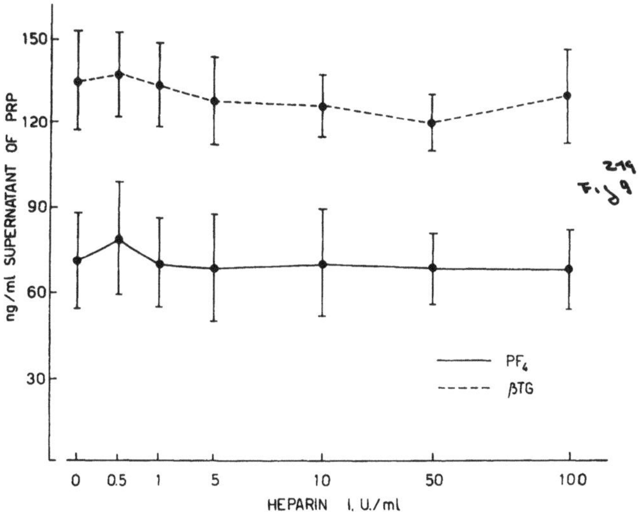

Fig. 9. ßtg and PF 4 release in vitro induced in PRP by increasing amounts of heparin (Liquemin, Roche). M ± SD of different experiments

Table 5. Behaviour of platelet serotonin, plasma and platelet ßtg and PF 4 after heparin injection (5,000 IU) Liquemin

Min. after heparin 5,000 IU iv	BTG		PF 4		5-HT
	ng/ml	ng/10^6 plat.	ng/ml	ng/10^6 plat.	nM/10^9 plat.
-15	39.9 ± 7.9	41.6 ± 5	16.6 ± 8.7	32 ± 12.5	2.65 ± 0.48
Basal	42.2 ± 10.8	31.9 ± 17.4	19.2 ± 9.1	28.5 ± 10.7	2.46 ± 0.20
5	46.3 ± 15.1	33.4 ± 11.4	152.3 ± 8.0	2.49 ± 10.2	2.49 ± 0.36
15	44.1 ± 10.6	35.7 ± 9.1	89.3 ± 13	31.9 ± 11.1	2.46 ± 0.29
30	44.9 ± 13.9	39.0 ± 3.0	50.7 ± 21.9	39.7 ± 17	2.93 ± 0.20
60	44.7 ± 14.1	44.0 ± 14.3	22.9 ± 16.1	30.1 ± 10.9	2.80 ± 0.44

Therefore, after injection, heparin, with a higher affinity for PF 4 than heparin sulphates, may displace PF 4 from endothelial cells increasing its concentration in the circulating blood. In the absence of appreciable amounts of heparin, endothelial cell-heparan sulphate may effectively bind PF 4 and therefore account for its very short half-life.

PF 4 determination, per se, may have little value as an indicator of in vivo platelet release or activation.

However, we think that the *heparin provocative test* proposed by us may be a useful tool in the investigation of heparin-endothelial interaction, namely, in the pathogenesis of one aspect of the thrombotic process.

References

1. Baird, A. R., Concery, F. R.: Arterial thromboembolism in patients receiving systemic heparin therapy. A complication associated with heparin induced thrombocytopenia. J. Bone Jt. Surg. Am. 59 A 1961-1964 (1977).

2. Bell, W. R., Royal, R. M.: Thrombocytopenia induced by heparin. A comparative study of three different heparin preparations. Blood 1979, supp. 1, 2332-2339.

3. Bush, W. R., Dawes, J., Pepper, D. S., Wasteson, A.: Binding of platelet factor four to cultured human umbilical vein endothelial cells. Thromb. Res. 19, 129-137 (1980).

4. Cella, G., Casonato, A., Visentin, L., Girolami, A.: Heparin and release. Thromb. Haemost. 44, 105 (1980).

5. Cella, G., Menardo, A., Girolami, A.: Effect of heparin in vivo. Platelet factor four (PF 4) release and platelet aggregation after aspirin administration. Clin. Lab. Haemat. 2, 333-338 (1980).

6. Crosti, P. F., Lucchelli, P. E.: An easy method to determine the serotonin content of human platelets. J. Clin. Pathol. 15, 191-198 (1962).

7. Dawes, J., Smith, R. C., Pepper, D. S.: The release, distribution and clearance of human ß-thromboglobulin and platelet factor 4. Thromb. Res. 12, 851-861 (1978).

8. De Marco, L., Fabris, F., Molaro, G., Girolami, A.: The effect of heparin on the interaction of factor VIII and human platelets in vitro. Haemostasis 6, 163-170 (1977).

9. Eika, C.: Anticoagulant and platelet aggregation activities of heparin. Thromb. Res. 2, 349-356 (1973).

10. Eika, C.: The platelet aggregation effect of eight commercial heparins. Scand. J. Haemat. 9, 480-487 (1977).

11. Fabris, F., Fussi, F., Casonato, A., Visentin, L., Randi, M. L., Smith, M. R., Girolami, A.: Normal and low molecular weight heparins: interaction with human platelets. In preparation.

12. Fabris, F., Randi, M. L., Casonato, A., Girolami, A.: The effect of normal and abnormal (AT III Padua) antithrombin-heparin complex on platelet function in vitro and in vivo. In preparation.

13. Girolami, A., De Marco, L., Virgolini, L., Peruffo, R., Fabris, F.: The effect of heparin on platelet aggregation by common inductors and by ristocetin in congenital bleeding disorders due to factor VIII or fibrinogen defects. Blut 31, 219-226 (1975).

14. Girolami, A., De Marco, L., Virgolini, L., Peruffo, R., Fabris, F.: Platelet aggregation and adhesiveness in congenital afibrinogenemia. Blut 30, 87-1000 (1975).

15. Gollub, S., Wein, A. W.: Heparin induced thrombocytopenia in man. J. Lab. Clin. Med. 59, 430-435 (1962).

16. Han, P., Ardle, N. G.: Heparin, platelets and blood coagulation: implications for low dose heparin prophylaçtig regimens in venous thrombosis. Brit. J. Haemat. 27, 253-272 (1974).

17. Heptinstal, S., Graham, P. M.: Adenosine diphosphate induced platelet aggregation and release reaction in heparinized platelet rich plasma and the influence of added citrate. Brit. J. Haemat. 36, 565-571 (1977).

18. Kaplan, K. L., Broekman, M. J., Chernoff, A., Lesznik, G. R., Drillings, M.: Platelet alfa granules proteins: studies on release and sub-cellular localization. Blood 53, 604-613 (1979).

19. Kirby, E. P., Millis, D. C. B.: The interaction of bovine factor VIII with human platelets. J. Clin. Invest. 56, 306-313 (1975).

20. Lindon, J., Rosenberg, R., Merril, R., Salzman, E.: Interaction of human platelets with heparinized agarose gel. J. Lab. Clin. Med. 91, 47-59 (1978).

21. MacFarlane, D. E., Walsh, P. N., Mills, D. C. B., Holmes, H., Day, H. J.: The role of thrombin in ADP induced platelet aggregation and release: a critical evaluation. Brit. J. Haemat. 30, 453-461 (1975).

22. Moore, S., Pepper, D. S., Cash, J. D.: The isolation and characterization of a platelet specific ß-globulin (ß-thromboglobulin) and the detection of anti-urokinase and antiplasmin released from thrombin-aggregated washed human platelets. Biochim. Biophys. Acta 379, 360-382 (1975).

23. Morgan, F. J., Begg, G. S., Chesterman, C. N., Pepper, D. S.: Partial aminoacid sequence of human ß-thromboglobulin: structural relationship with platelet factor 4. Thromb. Res. 12, 171-175 (1977).

24. Niewiarowski, S., Poplawski, A., Lipinski, B., Fabrizewski, L.: The rleease of platelet clotting factors during aggregation and viscous metamorphosis. Exp. Biol. Med. 3, 121-134 (1968).

25. O'Brien, J. R., Shoobridge, S. M., Finch, W. J.: Comparison of the effect of heparin and citrate on platelet aggregation. J. Clin. Path. 22, 28-35 (1960).

26. Pumphrey, C. W., Pepper, D. S., Dawes, J.: Heparin PF 4 pulsing as a measure of platelet-endothelial cells reaction in vivo. Thromb. Haemost. 42, 43 (1979) (abstract).

27. Roberts, B., Rosato, F. E., Rosato, E. F.: Heparin a cause of arterial emboli? Surgery 57, 131-137 (1965).

28. Salzman, E., Rosenberg, R. D., Smith, M. H., Lindon, J. N.: Effect of heparin fractions on platelet aggregation. J. Clin. Invest. 65, 64-73 (1980).

29. Thompson, C. C., Forbes, C. D., Prentice, C. R. M.: The potentiation of platelet aggregation and adhesion by heparin in vitro and in vivo. Clin. Sci. Mol. Med. 45, 485-494 (1973).

30. Zucker, M. B.: Biological aspects of heparin action. Heparin and platelet function. Fed. Proc. 36, 47-49 (1977).

Discussion

Dawes agreed with *Fabris* as far as the release of platelet factor 4 in vitro is concerned. She did the experiment with whole blood. The release was induced by thrombin and heparin did not increase the release of platelet factor 4 and β-thromboglobulin.

She would like to have agreed with *Fabris'* conclusions but she did not feel that there was any convincing evidence. The platelet content of plasma was unchanged. But the platelets contain such high amounts of these proteins compared with the content in plasma that the decrease in platelet count which would be associated with the increase in the plasma content of these proteins would not be detectable.

Concerning the effect of aspirin on the release reaction in vivo *Dawes* and *Fabris* achieved different results. Whereas *Fabris* found that the release of β-thromboglobulin and platelet factor 4 induced by thrombin, collagen or arachidonic acid is blocked by aspirin *Dawes* had confirmed these results only in vitro but not in vivo.

Characterization of a New Potent Heparin

Akhil S. Bhargava, Peter Günzel
Research Laboratories, Schering AG,
D-1000 Berlin

Introduction

In some of our previous reports we have described a new potent heparin preparation* which possesses 1.32 to 2.52 times higher activity than commercially available heparin, depending upon the test system used to assay the anticoagulation activity (1, 2, 3). The tests used so far to characterize this heparin preparation (Schering) were based on the determination of thrombin time, activated partial thromboplastin time, whole-blood clotting time, protamine neutralization, as well as amidolytic methods involving inactivation of specific factors like thrombin and factor Xa, using synthetic substrates. We would like to present some of the results obtained with this heparin by thrombelastography in vitro as well as by affinity chromatography on antithrombin-III-sepharose in comparison to commercially available heparin (4, 5). In addition, the recent results of a comparative study of this heparin in humans after a single intravenous application will be reported.

Thrombelastography

500 µl citrated blood was mixed with 50 µl solutions of heparin in 0.9 % W/V sodium chloride to give heparin concentrations for the new heparin (Schering) as well as for the commercial heparin ranging from 0.5 - 1.0 µg/ml for dog blood and 1.0 - 3.0 µg/ml for human blood. After 2 min of prein-

*German patent 2652272 (1978)

Heparin · New Biochemical and Medical Aspects

cubation of citrated blood with heparin at 37 °C, the thrombelastography was performed according to Hartert (6) and Keck and Lam (7) with the thrombelastograph (Fritz Hellige and Co., Freiburg). The speed of the photographic film of the instrument used was 2 mm/min. Reaction time (r in min), coagulation time (k in min), maximum amplitude (ma in mm) and tg α were evaluated after development of the thrombelastograms.

Regression analysis and parallel-line assay were performed using double log transformation to estimate the relative potencies of the new heparin preparation.

A concentration dependent prolongation of reaction time, coagulation time and a decrease in maximum amplitude and tg α was observed for heparin Schering as well as for commercial heparin used as a standard. However, when the effects of both heparin preparations were compared, the heparin Schering exerted a much greater anticoagulant effect than commercial heparin as estimated on the basis of thrombelastographic parameters. The typical thrombelastograms obtained using human citrated blood with heparin preparations are illustrated in Fig. 1. This shows that the anticoagulant effect of 2 μg heparin Schering was much more pronounced than 2.5 μg commercial heparin/ml citrated blood.

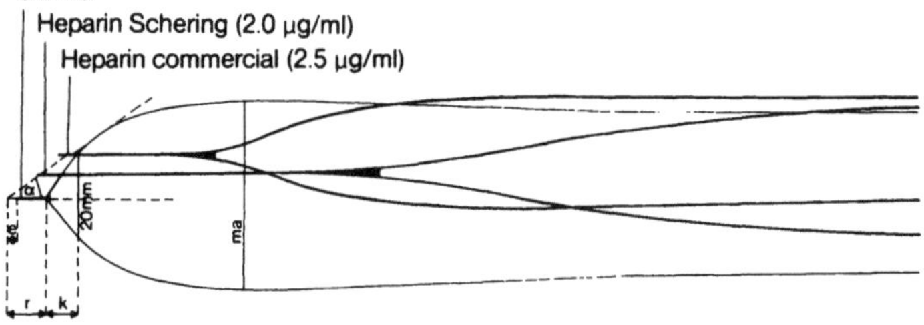

Fig. 1. Effect of heparin preparations on the thrombelastogram in vitro using human citrated blood

The relative potency of the heparin Schering was found to be 1.45 to 1.77 with dog citrated blood and 1.77 to 2.41 with human citrated blood on the basis of different thrombelastographic parameters as evaluated by parallel line assay (Table 1).

Table 1. Relative potency of heparin Schering as determined by thromblastography in vitro. ( ) = lower and upper confidence limit at the 95 % level.

Species	Reaction time (r) in min	Coagulation time (k) in min	Maximal amplitude (ma) in mm	tg α
Dog	1.45 (1.22 - 1.89)	–	1.59 (1.34 - 2.06)	1.77 (1.52 - 2.20)
Human	2.41 (1.83 - 3.78)	2.16 (1.71 - 3.05)	1.77 (1.34 - 2.74)	2.28 (1.71 - 3.66)

The potencies of the heparin preparation were calculated by parallel line assay using double log transformation where a commercial preparation containing 150 USP units/mg served as a standard and defined as 1.0.

Affinity chromatography

1 mg each of heparin (Schering) and commercially available heparin was applied separately to a column containing antithrombin-III-sepharose gel (10 ml), equilibrated with 0.2 mol/l NaCl-1/150 mol/l phosphate buffered, pH 7.4 at 4 °C. The column was first eluted with 40 ml buffered 0.2 mol/l NaCl and then with a linear salt gradient from 0.2 to 3 mol/l in buffer. Fractions of 2 ml each were collected. Effluent fractions were analyzed for uronic acid by the carbazole reaction. Fractions 1 to 9 (low affinity fraction) and 25 to 34 (high affinity fraction) were pooled separately, dialyzed against water and lyophilized. The low and high affinity fractions were then analyzed for uronic acid content and for their biologic activities in activated partial thromboplastin time and factor Xa assays using a heparin standard containing 133.5 USP units/mg.

Sepharose coupled to antithrombin-III for affinity chromatography was kindly provided by Dr. E. Holmer, KABI AB, Stockholm. The binding capacity of the material was 0.2 mg heparin/ml gel.

The elution pattern of 1 mg of the heparin Schering as well as commercial heparin is shown in Fig. 2. Most of the uronic acid content of the heparin Schering was eluted between 0.4 to 1.1 mol/l salt gradient while less of the commercial heparin was eluted at this range and more at 0.2 mol/l NaCl.

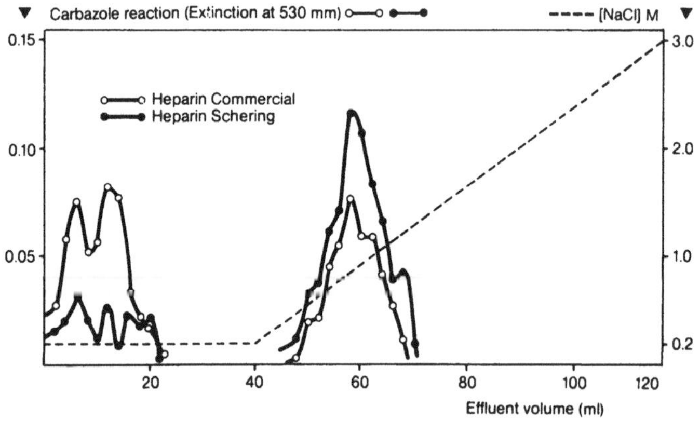

Fig. 2. Affinity chromatography of heparin preparations on antithrombin-sepharose.

The commercial heparin consisted of 60 % low affinity heparin and 40 % high affinity heparin whereas the heparin Schering had 83 % high affinity heparin and only 17 % low affinity heparin on the basis of uronic acid distribution.

The specific activity per µg uronic acid for high affinity fractions on the basis of activated partial thromboplastin time as well as factor Xa assay was of similar order for both heparin preparations, suggesting that the heparin Schering consists mostly of high affinity fraction, which is also present to 40 % in commercial heparin. This is further supported by the identical pattern of high affinity fractions of the heparin Schering as well as commercial heparin eluted from antithrombin-III-sepharose by a salt gradient.

Comparative study in humans after intravenous application

20 male and 20 female normal adult subjects participated in this study. 2 male and 2 female subjects per group were treated intravenously with doses ranging from 18.3-218.3 µg for heparin Schering and 40.3-483.0 µg for commercial heparin per kg body weight (see Table 2).

Table 2. Treatment scheme for single intravenous application of heparin preparations to 2 male and 2 female normal adult subjects per group.

Group	Heparin preparation	Doses in I.U./kg bodyweight (on the basis of manufacturer's stated potency)	Doses in U/kg bodyweight (on the basis of factor Xa inactivation assay)	Doses in µg/kg bodyweight (on the basis of the dryweight)
1	Heparin (Commercial)	6.25	5.62	40.3
2		12.5	11.25	80.5
3		25	22.5	161.0
4		50	45.0	322.0
5		75	67.5	483.0
6	Heparin (Schering)	–	5.62	18.3
7		–	11.25	36.5
8		–	22.5	73.1
9		–	45.0	146.2
10		–	67.5	218.3

Determinations of thrombin time, whole blood clotting time, activated partial thromboplastin time and plasma heparin levels using factor Xa inactivation assay were performed before and 5, 10, 15, 30 and 60 min after heparin application. The regression analysis and parallel line assay were performed using log dose or double log transformation or log dose and square root transformation of areas under the curve to estimate the relative potencies of heparin Schering.

In addition, biological activity of heparin Schering and commercial heparin solutions were also determined on the basis of factor Xa inactivation assay. However, the doses used in this experiment will be referred to in µg/kg body weight, which was calculated for commercial heparin on the basis of dry weight determinations (155 IU/mg dry weight). Furthermore, clinical chemistry (glucose, alkaline phosphatase, GOT, GPT, LDH, γ-GT, α-amylase, cholesterol, triglyceride, bilirubin, uric acid, creatinine, urea nitrogen, inorganic phosphorus, sodium, potassium, calcium, chloride determinations and protein electrophoresis in serum), coagulation studies (fibrinogen, thromboplastin time, partial thromboplastin time) and haematological examination (erythrocyte, haemoglobin, haematocrit, thrombocyte, reticulocyte, leucocyte and differential counts) were carried out before and 24 h after heparin application to check the values before and side effects which might occur after heparin application.

A dose dependent prolongation of whole-blood clotting time, thrombin time and activated partial thromboplastin time was observed following i. v. applications of both heparin preparations to human subjects. As evident from Fig. 3, the heparin Schering showed more pronounced effect when compared to commercial heparin, considering lower doses of the heparin Schering required for comparable prolongation of the whole blood clotting time.

The relative potencies of the heparin Schering were calculated by parallel line assay using 5, 10 and 15 min values as well as areas under the curves up to 30 and 60 min. As can be seen from Table 3 a relative potency between 1.5 to 2.0 was found for the heparin Schering compared to the commercial preparation on the basis of thrombin time and whole-blood clotting time. However, a calculation of relative potency on the basis of activated partial thromboplastin time was not possible due to the highly significant deviation from linearity ($p < 0.01$) in regression analysis for the heparin Schering response at 5, 10 and 15 min as well as for both preparations using area under the curves up to 30 and 60 min.

Determinations of plasma heparin levels, based on inactivation of factor Xa, showed a dose dependent increase with the maximum plasma concentration measured at 5 min (Fig. 4). Lower i. v. doses of the heparin Schering than of commercial heparin gave a comparable rise in plasma heparin concentration.

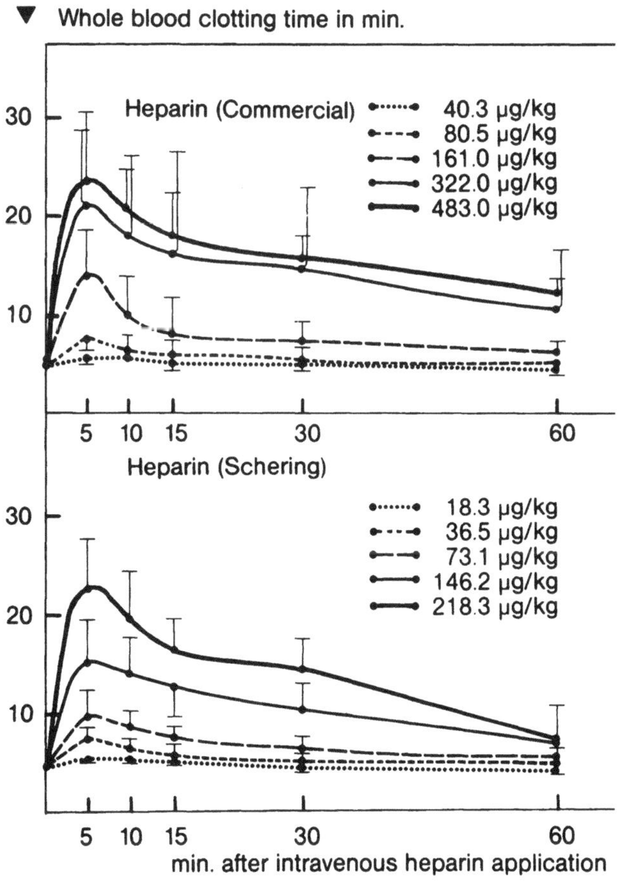

Fig. 3. Effect of a single intravenous application of heparin preparations on whole blood clotting time in humans (N = 4, M/SD).

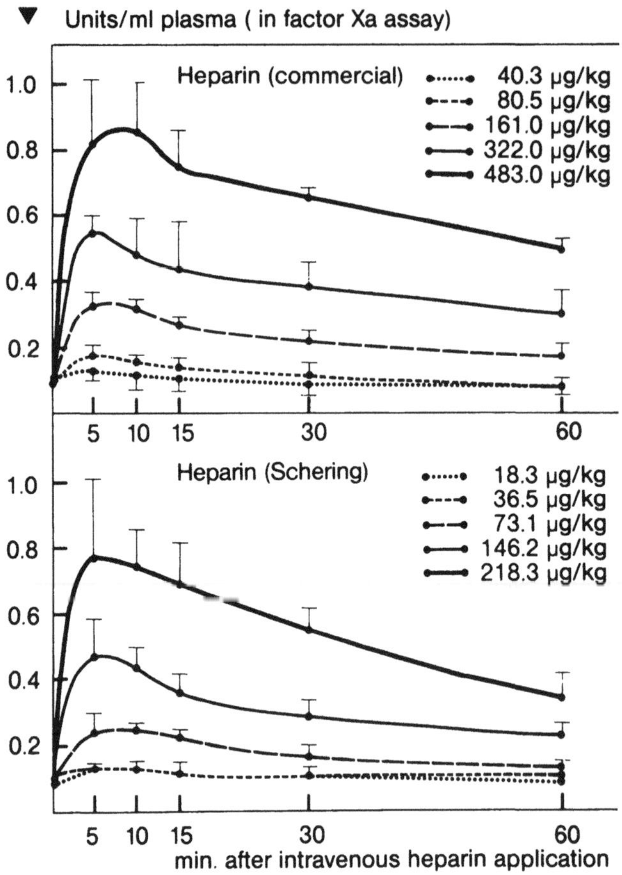

Fig. 4. Heparin levels after a single intravenous application of heparin preparations in humans (N = 4, M/SD).

As indicated in Table 3, the heparin Schering was 1.7 to 1.8 times more effective than commercial heparin, also on the basis of increase in heparin levels as measured by amidolytic assay.

Table 3. Relative potency of heparin (Schering) after a single intravenous application in humans.

Coagulation Indices	Calculated from values obtained at min.			Calculated from area under the curve till min.	
	5	10	15	30	60
Thrombin time	2.0	1.7	2.0	1.8	1.8
Whole blood clotting time	1.7	1.8	1.7	1.6	1.5
Amidolytic assay (Factor Xa inactivation)	1.7	1.8	1.7	1.8	1.7

Potencies of heparin (Schering) were calculated by parallel line assay where a commercial heparin preparation containing 155 I.U./mg on dry weight basis served as a standard (1.0).

Determinations of clinical chemical and haematological parameters, 24 h after heparin application in all human subjects, revealed no signs of any adverse effect for both heparin preparations as all values remained within the normal range.

Conclusion

From the thrombelastographic results presented in this communication, it is quite evident that the heparin Schering is a more potent anticoagulant than a commercial heparin preparation containing 150 USP U/mg.

Considering the effect of heparin preparations on tg α to be the resultant of all thrombelastographic indices, the relative potencies of heparin Schering were found to be 1.77 for dog and 2.28 for man. The relative potency of heparin Schering on human citrated blood (2.28), on the other hand, correlates well with the results obtained using chromogenic substrates for factor Xa (2.14) and thrombin inactivation (2.37) as reported earlier (3).

The characterization by affinity chromatography on antithrombin-III-sepharose revealed that the heparin Schering consists of 83 % high affinity heparin and 17 % low affinity heparin whereas commercial heparin contains only 40 % high affinity heparin and 60 % low affinity heparin. The amount of high affinity fraction present in commercial heparin is in good correlation with the findings of Höök et al. (8), who also described that 38 % of the uronic acid content of a heparin preparation emerged during gradient elution on antithrombin-sepharose with the high affinity fraction.

Thus it is concluded that the 2 times more potent anticoagulant activity of the heparin Schering is due to the presence of 83 % of high affinity fraction.

The comparison of the anticoagulant effect of this heparin with commercial heparin following a single i. v. dose to humans, showed that the heparin Schering is 1.5 to 2.0 times more potent depending upon the coagulation tests used and the length of the observation period. The relative potency of the heparin Schering in a range of 1.7 - 1.8 compared to the commercial preparation in humans after i. v. application is of a similar order as that previously found in different in vitro tests and in vivo using the dog as experimental animal (1, 2, 3, 4).

References

1. Bhargava, A. S., Heinick, J., Schöbel, Chr., Günzel, P.: Arzneim.-Forsch./Drug Res. 30 (I), 993-996 (1980).

2. Bhargava, A. S., Heinick, J., Schöbel, Chr., Günzel, P.: Thrombos. Haemostas. 42, 381 (1979).

3. Bhargava, A. S., Heinick, J., Günzel, P.: Arzneinm.-Forsch./Drug Res. 30 (II), 1071-1074 (1980).

4. Bhargava, A. S., Freihube, G., Günzel, P.: Arzneim.-Forsch./Drug Res. 30 (II), 1256-1258 (1980).

5. Bhargava, A. S., Freihube, G., Günzel, P.: Arzneim.-Forsch./Drug Res. 30 (II), 1621-1623 (1980).

6. Hartert, H., Z. ges. Exp. Med. 117, 189-203 (1951).

7. Keck, G., Lam, A., Kleintierpraxis 17, 1-6 (1972).

8. Höök, M., Björk, I., Hopwood, J., Lindhal, U.: FEBS Lett. 66, 90-93 (1976).

Side Effects of Heparin

Ellen Weber, Erhard Walter, Job Harenberg
Abteilung Klinische Pharmakologie
der Medizinischen Universitätsklinik Heidelberg
D-6900 Heidelberg

Besides sequels due to its anticoagulatory effect severe adverse reactions of heparin are rather seldom. This is an astonishing fact considering that this endogenous substance, even in small concentrations in vitro and in vivo, is able to influence a variety of actions (Table 1; see also the contribution of Dawes).

In Table 2 some effects of heparin are summarized which are not related to its anticoagulatory action. Not all of them will be discussed.

Haemorrhage due to heparin

One of the greatest difficulties even under otherwise comparable conditions is a definition of the phenomenon *bleeding*, in order to obtain valid results. Therefore it is obvious that the frequency of bleeding due to heparin cannot be given in a definite way. Table 3 shows an arbitrary selection of examples. In these few analyses the incidence of bleeding events due to heparin lies between 0.8 and 36 %. Indeed, the bleeding events can only be compared under equal conditions because they are extremely dependent on the circumstances. It is not unimportant whether the patient is under medical or surgical therapy, in the latter case the kind of operation also being decisive. Obviously, the dosage and mode of application are further important factors. Risk factors in patients are more important than the external situation. An example confirming these findings is given in Table 4, which has been taken from a publication by Walker and Jick (1).

Heparin · New Biochemical and Medical Aspects

Table 1
Some effects of heparin on biological systems* (12)

	inhibits	stimulates
Hematological	blood clotting	fibrinolysis
Enzymes	cortisone reductase	lipoprotein lipase
	fumarase	
	trypsin	
	proteases	bone collagenase
	acid and alkaline ribonuclease	
	acid and alkaline phosphatase	scorbutism
	beta glucuronidase	
	lysozyme	
Allergic response	Arthus phenomenon	
	Schwartzmann reaction	
	complement (in vitro)	
Endocrine	steroid induced leucopenia	positive nitrogen balance
		parathyroid hormone in tissue culture
Cellular activity	cell division (mitosis)	pinocytosis
	fibroblast growths in tissue culture	
Wound repair	wound healing	wound healing
	keloid formation	
	fracture healing	
	bone formation	osteoporosis
Miscellaneous	serotonin effects	aggregation of collagen fibers in vitro
	histamine effects	

*Some known effects are not listed due to limited space. The effects listed give some indication of the variety of studies that have been carried out and the extent of the inhibitory effects.

It can be derived that in medical patients the risk of major bleeding due to heparin is greater in elderly women, severely ill individuals, and those with uraecemia, alcohol abuse, concurrent aspirin administration, and also in cases in which gastrointestinal bleeding had occurred beforehand.

Table 2
Non coagulatory effects of heparin (19)

Endocrine, metabolic

- clearing action on postprandial lipidaemia
- \- insulin secretion

Mineral and fluid balance

- \+ natriuresis
- mobilization of calcium and inorganic phosphate

Renal

- antialdosterone effect

Haematological

- decrease in the number of circulating platelets

Skin and appendages

- allergic reactions
- local stinging sensations or pruritus
- lipodystrophy
- temporary alopecia

Table 3
Haemorrhage due to heparin

n	%		ref.
374	0.8	wound hematomas requiring surgical treatment and/or prolongation of hospitalisation	38
575	1.2	major GI bleeding complications	39
407	2.2	abnormal bleeding	40
206	2.5	major bleeding	41
	5.0	retroperitoneal haemorrhage	3
68	10.3	severe bleeding (total hip replacement)	42
76	13.0	severe bleeding	4
100	21.0	major bleeding	43
76	21.0	bleeding of surgical wounds	4
42	26.2	major bleeding episode	44
135	27.0	bleeding and wound complications	45
86	36.0	wound haematoma in herniorrhaphy	46

Table 4
Indicators of risk for bleeding among 2,656 hospitalized patients receiving heparin sodium (1)

	Relative risk for bleeding[*]	
Comparison	minimal and moderate (n= 203)	major (n = 35)
Sex		
F vs M	1.5 (1.1, 1.9)[+]	2.1 (1.1, 4.0)
Age, yr		
40-59 vs <40	0.9 (0.7, 1.3)	2.3 (0.6, 8.7)
>60 vs <40	1.1 (0.8, 1.5)	3.1 (0.8, 11.4)
Dose, units/kg/dose		
50-99 vs <50	2.0 (1.2, 3.1)	1.3 (0.4, 4.3)
>100 vs <50	3.2 (2.0, 5.1)	2.6 (0.8, 8.2)
Frequency		
every 2 or 3 hr vs other	0.4 (0.1, 1.5)	0
Aspirin		
used vs not used	1.5 (1.1, 2.0)	2.4 (1.1, 5.1)
Survival		
died vs survived; [++] died this admission	1.6 (1.0, 2.6)	4.0 (2.0, 8.2)
Alcohol, drinks/day		
>5 or binge vs ≤5	0.7 (0.3, 1.5)	6.9 (2.2, 21.0)
BUN, mg/dl		
≥50 vs <50	1.0 (0.7, 1.7)	2.0 (0.9, 4.5)

[*] This is the ratio of *daily risks* between the comparison groups, as derived from a Cox life-table analysis. Each relative risk is adjusted for the effects of all other indicators listed as well as for interhospital variation and duration of therapy.

[+] Numbers in parentheses are the 90 % confidence intervals for the relative risk. These theoretical values of relative risk are consistent with the observed values at a one-sided P value of .05.

[++] Excluding deaths caused by hemorrhage.

On the other hand there are no definite data to conclude that a frequent occurrence of bleeding complications correlates with the material from which the heparin had been manufactured or with the cation of the heparin preparation.

Loeliger (2) summarized in 1975 those bleeding complications which have been encountered rarely (Table 5). In contrast, Curry and Bacon (3) and Mant et al. (4) observed as much as a 5 % incidence of retroperitoneal haematoma with, however, high conventional doses of heparin (see also 5).

Table 5
Rarely encountered bleeding complications in heparin therapy (19)

intramural haemorrhage of the intestinal wall
retroperitoneal haematoma
femoral nerve entrapment
subdural haematoma after lumbal puncture
bilateral adrenal haemorrhage
spontaneous rupture of the spleen
massive heaemothorax
haemarthrosis hip

Heparin and cardiac arrythmias

In 1970 the mechanism involved in developing arrhythmias, often seen in myocardial infarction, were discussed. The following were made responsible for the occurrence of such arrhythmias (see e. g. 6): rise in the plasma concentration of catecholamines as well as glucocorticoides and also growth hormone. All of these can induce an increase of free fatty acids in plasma. As it is known that heparin (see also Table 1 and 2) activates lipoprotein lipases and thus enhances free fatty acids in plasma, it was assumed that at least some of the cardiac arrhythmias in myocardial infarction are due to heparin therapy. This was a controversial topic for several years. Today, it is considered unlikely that heparin causes this kind of cardiac arrhythmias. So it could be shown that no more cardiac arrhythmias occurred in groups to which heparin was given compared with those without heparin (6, 7). Also, a rise in free fatty acids is no longer believed to increase the incidence of cardiac arrhythmias (8, 9). Moreover, Arnesen et al. (10) pointed out in 1980 that subcutaneously administered low-dose heparin does not lead to a rise in free fatty acids in plasma.

Osteoporosis

Today, it is considered likely that severe osteoporosis with spontaneous fracturing develops when more than 150 mg, i. e. about 20,000 units of heparin/day, are given for more than 4 months (2). Griffith et al. (11) already published in 1965 corresponding results. In 107 out of 117 patients on longterm sodium heparin therapy, no symptoms of osteoporosis developed. They received 10,000 units of sodium heparin once daily or less during a period of 1 to 15 years. In contrast to these results, 6 out of 10 patients treated daily with larger doses (15,000 - 30,000 units) for six months or longer, developed spontaneous fractures of vertebrae or ribs, biopsy disclosing soft, bony matrix.

A noxious influence on bone metabolism has been proven several times in animals (e. g. 12). Osteoporosis has been ascribed to the enhancement of collagenolysis by heparin (13). Others assumed an enzymatic inhibition (14) or a deprivation of ascorbic acid at the site of osteoblast activity. Recently Aarskog et al. (15), reported an interesting observation: Increasing lower back pain developed one week post partum in a 22 year old woman. Subcutaneous heparin injections were started 8 weeks before term in doses up to 15,000 units t.i.d. and continued after delivery at 5,000 units t.i.d. X-rays disclosed gross thoracolumbar spinal osteoporosis with compression fractures. Whereas the concentrations of 25-OH-vitamin D (OHD) and 24,25 $(OH)_2D$ were found in the normal range, the serum levels of 1.25-$(OH)_2D$ were well below normal (Table 6). The mechanism for the heparin induced osteopenia remains unclear; the authors assumed a relationship to PTH function. But more experience is necessary before pregnant women treated with subcutaneously administered heparin can be given $1,25\text{-}(OH)_2D$.

Table 6

Vitamin D metabolites and urinary cyclic AMP in relation to heparin (15)

Time	25-OHD nmol/l	$24,25\text{-}(OH)_2D$ nmol/l	$1,25\text{-}(OH)_2D$ pmol/l	Urinary cAMP µmol/24 h
On heparin	80.3	4.1	21.3	5.7
1 week after heparin	78.4	4.2	23.8	-
4 weeks after heparin	52.0	4.0	47.8	5.0
Normal range	38-99	0.8-5.5	42-145	2.5-6.5

Transaminase increase after heparin

Hypertransaminasemia with heparin therapy had been described by Sonnenblick et al. (16) and also by Olsson et al. (17). Recently Minar et al. (18) showed that heparin given to 46 patients in a dosage of 5,000 - 15,000 units induced a rise of GPT in 41 of them (89 %) and of GOT in 38 (82 %). The average maximal values of GOT were 39.7 ± 3.9 U/l at mean on the 5th day, and 67.0 ± 7.3 U/l in GPT on the 8th day. On reaching maximal values, enzyme activity decreased to the initial values despite continuance of heparin treatment. An increase in gamma-GT during subcutaneous administration occurred in 17 patients, i. e. 37 % (average maximal value 57.8 ± 8.4 U/l), while there was no significant change in alkaline phosphatase and LDH. A certain dependence of the incidence and/or extent of the transaminase increase on heparin dosage was noted, especially when comparing low-dose and full heparinization.

Heparin and allergy?

Loeliger (19) summarized phenomena after heparin treatment described in literature which are assumed to be of an allergic nature: urticaria, conjunctivitis, rhinitis, asthma, cyanosis, tachypnea, feeling of oppression, fever, angioneurotic oedema and anaphylactic shock. Considering differences in the origin of heparin like impurities of animal proteins in heparin preparations and added preservatives, it is feasible that allergies could develop.

Data on adverse drug reactions have been collected by the Department of Internal Medicine in Heidelberg from 1971 onwards (for methods see 20). 5 % of about 63,000 patients treated in the time period from 1971 - 1980 received heparin. 26 patients developed cutaneous phenomena, exanthemes and local necrosis which had been related to heparin allergy by the treating physicians. 16 (9 women and 7 men) of the 26 patients were examined recently (6 of the other 10 patients had died and 4 did not consent to reexamination).

At the time of heparin-treatment chronic haemodialysis was undertaken in 8 of the 16 patients. 10 of them had had intravenous heparin, 6 subcutaneously. The dosage was 8,000 - 25,000 units/day. The observed phenomena were as follows:

pruritus	1
pruritus ubiquitare	3
exantheme	9
necrosis	2
shivering after dialysis	1
	16

The observed reactions began in 8 patients during the first 6 hours after the first administration of heparin. In each of 2 patients reactions occurred for the first time on the 3rd, 4th and 10th day, and in one patient both on the 6th and 9th day after commencing heparin therapy.

In these 16 patients with the positive history of heparin reactions two sodium and one calcium heparin from mucosa, sodium pyrosulfite and 4-chlor-m-kresol as preservatives were tested parallel with histamine. The scratch test was used as proof of an immediate reaction. If this test proved to be negative then an intracutan testing was carried out. If the intracutan test proved to be positive an epicutan test followed.

Only in one patient a questionable positive reaction in the intracutan test could be observed. The epicutan testing was negative. In the lymphocyte transformation test only the reaction to the preservative 4-chlor-m-kresol turned out to be positive. These results show that not heparin but its preservative was the cause of sensibilization in the patient (20 a).

Vasospastic reactions

Loeliger (19) described a special type of vasospastic reaction after heparin. It is characterized by local pain, local cyanosis and ischaemia. Cyanosis can be generalized and is accompanied by tachypnea, a feeling of oppression and headache. Another variant is known as *dysesthesia pedis*, which is characterized by very severe itching and burning, especially on the plantar surface of the feet. Dysesthesia pedis starts 6 - 10 days after heparin therapy and lasts for 4 - 6 hours. Women prevail over men. If the patient is re-exposed the reaction is enhanced. The prognosis is good, but in two cases necrotic ischaemic reactions have been observed. The phenomenon is not related to the origin of the heparin.

It has been suggested that in vasospastic reactions heparin is a hapten in a heparin protein complex, which acts as an antigen. The antibodies induce an antigen antibody reaction as soon as heparin is given. The incidence of this phenomenon is not known, but it seems to be rather seldom.

Decrease of platelet counts - The White-clot syndrome

The most fascinating development in the domain of adverse drug reactions of heparin nowadays deals with the decrease in the number of platelets, sometimes connected with heparin therapy.

A question often discussed is, how far does heparin reduce the platelet count. This phenomenon is to be expected as we know from in vitro investigations that heparin enhances the aggregation of platelets, induced by other agents. This action of heparin is blocked by substances which raise the content of platelet cyclic AMP and by EDTA, but not by inhibitors of platelet cyclooxygenase. The effect is not ADP- or platelet phospholipase-dependent (21). Heparin is also able to abolish the antiaggregating effect of prostaglandin I_2 and D_2 (22).

The international committee on thrombosis and haemostasis published a report on thrombocytopenia and heparin in 1980 (23). 9 prospective studies on heparin-associated thrombocyctopenia comprising a total of 770 patients were revised. In one study a fall in platelet count below 100,000/µl was found in 16 out of 52 patients (24). In the other 8 studies with a total of 718 patients the incidence of thrombocytopenia varied from 0 - 6 %. In 8 patients the platelets fell below 100,000/µl and in 27 patients counts between 150,000 and 100,000/µl were determined. In all 770 patients 4 spontaneous bleedings occurred and no thrombotic complications were observed. Furthermore, the bleedings were not serious. The fall in blood platelet count occurred during the first 5 - 7 days of treatment and cases of disseminated intravascular coagulation were observed. Beef lung heparin was used in the study in which an incidence of 31 % of thrombocytopenia was found (24). But this high incidence could not be confirmed in another prospective study with beef lung heparin (25).

In contrast to this transient fall in platelet count the *white-clot syndrome* presents a probably completely different type of event. The first report was by Weissmann and Tubin (26) in 1968, who described embolie under therapy with heparin. The *white-clot syndrome* consists of *thrombocytopenia*, *thrombo-haemorrhagic complications* and *skin necrosis*. Towne et al. (27) proposed the name white-clot syndrome because of the pale thrombie or embolie, which consist of thrombocytes and fibrin. Recently a short survey of the syndrome was given by Loeliger (28) in 1981:

The white-clot syndrome does not occur until the 6th day of treatment and seems to be independent of the type, the dosage and mode of administration of heparin. A sudden fall in platelet count leads to values below 100,000/µl, on the average 30,000/µl. There is an absence of pronounced disseminated intravascular coagulation and therefore no definite fall in fibrinogen. However, new and also recurring arterial thrombembolic complications occur. They are frequently localised in the distal aorta or in a lower extremity. But also myocardial infarction, hemiplegia, pulmonary embolism and/or progression of deep vein thrombosis can be found. Haemorrhagic symptoms such as petechiae, ecchymoses, oozing from vein puncture sites, epistaxis, haemoptysis and intracerebral haemorrhage are frequently observed. Also skin necrosis occurs. This was described for the first time in 1973 by O'Toole (29) in 2 patients after subcutaneous administration of heparin. A re-exposition of one of the two patients with intravenous heparin produced an anaphylactic shock. White et al. (30) described 6 further impressive cases of heparin-induced skin necrosis.

First signs of the *white-clot syndrome call for an immediate discontinuance of heparin therapy*. A few re-exposition trials induced a severe to excessive decrease in platelet count, in general during the first 48 hours after administration (e. g. 31, 32).

It is now believed that the cause of the syndrome is the development of heparin-dependent platelet membrane antibodies in *predisposed* patients. Detection of these antibodies can be determined by performing thrombocyte aggregation tests. Using the plasma of patients suffering from the white-clot syndrome, the platelets of normal donors are aggregated. The test can not be used to predict thrombocytopenia since aggregation only occurs when the platelet count falls. Patients with myeloproliferative diseases seem to be at a higher risk.

It is not as yet clear to what extent this syndrome prevails. Powers et al. (33) found it in less than 2 % of 120 patients. Gallus et al. (34) observed the syndrome in 5.4 % of 166 patients. These authors express the opinion that this syndrome is most likely caused by heparin in 3 % of the total number of patients. Of interest are the observations of Ansell et al. (35), who noted a fall in platelet count with *nadirs not below 100,000 platelets/µl plasma* in 5 of 43 patients (11.6 %). Furthermore they observed that blood samples of these patients induced a high release of serotonin from normal platelets or caused normal platelets to aggregate in the presence of additional heparin. In contrast to the white-clot syndrome (28), the thrombocytopenia - not below 100,000 platelets/µl plasma - did not result in haemorrhagic complications, and thrombembolic events are not mentioned. The fall of platelet-count in 4 of the 5 cases did not oocur before the 6th day of heparin treatment. The study suggests that the etiology of *delayed onset thrombocytopenia*, whether mild or severe, is similar in that a platelet aggregating factor can be identified. Perhaps the most important feature is the time of onset of the fall in platelet count.

Drug interactions with heparin

Considering the highly negative-charged molecule of heparin, one could assume that heparin often leads to drug interaction. Heparin, however, is not very often involved in important clinical drug interactions. Indeed, only a few drug interactions of heparin have been reported; they can be ascribed to 2 types:

Type 1: Enhancement of bleeding tendencies in all combinations of heparin with drugs which lead to bleeding such as non-steroidal anti-rheumatics, glucocorticoids, platelet antiaggregating substances and oral anticoagulants.

Type 2: Decreasing of the plasma protein binding by heparin of endogenous substances or of drugs.

Wiegand and Levy (36) showed that intravenous heparin injection significantly increased the free bilirubin and salicylate fraction in the plasma of rats beginning with the second minute after administration and lasting until the 45th minute. The authors assume that free fatty acids liberated by the activation of lipoprotein lipase by heparin misplace bilirubin and salicylic acid from their protein binding. Possibly significant alterations in the plasma protein binding of bilirubin are produced by considerably lower heparin doses than those required to decrease the plasma protein binding of this compound in rats. Desmond et al. (37) showed that in normal non-fasting subjects heparin caused a rapid 150 - 250 % rise in the free fraction of diazepam, chlordiazepoxide and oxazepam but no change in that of chlorazepam. The changes were slightly smaller but still significant when the subjects were in a fasting state. This change occurred within 90 seconds of administration of heparin and binding had returned to baseline by 30 - 45 min. However, this result can be of importance when heparin is used during drug disposition studies because estimation of the pharmacokinetic parameters and also pharmacological effects could be affected.

Other effects ascribed to heparin

A multitude of other effects have been claimed for heparin, for instance metastatic calcifications and inhibition of the development of haematogenic metastases (see 19).

Heparin effects on blood tests

Drug therapy can be a source of misleading laboratory results due to interference with the testing procedure. The most important example is the elevation of serum thyroxine as measured by competitive protein binding (CPB), especially in non-fasting subjects. The mechanism involved is the increase of serum fatty acids caused by the activation of lipoprotein lipase. The free fatty acids compete with thyroxine for binding on thyroxine-binding globuline (TBG) (see 19).

References

1. Walker, A. M., Jick, H.: JAMA 244, 1209-1212 (1980).

2. Loeliger, E. A.: in: M. N. G. Dukes (Editor) Meyler's Side Effects of Drugs, Volume 8, Excerpta Medica, Amsterdam - Oxford 1975, p. 764-790.

3. Curry, P. V. L., Bacon, P. A.: Postgrad. Med. J. 50, 37 (1974).

4. Mant, M. J., O'Brien, B. D., Thong, K. L., Hammond, G. W., Birthwhistle, R. V., Grace, M. G.: Lancet I, 133-1335 (1977).

5. Loeliger, E. A.: in: M. N. G. Dukes (Editor) Side effects of drug annual 4. A worldwide yearly survey of new data and trends. Excerpta Medica Amsterdam - Oxford - Princeton 1980, p. 245-251.

6. Russo, J. V., Margolis, S., Friesinger, G. C., Russ, R. S.: Lancet II, 1271-1275 (1970).

7. Nelson, P. G.: Brit. Med. J. 3, 735-737 (1970).

8. Gupka, D. K., Jewitt, D. E., Young, R., Hartog, M., Opie, L. H.: Lancet II, 1209-1213 (1969).

9. Rutenberg, H. L., Pamintuan, J. C., Soloff, L. A.: Lancet II, 559-564 (1970).

10. Arnesen, H., Skjaeggestad, Ø, Wik, B.: Act. Med. Scand. 207, 21-25 (1980).

11. Griffith, G. C., Nichols, jr., G., Asher, J. D., Flanagan, B.: JAMA 193, 85-88 (1965).

12. Thompson jr., R. C.: J. of Bone and Joint Surgery 55, 606-612 (1973).

13. Jaffe, M. D., Willis, P. W.: JAMA 193, 158-160 (1965).

14. Schlachtzki, J.: Fortschr. Med. 87, 119-122 (1969).

15. Aarskog, D., Aksnes, L., Lehmann, V.: Lancet II, 650-651 (1980).

16. Sonnenblick, M., Oren, A., Jacobsohn, W.: Brit. Med. J. 3, 77 (1975).

17. Olsson, R., Korsan-Bengtsen, B.-M., Korsan-Bentsen, K., Lennartsson, J., Waldenström, J.: Act. Med. Scand. 204, 229-230 (1978).

18. Minar, E., Ehringer, H.; Hirschl, M., Ingerle, H., Konecny, U., Marosi, L., Endler, T., Gabl, F., Deutsch, E.: Dtsch. Med. Wschr. 105, 1713-1717 (1980).

19. Loeliger, E. A.: in: M. N. G. Dukes (Editor) Meyler's Side Effects of Drugs, 9th edition. Excerpta Medica Amsterdam - Oxford - Princeton 1980, p. 587-613.

20. Weber, E., Gundert-Remy, U., Walter, E., Ding, R., Harenberg, J., v. Kenne, H., Spohr, U.: in: H. Ducrot, M. Goldberg, R. Hoigné, P. Middleton: Computer aid to drug therapy and to drug monitoring. North Holland Publ. Co. Amsterdam, New York, Oxford, 1978, p. 35-42.

20a.Harenberg, J., Schulze, F., Sheik, H., Zimmermann, R., Mörl, H., Weber, E.: Vasa Suppl. 8, abstr. No. 162, p. 84 (1981).

21. Salzmann, E. W., Rosenberg, R. D., Smith, M. H., Lindon, J. N., Favreau, L.: J. clin. Invest. 65, 64-73 (1980).

22. Eldor, A., Weksler, B. B.: Thromb. Res. 16, 617-628 (1979).

23. Godal, H. C.: Thrombosis and Haemostasis 43, 222-224 (1980).

24. Bell, W. R., Tumasulo, P. A., Alving, B. M., Duffy, T. P.: Ann. Intern. Med. 85, 155-160 (1976).

25. Eika, C., Godal, H. C., Laake, K., Hamborg, T.: Scand. J. Haematol. 25, 19-24 (1980).

26. Weismann, R. E., Tobin, R. W.: Arch. Surg. 76, 219 (1958).

27. Towne, J. B., Bernhard, V. M., Hussey, C., Garancis, J. C.: Arch. Surg. 114, 372-377 (1979).

28. Loeliger, E. A.: in: M. N. G. Dukes (Editor) Side effects of drugs annual 5. A worldwide yearly survey of new data and trends. Excerpta Medica Amsterdam - Oxford - Princeton 1981, p. 323-332.

29. O'Toole, R. D.: Ann. Int. Med. 79, 759 (1973).

30. White, P. W., Sadd, J. R., Nensel, R. E.: Ann. Surg. 190, 595-608 (1979).

31. Rhodes, G. R., Dixon, R. H., Silver, D.: Ann. Surg. 186, 752-758 (1977).

32. Rector, T. S., Cipolle, R. J., Seifert, R. D., Ramirez-Lassepas, M.: Amer. J. Hosp. Pharma. 36, 1561-1565 (1979).

33. Powers, P. J., Cuthbert, D., Hirsh, J.: JAMA 241, 2396-2397 (1979).

34. Gallus, A. S., Goodall, K. T., Beswick, W., Chesterman, C. N.: Aust. N. Z. J. Med. 10, 25-31 (1980).

35. Ansell, J., Slepchuk jr., N., Kumar, R., Lopez, A., Southard, J., Deykin, D.: Thrombosis and Haemostasis 43, 61-65 (1980).

36. Wiegand, U. W., Levy, G.: J. Pharmaceutical Sciences 68, 1483-1486 (1979).

37. Desmond, P. V., Roberts, R. K., Wood, A. J. J., Dunn, G. D., Wilkinson, G. R., Schenker, S.: Brit. J. Clin. Pharmacol. 9, 171-175 (1980).

38. Baumgartner, G., Fehr, H.: Schweiz. Rundschau Med. (Praxis) 63, 640-645 (1974).

39. Jick, H., Porter, J.: Lancet II, 87-89 (1978).

40. Stillman, R. M., Chapa, L., Stark, M. L., Malik, L. N., Keates, J. R. W., Sawyer, P. N.: Surgery, Gynecology and Obstretics 145, 193-197 (1977).

41. Sessner, H. H., Brockhaus, W., Kunzmann, G., Stingl, J.: Med. Welt 27, (N. F.), 187-191 (1971).

42. Mannucci, P. M., Citterio, L. E., Panajotopoulos, N.: Thrombosis and Haemostasis 36, 157-164 (1976).

43. Salzmann, E. W., Deykin, D., Mayer-Shapiro, R., Rosenberg, R.: New Engl. J. Med. 292, 1046-1050 (1975).

44. Vieweg, W. V. R., Piscatelli, R. L., Houser, J. J., Proulx, R. A.: JAMA 213, 1303-1306 (1970).

45. Pachter, H. L., Riles, Th. S.: Annals of Surgery 186, 669-674 (1977).

46. Dommering, M.: Arch. Chir. Neerl. 31, 51 (1979).

Supported by Bundesministerium für Forschung und Technologie, Bonn and Bundesgesundheitsamt, Berlin.

Discussion

Aronson asked if the antibodies against heparin preparations are directed against heparin itself or something else in the preparation.

Weber answered that it is not heparin by itself but heparin bound to something. It is interesting, however, that no antibodies are formed if heparin is not present. It can be an impurity of the heparin preparation.

Rosenberg pointed out that in the best studies on antibodies in patients developing thrombocytopenia, the antibodies could be detected before the heparin was given. It is unclear what the antibodies are directed against. The best studies have been done at the University of Pennsylvania. In the patients studied there the antibodies were clearly present in all cases. It is, however, unclear whether the antibodies are directed to some extent against heparan sulfates in vivo.

Weber agreed. She said that one can imagine that negative charged molecules are also able to do the same thing. There is only a small percent of perdisposed persons who develop antibodies.
Molecules with properties similar to those of heparin can do the same thing.

Rosenberg recalled the fact that some of the first studies were performed by *Heidelberger*, who showed that antibodies are made against glucuronic acid, which is the major constituent of heparin. These antibodies were studied in 1930.

Dawes reported that they had examined a lot of sera from such patients looking for an antibody against heparin. They were unable to find one in solution; it appears that there may be one attached to platelets. This may in fact be directed against heparin. They have not demonstrated with certainty antibodies against heparin in any of these patients.

Weber said that this may not be so in every case because one can also provoke aggregation of platelets in patients who have no antibodies. Perhaps there may be several mechanisms.

Bhargava made a comment on the allergic reaction. From his studies he concludes that heparin in sensitized persons can work as an adjuvans.

Weber pointed out that what one calls "heparin sensitization" is not provoked by heparin in all cases.

Bhargava said that there are few reports in the literature on the heparin side effect: osteoporosis. He wondered if there is a correlation with a particular kind of heparin (salt or source).

Weber answered that this is unknown. She believes that there is no great incidence of osteoporosis. Most people are treated with heparin only for a short time. Patients who receive heparin for more than four months are treated only with small amounts.

Bhargava asked if there is an age dependency.

Weber replied that this cannot clearly be answered. There are some observations of osteoporosis in young women during pregnancy when they were treated with heparin. She believes that it is not as age-related as the bleeding complications.

Fussi mentioned that one has to differentiate between two types of thrombocytopenia:
- the transient form which is very common
- the severe thrombocytopenia, which occurs after arterial thrombosis. The latter is predominantly observed in the United States and not in Europe. One has to consider that in the States 80 % of the heparin used is from beef lung, whereas in Europe nearly 100 % of it is pig mucosal heparin. It is, however, apparently not a question of the kind of heparin but a question of the impurity of the preparations. The preparation of beef lung heparin is very delicate.

Fussi believes that the severe type of thrombocytopenia is due to special impurities in the beef lung heparin preparations. With more careful prepared beef lung heparin this effect is no longer observed.

Weber is not sure that this has been shown definitely. She agrees that there is some evidence and that it is a good hypothesis but that further information is needed.

Schmitz-Hübner asked if there is any information concerning the molecular weight of the impurities mentioned.

Weber answered that there is no information.

Spaethe wondered if the extent of the aggregating effect depends on the dosage of heparin.

Weber felt that it probably does not.

Spaethe reported observations, known from the literature, that a decrease in the platelet count after heparin administration could be reversed by administration of antithrombin, antithrombin thus appearing to have a disaggregating effect. He wondered if it is possible that the aggregation is caused by low antithrombin levels and high heparin concentrations in plasma.

Weber's opinion is that this has not yet clearly been shown.

Wenzel inquired if there is something known about the conditons which elevate the risk of patients to suffer from the white clot syndrome.

Weber stated that the numbers of patients studied are still too small. If this syndrome is observed, she said that it is important to change the anticoagulant quickly.

Wenzel commented that in five years of experience with nearly 100000 patients treated with heparin, he has seen eight patients with allergic skin reactions (urticaria). In all these patients they changed the heparin preparation and could not reproduce the skin reaction.

Verstraete asked *Rosenberg* concerning the patients who had antibodies against heparan sulfates before they got the first shot of heparin: if he knew when they had received heparin and if the thrombocytopenia or the thrombotic complication had appeared in the first days or after an interval of one or two weeks.

Rosenberg explained that it is commonly believed that the severe thrombocytopenia occurs on the sixth day. Clinical data, however, indicate that this is not always true. The reaction can already start on the second or third day. Antibodies can actually be demonstrated and they can be observed for up to 20 days.

Weber confirmed this statement.

Rosenberg reported about sensitive techniques by which antibodies could be demonstrated present on the platelets prior to heparin therapy. They dramatically increased after heparin application: this was published by Schreiber et al. in J. of Medicine, eight months ago.

Weber conjectered that there might be people who have antibodies which are inactive. As soon as the patients receive heparin as an additive, however, then this sort of antibody can bind with membranes of platelets. She thinks that this is the desaster. This probably has nothing to do with platelets. The antibody - as soon as heparin comes in - can be bound together with the complement to platelet membranes.

Rosenberg affirmed that this is probably true: in some of those cases the situation is much like that in haemolytic anemias, where one can detect small amounts of antibodies on the red cells, and yet there are no clinical findings until the amount of antibodies increases.

Heene asked if corticoids can interfere with these reactions.

Weber believes that it is not necessary to give corticoids at all, because as soon as heparin is withdrawn the platelet count increases.

Bender wanted to know if there is a shape change of the platelets at the beginning of the heparin therapy.

Weber stated that there is astonishingly little information in the literature concerning these questions. More studies should be performed.

Role of Heparin-Like Molecules in Atherogenesis*

Robert D. Rosenberg
Department of Biology
Massachusetts Institute of Technology
Cambridge, Massachusetts, U.S.A. 02139 and

Department of Medicine
Harvard Medical School, Boston
Massachusetts, U.S.A. 02115

John J. Castellot, Jr., Morris J. Karnovsky
Department of Pathology
Harvard Medical School, Boston
Massachusetts, U.S.A. 02115

The healthy arterial wall consists of the intimal endothelial cells which line the lumen and the underlying medial smooth muscle cells which remain in a quiescent growth state (1). A variety of data generated via both in vivo as well as in vitro experiments indicate that endothelial cells function as important regulators of smooth muscle cells within the vascular wall. However, little is known of the cellular or molecular mechanisms that govern this process.

Ross (2, 3) and others (4, 5) have demonstrated that platelet-derived growth factor are required for smooth muscle cell growth in vivo and in vitro. Marcrophages (6) and endothelial cells (7) have also been shown to produce smooth muscle cell mitogens. However, it has been found that heparin (8, 9) and heparin-like molecules (10) may prevent the action of the

*Supported by Grants from the National Institutes of Health HL-2862501 and HL-25066 and The National Foundation for Cancer Research, Bethesda, Maryland, U.S.A.

Heparin · New Biochemical and Medical Aspects

growth factor upon smooth muscle cells. In the sections below, we outline data that supports this hypothesis and propose a simple model for growth regulation within the vascular.

Twenty-two male Sprague Dawley rats were utilized to test whether heparin inhibits the proliferation of intimal smooth muscle cells in vivo. For this purpose, the rat was anesthetized with intraperitoneal pentobarbital. The right common carotid artery was exposed and ligated at two points 1.5 cm apart. A 30 gauge hyperdermic needle was inserted into the proximal end of the segment. An exit hole was punctured at the distal end of the segment either by passing the same needle down the lumen and out through the wall or by puncturing with an additional needle from the outside. After the lumen had been rinsed with phosphate buffered saline, dry (compressed) air was allowed to flow through the segment for 3.5 minutes at a rate of 50-60 ml/min. Ligatures were then removed and hemostasis was obtained by pressure. Within minutes to a few hours after re-establishment of blood flow in the arterial segment, desiccated endothelial cells detached from the arterial wall and were swept away. The completeness of the endothelial denudation was monitored by the perfusion silver staining technique of Fishman et al. (11).

Twenty-four hours after the administration of the carotid air-drying injury, either buffer, or anticoagulantly active heparin, or unfractionated commercial heparin (Upjohn), or non-anticoagulant heparin (~0.5-0.65 mg/kg/hr) was administered to four experimental groups as shown in Fig. 1. Myointimal growth, determined two weeks after air-drying carotid injury, showed that plaque size was maximal at this time. Blood for tests was drawn and animals were fixed by perfusion. Carotids were sectioned midway between the original needle puncture sites and embedded in Epon 812. Two-micron sections were cut perpendicular to the vessel axis at 500 μm intervals to a depth of 5 mm in each half of the original carotid segment. This process yielded 22 sections for plaque volume analysis. Because the plaque tended to grow largest at the midportion of the denuded segment and because of shrinkage of tissue during processing, essentially all of the intimal plaque volume was contained within this distance. Sections were stained with toluidine blue, then projected at approximately 200 fold magnification onto bond quality typing paper which varied in weight per unit area by ± 1 %. The outlines of intima and media were traced, and the paper was cut and weighed. Repeated area determinations for individual samples of intima and media from 20 sections showed good reproducibility, with an intraclass correlation coefficient of 1.00. The total weight of tracings of intima was divided by the total weight of tracings of media to give an index of plaque volume in each animal (8).

Our data shows that the unfractionated heparin and the non-anticoagulant heparin inhibits the proliferation of intimal smooth muscle cells which occurs after denudation of endothelium by air-drying injury in the rat carotid artery. Indeed, as shown in Fig. 1, the level of inhibition with these glycosaminoglycans is ≅77 % of that observed in the absence of mucopolysaccharide. We have also considered the possibility that the antiproliferative effect of heparin is secondary to effects on platelet adherence to subendo-

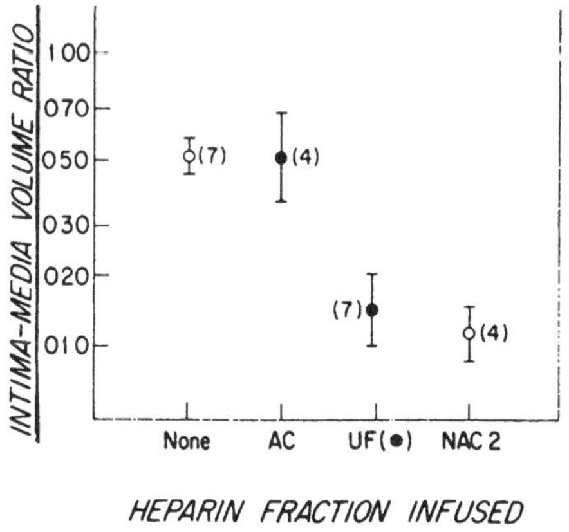

Fig. 1. Intima-media volume ratios two weeks after air-drying carotid injury in rats continuously infused with various forms of heparin. Numbers of rats in groups are shown in parentheses. Means ± SEM were obtained after transformation of individual data to the fourth root. None, indicates the control group receiving no heparin, AC designates the group injected with anticoagulantly active heparin; UF refers to the group infused with unfractionated commercial heparin; and NAC constitutes the group receiving non-anticoagulant mucopolysaccharide.

thelium or endothelial regeneration. Morphometric examination by scanning electron microscopy showed that heparin did not alter platelet adherence 5 days after arterial injury and had little or no effect on endothelial regeneration at 5 and 10 days. Thus our data would suggest that inhibition of arterial smooth muscle cell proliferation by heparin is not mediated by effects on other cells at the level of the arterial wall or by antithrombin (8).

We have also studied the in vitro effects of heparin on the growth of rat aortic smooth muscle cells. Measurements of growth were monitored by changes in cell number over a 3 day period. Our results show that heparin - highly anticoagulant or non-anticoagulant - significantly inhibits growth of both exponentially increasing or growth arrested smooth muscle cells. We have also demonstrated that this is a highly specific interaction with regard to mucopolysaccharide: i. e. other glycosaminoglycans do not have the same effect on growth (9), Fig. 2.

It might be argued that the heparin molecule acts by binding non-specifically to the platelet derived growth factor and thereby interferes with the function of this mitogen. To exclude this possibility, we have preincubated the smooth muscle cells in heparin followed by two washes with buffer prior to the addition of a crude preparation of the growth factor. If preincubation is carried out for 24 hours, the inhibitory effect of the mucopolysaccharide is almost identical to that observed when heparin is admixed with the crude growth factor at the inception of the experiment. Furthermore, we have also noted that passing crude platelet extracts over a heparin-Sepharose column did not remove mitogenic activity. These two types of experiments indicate that the mucopolysaccharide directly inhibits smooth muscle cell proliferation.

The above data suggests that non-anticoagulant heparin might serve as a useful pharmacologic agent for inhibiting atherogenesis. However, it is also possible that this molecular species might function as a physiologic agent in a similar fashion. Using cultured cells from bovine and rat aortas, we have examined the possibility that endothelial cells might regulate the growth of smooth muscle cells via the release of heparin-like molecules. Our data shows that conditioned medium from confluent bovine aortic endothelial cells inhibited the proliferation on growth-arrested smooth muscle cells. Conditioned medium from exponential endothelial cells, and from exponential or confluent smooth muscle cells and fibroblasts, did not inhibit smooth muscle cell growth. Conditioned medium from confluent endothelial cells did not inhibit the growth of endothelial cells or fibroblasts, Table 1.

In addition to the apparent specificity of both the producer and target cell, the inhibitory activity was heat stable and was not affected by proteases. It was sensitive to *Flavobacterium* heparinase but not altered by hyaluronidase or chondroitinase sulfate ABC lyase. Thus the inhibitory component appears to be a heparin-like substance.

It should be noted that small amounts of serum are required for liberation of the heparin-like inhibitor from bovine aortic endothelial cells. We have attempted to identify the serum component responsible for release of the heparin-like substances from these cellular elements. Our data showed that much less inhibitory activity was liberated by platelet poor plasma than by serum. Indeed, at least twenty times as much platelet poor plasma was required to release the same amount of inhibitory activity as was liberated with 0.4 % serum. Thus it seemed likely that a platelet factor was required to release the inhibiting substance from endothelial cells.

We have recently isolated an endoglycosidase which cleaves heparin or heparan sulfate from outdated human platelets by freeze-thaw solubilization, heparin-Sepharose chromatography, octyl-agarose chromatography, Concanavalin A-Sepharose chromatography and Sephacryl S-200 gel filtration. The overall extent of purification of the platelet heparitinase is about 240,000 fold and the overall yield of the enzyme is about 5.6 % as compared to the initial freeze-thaw solubilized preparation. The final product is physically homogenous as judged by disc gel electrophoresis at acidic pH as well as gel filtration chromatography and exhibits an apparent molecular weight of approximately 134,000. Furthermore, our results indicate that the above enzyme is present within platelet lysosomes (12).

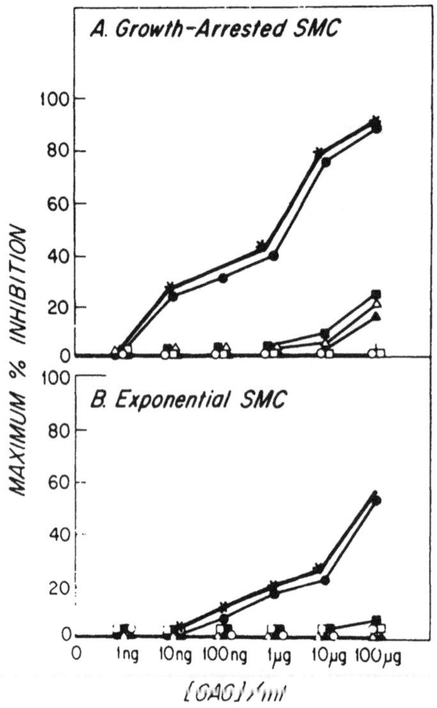

Fig. 2. Effect of glycosaminoglycans on rat smooth muscle cells growth. (*A*) Rat smooth cells were plated and growth-arrested. The cells were then exposed to RPMI + 20 % fetal calf serum containing the indicated concentrations of glycosaminoglycans. Cell number was measured at daily intervals. Data were expressed as maximum percent inhibition.

(*B*) Rat smooth muscle cells were plated at 6 x 10^3/16 mm well. After 24 hours, the medium was aspirated and replaced with fresh RPMI + 20 % fetal calf serum with or without the indicated concentrations of glycosaminoglycans. Data are expressed as maximum percent inhibition. 0—0, anticoagulantly active heparin; *—*, non-anticoagulantly active heparin; □—□ , bovine aortic heparan sulfate; ■—■ , beef lung heparan sulfate; Δ—Δ, dermatan sulfate; ▲—▲, chondroitin ABC sulfate; 0—0, hyaluronic acid. Data for the heparan sulfates are the average of three experiments; data for other glycosaminoglycans are the average of five or more experiments.

Table 1. Specificity of the Bovine Aorta Endothelial Cells-Culture Medium Effect

	Maximum Percent Inhibition			
Type of Culture Medium	BHK Fibroblasts	Bovine Aorta Endothelial Cells	Rat Smooth Muscle Cells	Rat Smooth Muscle Cells
None (normal growth medium)	0	0	0	0
Exponential BHK Fibroblasts	2	11	8	4
Confluent BHK Fibroblasts	13	3	16	10
Exponential Rat Smooth Muscle Cells	9	11	16	7
Confluent Rat Smooth Muscle Cells	8	15	1	12
Exponential Calf Smooth Muscle Cells	0	6	7	9
Confluent Calf Smooth Muscle Cells	0	8	13	18
Exponential Bovine Aorta Endothelial Cells	7	0	0	1
Confluent Bovine Aorta Endothelial Cells	6	2	63	> 80

The data are presented as maximum percent inhibition. 0 means that there was no inhibitory effect of culture medium. Exponential bovine aorta endothelial cells-culture medium stimulated cell growth when compared to normal growth medium. Experiments involving BHK fibroblasts or BHK culture medium were done twice. All other combinations were done four or more times. In all cases, cells in normal growth medium doubled four or more times, before reaching confluence.

When rat or bovine endothelial cells were incubated with RPMI-1640 containing 1 ng/ml platelet heparitinase, complete release of inhibitory activity into the supernatant was observed. Utilizing appropriate controls, we have shown that the material released is a heparin-like substance, and that the inhibitory effect is not an artifact of experimental manipulations. In addition, we have demonstrated that the release process is enzyme specific. Furthermore, we have proven that the platelet heparitinase does not convert prereleased material to an active component but directly liberates the active, heparin-like species from the endothelial cells. Dose response experiments indicate that only 20 pg/ml of platelet heparitinase are necessary to liberate 50 % of the heparin-like material from the endothelial cells (13).

Based on the above observations, we would like to propose a simple model for the possible role of heparin-like components and the endoglycosidase in the normal and injured vessel. In the normal (uninjured) artery, the intimal endothelial cells release heparin-like substances from their abluminal surface. The heparin-like material remains in the intracellular matrix of the intima and inner media, and prevents the medial smooth muscle cells from proliferating. The platelet heparitinase has been detected in the lysosomal fraction of many cell types. It is likely that smooth muscle cells and endothelial cells also contain this enzyme in their lysosomes. It is appreciated that these molecular species can be transported into the external milieu. Thus the endoglycosidase may be present in the intima and media, where it could function to release antiproliferative heparin-like components from endothelial cell surface. Another possible source of heparin-like molecules are the mast cells which are occasionally found in the intima. A variety of substances are known to induce mast cell release and these materials could represent an additional system for modulating smooth muscle cell proliferation.

If the endothelial cells are injured or removed, the exposed vessel wall is no longer non-thrombogenic. Platelets adhere, aggregate, and subsequently release their cellular contents. Included in the platelet products present at the site of injury are platelet heparitinase, platelet-derived growth factor, and platelet factor 4. The latter protein has a very high affinity for heparin (14), and has been shown to penetrate into the media after endothelial denudation (15). Macrophages are also found in the injured area, and are a likely source of smooth muscle cell mitogens (6). A critical aspect of this model is the fact that the presence of mitogens is not sufficient to stimulate smooth muscle cell migration and proliferation. The inhibitory effect of heparin-like components must be overcome before the smooth muscle cell can respond to those stimuli. This hypothesis is based on our observations that even in the presence of large amounts of serum or platelet extract (up to 20 %), heparin is capable of inhibiting smooth muscle cell growth in vitro. There are at least three possible mechanisms for overcoming the inhibitory phenomenon:

1. endoglycosidases from adherent platelets present in the vessel wall might cleave heparin-like substances into fragments, which diffuse away since the injury has removed both the physical barrier to diffusion and the source of heparin-like material;
2. the local concentration of mitogens may be so high that smooth muscle cells can proliferate despite the presence of heparin-like components; and
3. platelet factor 4 could inactivate heparin-like molecules to a sufficient degree.

Preliminary experiments suggest that platelet factor 4 can prevent the inhibitory effect of heparin on smooth muscle cells in vitro. Once the inhibitory effect of heparin is negated, the smooth muscle cells can migrate into the intima and proliferate. However, as soon as the damaged area is re-endothelialized, smooth muscle cell growth ceases (16). This could be due to the presence of heparin-like substances released by the endothelial cells behind the regenerating front. The observation of Wright et al. (17) support this hypothesis.

The cellular and molecular mechanisms of growth regulation in blood vessels are undoubtedly more complicated than the simple model presented above. However, alterations in the biosynthesis of heparin-like molecules by endothelial cells; changes in the production or release of endoglycosidases by platelets; smooth muscle cells or endothelial cells; and alterations in the response of smooth muscles to these complex carbohydrates could in part be responsible for the initiation of the atherosclerotic process.

References

1. Chamley-Campbell, J., Campbell, G. R., Ross, R. Physiological Reviews 59, 1-61 (1979).

2. Harker, L. A., Ross, R., Slichter, S. J., Scott, C. R. J. Clin. Invest. 58, 731-741 (1976).

3. Ross, R., Glomset, J., Kariya, B., Harker, L. Proc. Natl. Acad. Sci. U.S.A. 71, 1207-1210 (1974).

4. Fuster, V., Bowie, E. J., Lewis, J. C., Fass, D. N., Owen, C. A., Brown, A. L. J. Clin. Invest. 61, 722-730 (1978).

5. Moore, S., Friedman, R. J., Singal, D. P., Gauldie, J., Blajchman. Thromb. Diath. Haemorrh. 35, 70-81 (1976).

6. Martin, B. M., Baldwin, W. M., Gimbrone, M. A., Unanue, E. R., Cotran, R. S. J. Cell Biol. 83 (2. Pt. 2): 376 a (Abst). (1979).

7. Gajdusek, C., Dicorleto, P., Ross, R., Schwartz, S. M. J. Cell Biol. 85, 467-472 (1980).

8. Guyton, J. R., Rosenberg, R D., Clowes, A. W., Karnovsky, M. J. Circ. Res. 46, 625-634 (1980).

9. Hoover, R L., Rosenberg, R. D., Haering, W., Karnofsky, M. J. Circ. Res. 47, 578-583 (1980).

10. Castellot, J. J., Jr., Addonizio, M. L., Rosenberg, R. D., Karnovsky, M. J. J. Cell Biol. 90, 372-379 (1981).

11. Fishman, J. A., Ryan, G. B., Karnovsky, M. J. Lab. Invest. 32, 339-351 (1975).

12. Oosta, G. M., Favreau, L. V., Rosenberg, R. D. Submitted for publication.

13. Castellot, J. J., Jr., Favreau, L. V., Karnovsky, M. J., Rosenberg, M. D. Submitted for publication.

14. Handin, R. I., Cohen, H. J. J. Biol. Chem. 251, 4273-4282 (1976).

15. Goldberg, I. D., Stemerman, M. B., Handin, R. I. Science 209, 611-612 (1980).

16. Schwartz, S., Haudenschild, C., Eddy, E. Lab. Invest. 38, 568-580 (1978).

17. Wright, T. N., Ross, R. J. Cell Biol. 67, 675-686 (1975).

Discussion

Aronson stated that in his experience development of atheroma is not only a simple proliferation of muscle cells but probably a clone of certain muscle cells which has undergone change. He wanted to know if these muscle cells respond to heparin.

Rosenberg said that there is considerable argument as to whether it is a clonal response or not. He had no information about that. It would be interesting to know if they respond to mucopolysaccharides.

Wenzel asked if Rosenberg had found an inhibitory activity against the heparinase of the platelets in healthy subjects or in patients suffering from atherosclerosis.

Rosenberg answered that almost anything that would bind the mucpolysaccharides would probably be inhibitory.

A lot of candidates are possible. It is a complex process because there are many proteins in the endothelium which bind the mucpolysaccharides, for instance, fibronectin. There are a lot of protein interactions which could probably have physiological or pathological importance.

Aronson wished to look at smooth muscle cell proliferation as a physiological need. What *Rosenberg* had described was something essentially pathological. *Aronson* wondered if abrogation of this activity may also be needed to control smooth muscle cell proliferation under physiological conditions.

Rosenberg conceded that Ross' concept of atherogenesis seems to be based on a rather simplistic assumption, the injury of endothelial cells. He stressed that the real question is whether denudation of endothelial cells necessarily takes place in atherogenesis early on.

Rosenberg feels that the mechanism he described may present a basal way of controlling smooth muscle cell proliferation because this enzyme is present not merely in the platelets but also in smooth muscle cells. He thinks that there might be a release of enzyme from smooth muscle cells cleaving off mucopolysaccharides in the region of the smooth muscle cells and hence controlling proliferation without injury of the endothelium.

This would be a basal way of maintaining smooth muscle cells in a resting state. This goes around the endothelial denudation aspects. There are a variety of systems in biology which seem to be similar to this. It is a kind of general control mechanism which will maintain cells in resting states.

Heene said that the heparinase splits heparin at a very specific site. This might change the amount of negative charge at the heparin molecule. He wanted to know if this altered heparin might change the heparin receptors in the smooth muscle cells.

Rosenberg reported about his binding studies with smooth muscle cells and radioactive labelled heparin. He said that the results are very difficult to interpret for two main reasons:
Heparin binds to a lot of things. One can make Scatchard plots but one does not know what they mean.

Many of the binding constants obtained seem to have relatively little relevance to the biologic state. One can modify heparin in some special ways and eliminate the reactive proliferative activity and yet it seems to bind to smooth muscle cells.

There are reasons to believe that there are specific binding sites at the smooth muscle cells, but they are difficult to detect. There are a lot of non-specific interactions and relatively few specific ones.

Rosenberg believes that it is primarily the unspecific one which are measured.

Bhargava had a question concerning the purification of the heparinase. He wanted to know if there are differences between the glucuronidase from the lysosomes of liver and from the lysosomes of platelets.

Rosenberg explained that glucuronidase has been found in many tissues, for instance spleen and liver. They have been well characterized. The enzyme from the platelets has a specific role. Its pH-optimum is 7.4, which is somewhat unusual for a lysosomal enzyme. They have normally a pH-optimum of 6.5. So it is an interesting candidate for physiological controls.

The use of non-anticoagulant heparin is an interesting approach to a variety of potential clinical problems.

Bhargava asked for the definition of the non-anticoagulant heparin.

Rosenberg explained that it is heparin which does not bind to antithrombin. It is a no-affinity heparin! If the preparation has any affinity, it is due to contamination with an active fraction.

Witt raised the question if under these aspects heparin could have an positive effect in arterial thrombosis.

Rosenberg said that one could ask whether all the numerous studies which have been done on the effect of heparin on atherosclerosis also work in human subjects. It would be interesting to reconsider that possibility and to see whether non-anticoagulant heparin has an effect in humans if it is given over a long period of time.
It remains to be shown that it is an important control mechanism.

Marbet stated that haemodialysis patients with renal insufficiency receive heparin repeatedly. These patients often have extensive atherosclerosis. He asked for *Rosenberg's* comment.

Rosenberg felt the reason to be that these patients receive the heparin over a rather short period of time.

Unresolved Problems in the Use of Heparin

Marc Verstraete
Centre for Thrombosis and Vascular Research
Department of Medical Research
University of Leuven
Campus Gasthuisberg
3000 Leuven, Belgium

I was most pleased to receive the invitation to this symposium for at least two reasons. The closed-door workshop was to be attended by the Gods of the heparin-Olympus, who agreed to cross the ocean or the channel to land at the Titisee, a most enjoyable vacation resort. In addition, I was given a topic which did put me at ease as in this setting of experts there would not be many problems unresolved. To my dismay, it now appears that still a number of questions were not discussed which merit more attention.

Route of Heparin Administration

Some patients require long-term heparin anticoagulation e. g. those with lowered antithrombin III levels or high risk pregnant patients. Repeated subcutaneous injection may be cumbersome and painful and one wonders why the intrapulmonary route of heparin administration by Jaques (1) has not been further explored. An initial large dose of 15 mg/kg body weight inhaled from an ultrasonic nebuliser followed by a maintenance dose of 12 mg/kg weekly or 15 mg/kg once a fortnight results in sustained blood levels between 0.6-2.5 units/ml of plasma. Inhaled heparin is rapidly adsorbed and taken up by the macrophages of the lung and apparently held by these cells without degradation or release, until disintegration of the macrophages.

Heparin · New Biochemical and Medical Aspects

Printed in Germany

Heparin is poorly absorbed from the small intestine as there seems to be no active transport for this molecule. Hence, its absorption depends on passive transport which is mainly determined by the lipid solubility of the substance and molecular size. This alternative route of administration was not discussed although there are clinical indications for regional anticoagulation in the portal venous system.

Ultra-low Doses of Heparin

Not a single word has been said so far about ultra-low doses of heparin (1 IU $kg^{-1}h^{-1}$ given intravenously). Negus et al. (2) suggested that ultra-low doses of heparin may act by releasing heparin (heparitin) sulphate from cell surface. Years ago Pulver (3) demonstrated that the heparinoid G 31150 acted as an anticoagulant in vivo by releasing up to 0.5 units of protein bound heparin per ml plasma and suggested a similar effect produced by the non-anticoagulant fraction of commercial heparin. This was indeed the case as Raby et al. (4) found that after I.V. injection of commercial heparin, the heparin isolated from the blood had a much higher specific antithrombotic activity.

After ultra-low doses of heparin, no anticoagulant activity in the plasma is measured (theoretical level 0.007 IU/ml) but apparently an effective prevention of postoperative deep-vein thrombosis is offered (2). It was also shown by the same group of investigators that 1 IU heparin per kg body weight is enough to release lipoprotein lipase, reducing platelet adhesion (5).

It is most surprising that a dose and mode of administration which would result in a substantial improvement in the cost/benefit ratio of prophylaxis against venous postoperative thromboembolism has not stimulated further clinical research of this intriguing prospect.

Is the Antithrombotic Property of Heparin Rather Correlated with its Anti-Xa than with its Antithrombin Effect?

The main untoward effect of heparin is haemorrhage. Once upon a time the anticoagulant, antithrombotic and bleeding inducing effects of heparin were considered in one term. We learned in the last years to dissociate an anti-Xa activity from an antithrombin effect and we now tend to believe that the antithrombotic property of heparin closely follows its antifactor Xa property (6).

Whether the assumption that a high anti-Xa activity indeed correlates in experimental models and in man with antithrombotic activity was not discussed, not even challenged during this meeting.

There ist still a distressing ignorance about the direct cause of bruising during heparin treatment. Thrombocytopenia and inhibition of platelet aggregation by unfractionated heparin is only a partial answer. The suggestion that heparin competes with myosin adenosine triphosphate in the vessel wall explaining the haemorrhagic effect observed when blood vessels of an heparinized individual are punctured or cut, has never been seriously explored (7).

Clinical Relevance of the Determination of Intravascular Heparin

Heparin is avidly taken up by the vascular endothelium against a concentration gradient, the concentration of extracted heparin in endothelium being over 100-fold that in plasma (8). The increase in negative charge of the vessel wall accounts for a large part of the clinical effectiveness of heparin in preventing thrombosis. One therefore wonders what clinical relevance the intravascular levels of heparin may have in terms of its antithrombotic effect.

Preparation of Stabilised Heparin-Antithrombin III Complexes

The half-life of the anticoagulant activity of heparin in plasma following intravenous injection in man varies between 23 min and 2.5 hours, whereas that of antithrombin III was found in our laboratory to be 2.7 days (9). At present it is not clearly established whether the anticoagulant activity disappears from the blood due to clearing of the intact complex or to dissociation of the complex in the blood. Following intravenous injection of a mixture of heparin and ^{125}I-labeled antithrombin III in a patient, we observed a marked difference in the disappearance rates of the anticoagulant activity and the label (10), suggesting that dissociation of the complex occurred. On the basis of this finding we anticipated that stabilized active antithrombin III-heparin complexes might circulate longer in the blood and be cleared with a half-life between that of free heparin and free antithrombin III.

We therefore undertook a study to validate this hypothesis. High affinity heparin obtained by chromatography of clinical grade heparin on antithrombin III-Sepharose was covalently coupled to antithrombin III using a three step procedure: 1. introduction of free amino groups in the heparin molecule; 2. reaction of these amino groups with the difunctional reagent tolylene-2,4-diisothiocyanate; and 3. reaction of the remaining isothiocyanate group with amino groups of antithrombin III. Amino groups were introduced in the heparin molecule by limited N-desulfation or by reaction of carboxyl groups with hexamethylenediamine with the use of a water soluble carbodiimide. On average between 1 and 2 moles of NH_2 groups were introduced per 15,000 g heparin and the yield of the coupling procedures was 25 to 30 percent. The specific anticoagulant activity of the complexes (expressed per mg heparin) was approximately 57 percent of that of the original high affinity heparin. The half-life of these complexes in blood following intravenous injection of about 100 heparin equivalents in rabbits was 0.68 ± 0.08 hours for the N-desulfated heparin-antithrombin III complex and 0.99 ± 0.27 hours for the hexamethylenediamine substituted heparin-antithrombin III complex, which is 2.4 and 3.5 times longer than the half-life of free heparin in blood (10). Such complexes could therefore be of clinical importance as the fequency of heparin injections may be reduced. The yield of the present coupling procedure has to be improved in order to produce an inexpensive pharmaceutical form.

Semisynthetic Heparin

The semisynthetic heparin analogue SSHA-73025 has virtually no in vitro anti-factor Xa activity nor does it prolong the activated partial thromboplastin time; however, it induces after subcutaneous or intravenous injection a higher anti-factor Xa activity than the same amount of unfractionated heparin (11, 12). The heparin analogue also releases lipoprotein lipase activity and platelet factor 4 antigen (13). Moreover, the heparin analogue administered subcutaneously prolongs the one-stage prothrombin time in a dose related manner (14). The hypothesis was raised that the synthetic heparin analogue was releasing endogenous glycosaminoglycan (possibly heparin sulphate) (13). Repetitive injections at 90 min or an increase in dose does not appear to increase the anti-Xa activity level. This state of relative or limited responsiveness is further to be elucidated; one also would like to know the mechanism by which the prothrombin times are prolonged.

Chloromethyl Ketone Derivatives, In Vivo Inhibitors of Thrombin

The group of Shaw (15, 16) has investigated chloromethyl ketone derivatives as inhibitors of serine proteinases and has observed that thrombin is most sensitive to arginine derivatives tailored from sequence preceding the scissile bond in physiological substrates. In a recent study, D-Phe-Pro-Arg-chloromethyl ketone, a tripeptide sequence which does not occur in physiological thrombin substrates, was found to be an extremely efficient inhibitor (17). In our laboratory D-Val-Leu-Lys-CH_2Cl was also found to be a very efficient inhibitor of thrombin (18).

Our group has shown that D-Phe-Pro-Arg-CH_2Cl appears to be an efficient inhibitor of intravascular coagulation caused by thrombin or tissue thromboplastin in rabbits, and was well tolerated by these animals (19). Intravenous injections of 0.5 mg (circa 1,200 NIH units) of human thrombin over 5 min in seven anesthesized rabbits resulted in death due to massive thrombosis in the right heart in all animals. Six rabbits which had received an intravenous injection of 1 mg of D-Phe-Pro-Arg-CH_2Cl just before the thrombin infusion all survived without a significant drop in their plasma fibrinogen levels. Infusion of 12 ml of a brain thromboplastin suspension over 30 min in six rabbits resulted in extensive prothrombin activation (resulting prothrombin 21 ± 1.5 percent of preinfusion value) and virtually complete defibrination (residual fibrinogen 14 ± 4 percent). Subcutaneous injection of 1 mg of the tripeptide before and 30 to 60 min after the start of the thromboplastin infusion in four rabbits resulted in a comparable degree of prothrombin activation and a decrease of the fibrinogen level to 30 ± 5 percent of its preinfusion level. Intravenous injection of 1 mg of D-Phe-Pro-Arg-CH_2Cl before the start of the infusion followed by continuous infusion of 4 mg over 45 min in six rabbits resulted in a residual prothrombin level of 27 ± 7 percent and a fibrinogen level of 68 ± 3 percent of the preinfusion levels. By extrapolation these first in vivo data show that neutralization of trypsin-like serine proteases by specific and sensitive inhibitors of the chloromethyl ketone type is feasible. This approach could be useful to monitor or counteract enhanced formation of such enzymes in vivo; further studies are in progress.

References

1. Jaques, L. B., Mahadoo, J., Kavanagh, L. W.: Lancet II, 1157-1161 (1976).

2. Negus, D., Freedgood, A., Cox, S. J., Peel, A. L. G., Wells, B. W.: Lancet I, 891-894 (1980).

3. Pulver, R.: Arzneimittel-Forsch. 15, 1320-1323 (1965).

4. Raby, C., Bertrand, H.: In: McDuffie, N. M., ed., Heparin: Structure cellular functions, and clinical applications. Academic Press, London, 299-309 (1979).

5. Negus, D., Pinto, D. J., Slack, W. W.: Lancet I, 1202-1204 (1971).

6. Verstraete, M., Machin, S. J.: Scand. J. Haemat. 25, suppl. 36, 1-188 (1980).

7. Cruz, W. O., Dietrich, C. P.: Proc. Soc. Exper. Biol. Med. 126, 420-426 (1967).

8. Hiebert, L. M., Jaques, L. B.: Artery 2, 26-27 (1976).

9. Collen, D., Schetz, J., De Cock, F., Holmer, E., Verstraete, M.: Eur. J. Clin. Invest. 7, 27-35 (1977).

10. Collen, D., Ceustermans, R., De Mol, M., Hoylaerts, M.: Thrombos. Haemostas. 478, 185 (abstract) (1981) and submitted for publication.

11. Thomas, D. P., Michalski, R., Lane, D. A., Johnson, E. A., Kakkar, V. V.: Lancet i, 120-122 (1977).

12. Lane, D. A., Michalski, R., van Ross, M. E., Kakkar, V. V.: Br. J. Haemat. 37, 247-256 (1977).

13. Thomas, D. P., Barrowcliffe, T. W., Merton, R. E., Stocks, J., Dawes, J., Pepper, D S.: Thromb. Res. 17, 831-840 (1980).

14. Kakkar, V. V., Djazaeri, B., Scully, M., Weeraginghe, K.: Lancet I, 1167 (1981).

15. Shaw, E.: Physiol. Rev. 50, 244-296 (1970).

16. Kettner, C., Shaw, E.: Thromb. Res. 14, 969-973 (1979).

17. Kettner, C., Shaw, E.: Biochemistry 17, 4778-4784 (1978).

18. Collen, D., Lijnen, H. R., De Cock, F., Durieux, J. P., Loffet, A.: Biochim. Biophys. Acta 165, 158-166 (1980).

19. Collen, D., Matsuo, O., Stassen, J. M., Kettner, C., Shaw, E.: Submitted for publication.

Discussion

Weber wondered if *Verstraete* thought that the liver is degrading or metabolizing heparin in an essential way and that one cannot predict a consistent effect of heparin if it is given orally.

Verstraete does not think that there is evidence to say so. What he wanted to imply was that if heparin is present in the vena portae, there will be a higher concentration in the liver which is then diluted out in the body and surpasses the liver. That might be a useful condition in some patients, for instance, in patients with liver disorders when one has some limited intravascular coagulation and when one would like to give heparin to prevent part of this intravascular coagulation. This could be a useful approach. It is not yet proven

Wenzel referred to the variation of the individual response of patients on a standardized heparin dosage. This was already shown by *Estes* about ten years ago.
He demonstrated how one can decrease this variation by simply calculating the half life of heparin in those individuals and adjusting the dosage accordingly.

Wenzel conjectered if this had been done in *Verstraete's* patients, the high variations might have been eliminated. *Wenzel* thinks that this would be in accordance with *Jacques'* hypothesis that heparin is first taken up by endothelial cells which would be the reason for individual variation. He asked if *Verstraete* had calculated the half life time of heparin and adjusted the dosage to eliminate variation.

Verstraete said that he had tried to reproduce the experiments of *Estes*, but that he had been unable to do so. He thinks the system is much more complicated than hitherto assumed. He wanted to draw attention to the fact that nobody really knows what happens with the patient when he is given heparin.

It is assumed that heparin will react in all patients in the same way after subcutaneous administration. This is not always the case. A certain number will be underdosed and a certain number overdosed.

In prevention, when very low doses of heparin are sufficient, it does not matter. Excess heparin is excreted in the urine. This seems to be true for the venous site but it is unknown for the arterial site.

The possibility of heparin inhalation was raised in the discussion, but apart from a few publications which appeared several years ago nobody has picked it up again. The situation is similar for the vitamin B_6 story.

Duckert expressed his opinion on the problem of subcutaneous heparin administration. He thinks that the absorption is the main problem. It is very variable for different patients. He also asked if the anticoagulatory action of protamine is a real problem or not.

Verstraete admitted that if too much protamine is given too rapidly fibrinogen can decrease, but this happens only with protamine sulfate and not with proamine chloride.

Schmitz-Hübner felt that there is a certain discrepancy between *Verstraete's* statement that the inhibition of coagulation does not necessarily correspond to thrombosis prophylaxis and his suggestion that thrombin antagonists might be potential antithrombotic drugs. He wanted to know if one really needs thrombin inhibitors.

Verstraete said that the assumption that anticoagulant agents are not necessarily antithrombotic agents might be explained by the possibility of different pathways which can lead to thrombosis. If one interferes with the final steps of coagulation then there is a fair chance of having an anticoagulant which is also an antithrombotic agent. If a substance interferes with one of the earlier steps of coagulation, it might inhibit thrombogenesis but not necessarily be an anticoagulant in the usual sense of the word.

As there are different pathways involved in the pathogenesis of thrombosis, it seems to be necessary to interfere at different levels, which is the major problem.

Weber referred to *Verstraete's* point that there are wide variations in the concentration or activity of heparin in different individuals. She wondered to what extent the uptake of heparin by the endothelial and the reticulum cells might be responsible for these individual differences.

Verstraete said that gravide rabbits with a loaded RES are more sensitive to heparin than non-gravide rabbits. There have also been experiments in which the RES has been loaded with Chinese ink, and higher intravascular heparin levels were found here too after injection of heparin.

Aronson made a comment to this question also. He studied the uptake of carbon and Latex particles as well as yeast by macrophages. There was a temporary decrease in heparin uptake because the receptors were occupied.

Verstraete wanted to know how long the clearing of carbon particles took.

Aronson explained that when others tried to find that out, they had to load the animals with tremendous amounts of carbon or thorotrast but nevertheless could not keep the activity for a long time in a depressed state.

Schöndorf asked if the hypercoagulability due to antithrombin III depression after the cessation of heparin administration had been observed after subcutaneous application and if it was dose related.

Verstraete replied that he thought that it had been after intravenous administration and that other groups had observed the same thing.

Róka wanted to know if the stabilized antithrombin III-heparin which *Verstraete* prepared had shown the same anti-Xa and anti-thrombin activity as the same heparin before fixation.

Verstraete answered in the affirmative.

Bhargava asked if this complex was injected intravenously.

Verstraete said that it was injected intravenously in rabbits.

Marbet was curious about the relationship between antithrombin III and heparin in cases where the concentration of antithrombin III is critically diminished, so that there is no longer an adequate heparin effect.

Verstraete stated that antithrombin III has to decrease to 40-50 % of the normal level to have thrombotic events as shown in congenital antithrombin III deficiency.

Concerning the question about the critical level of antithrombin III where heparin is no longer effective, *Verstraete* could only talk about experiments with animals. There 25 % of normal is a minimal level. If this is the same for the human system is not proven. *Verstraete* felt it amasing that these questions are still asked after 30-40 years of wide heparin usage.

IV. Experience with ”Monitoring of Heparin Therapy“

Heparin Treatment of Deep Venous Thrombosis: Correlation Between Clinical Effects and Heparin Assays

Hans Asbjørn Holm, Ulrich Abildgaard
Aker Hospital
Oslo 5, Norway

Our knowledge concerning the usefulness of different heparin assays is rather incomplete. Still, most clinicians wish to have some kind of assay, and a wide number of tests have been used for this purpose. Variations of coagulation tests, and especially the various APTT tests have gained a widespread popularity.

With the introduction of chromogenic assays, heparin concentration may be measured with methods which are well suited for clinical-chemical laboratories and which may be automated. In vitro studies, involving both normal and pathological plasma samples have shown that the determination of heparin concentration with the chromogenic substrate S-2222 is equal to or better than the best of the coagulation methods (1).

The present report concerns a clinical trial in which the main objective was to examine whether there is a correlation between the results of different heparin assays, and the effect of heparin treatment of deep venous thrombosis (DVT) with respect to clinical effects such as fate of the thrombus, bleeding complications, and local symptoms of the affected leg.

Heparin · New Biochemical and Medical Aspects

Patient Material

Included in the study were patients with clinical symptoms of DVT of less than 14 days duration. The diagnosis was confirmed by phlebography.

When the trial was terminated, 280 patients had been included. Of these 160 were men and 120 women with a mean age of 63 years (22-90). 243 were medical patients, 37 surgical patients.

Patients in medical departments with the diagnosis of DVT often have a major coexistent illness, as is shown in Table 1.

Table 1. Coexistent disease

Disease	Medical pts n = 243	Surgical pts n = 37
Heart disease	66 (27 %)	5 (14 %)
Malignancy	32 (13 %)	6 (16 %)
Diabetes	15 (6 %)	1 (3 %)

Operation bears a definite risk for development of DVT. 23 of the surgical patients (62 %) had been operated on less than four weeks before the diagnosis of DVT. The departments involved had a rather low prophile concerning prophylaxis.

Symptoms of DVT are often vague and insidious, and are therefore often overlooked, or the diagnosis is delayed. Table 2 shows number of days from onset of symptoms to phlebographic diagnosis.

Table 2. Number of days from onset of symptoms to phlebographic diagnosis

	not defined	Days < 1	1 - 3	4 - 6	7 - 14
Number of pts	22	3	122	70	63
Per cent of total	8	1	44	25	22
	Mean: 4.65		SD: 3.50		

Dose Regimen

The heparin used in this study was supplied by Nyegaard, Oslo, (heparin from porcine mucosa). One batch was ear-marked for this study.

Heparin was given for about seven days. The recommended dose was 150 U of heparin per kg body weight as intravenous injection, followed by 400 U/kg/day. It was recommended that the dose should be reduced by about one third in older people, especially in older women. Warfarin therapy was started on day 3. Since most of the clinics involved did not use any heparin assay for monitoring of therapy prior to this study, daily dose adjustment was mainly a question of clinical judgement. Table 3 shows the mean daily dose in the younger and the older part of the material. The recorded doses correspond well to the recommendation given, except that mean daily dose in the women is somewhat higher than recommended.

Table 3. Mean daily heparin dose in different age groups

	Units of heparin per kg body weight	
Age:	Below 50 years	Above 80 years
Males	400 (n = 18)	310 (n = 8)
Females	420 (n = 19)	370 (n = 11)
Total	411 (n = 37)	340 (n = 19)

Heparin Assays

Blood samples were drawn daily, and analysed for heparin activity with the following assays:

1. APTT with Cephotest from Nyegaard, Norway.
2. Calcium Thrombin Time (0.1 ml citrated plasma + 0.1 ml 0.15 M NaCl + 0.1 ml thrombin 5 U/ml in 0.05 M $CaCl_2$).
3. Thrombin Time of citrated plasma (0.2 ml citrated plasma + 0.1 ml thrombin 30 U/ml in 0.15 M NaCl).
4. Amidolytic assay with the chromogenic substrate S-2222 (Coatest heparin) from KABI, Sweden (2).

All tests were performed at 37 °C.

Empirically, the *therapeutic range* of heparin is defined as 0.2-0.7 U/ml plasma. The corresponding clotting test results, obtained in mixed normal plasma, were as follows:

APTT (Cephotest)	60 - 120 sec
Thrombin Time of citrated plasma	8 - 20 sec
Calcium Thrombin Time	20 - 120 sec.

Bleeding Complications

Bleedings were recorded in 36 patients, of which 8 (2 men and 6 women) were classified as *major bleeds* (2.9 %), 2 haematemesis, 5 retroperitoneal; and 1 thoracic bleeding which was the only fatal bleeding. This patient was a 75 year old woman who after gall bladder surgery developed signs of DIC and had a leg vein thrombosis. After less than 24 hours of heparin treatment, a thoracocentesis was followed by severe thoracic bleeding which necessitated thoracotomia. After a few days the patient died with symptoms of DIC and multi-organ failure. Only one blood sample was drawn from this patient, and she is not included in the statistical analysis.

In the remaining major bleeds symptoms of bleeding resulted in cessation of heparin treatment. Frank symptoms of major bleeding tended to occur after 4 or 5 days of heparin treatment. These patients received blood transfusions, and surgical evacuation of haematomas was performed in two patients (retroperitoneal bleeds).

The mean values of the blood tests are shown in Table 4. There is a slight tendency towards longer clotting times in patients with bleeding, and especially those with major bleeding, but the differences are not statistically significant. However, with the cromogenic assay, measuring heparin concentration, a statistically significant difference is found between the mean values of those without bleeding symptoms compared to those with recorded bleeding.

Table 4. Mean clotting times and heparin concentration in patients with and without bleeding symptoms

Assay	No bleeding (n = 241)	Bleeding all (n = 35)	Bleeding major (n = 7)
APTT (sec)	68	74	87
Thrombin Time Ca^{++} (sec)	25	36	56
Thrombin Time Ci (sec)	9	13	12
Heparin conc (U/ml)	0.38	0.51*	0.74

* p = 0.046

Phlebography

Whenever possible a repeat phlebography was performed at the time of cessation of heparin therapy. The initial and repeat phlebograms were evaluated and each patient assigned a *phlebography score* value as follows:

Increased thrombosis: score value 6. Unchanged: 4.
Partly cleared: 2. Cleared: 0.

Increased thrombosis was found in 49 patients (22 %), unchanged 85 patients (78 %), partly cleared 83 patients (37 %), and cleared 7 patients (3 %).

Table 5 shows the correlation between results of heparin assay and phlebography score. All but the thrombin time of citrated plasma show a significant correlation. However, the correlation coefficients are rather weak.

Table 5. Correlation between mean results of heparin assays and phlebography score

Assays	Correlation coeff.	p
APTT	- 0.153	0.023
Thrombin Time Ca^{++}	- 0.140	0.036
Thrombin Time Ci	0.010	0.877
Heparin conc	- 0.186	0.005

Thrombosis Score

Each patient was assigned a thrombosis score value (range 0-17) based on the above mentioned phlebography score, and edema, pain and discolouration at cessation of heparin therapy, and at a follow up three months later.

Table 6 shows the correlation between thrombosis score and the results of heparin assays. Again, the chromogenic assay shows the best correlation, but even APTT and the Calcium Thrombin Time correlate significantly to the thrombosis score.

Table 6. Correlation between mean results of heparin assays and thrombosis score

Assays	Correlation coeff.	p
APTT	- 0.167	0.018
Thrombin Time Ca^{++}	- 0.178	0.011
Thrombin Time Ci	- 0.083	0.237
Heparin conc (U/ml)	- 0.223	0.001

Pulmonary Embolism

The diagnosis of pulmonary embolism, mainly based on clinical symptoms, was recorded in 13 patients while on heparin treatment. None was fatal.

Mean clotting time and heparin concentration were lower in patients with recorded pulmonary embolism than for the remaining material (Table 7). The difference reached statistic significance with the Calcium Thrombin Time and the chromogenic assay.

Table 7. Mean clotting times and heparin concentration in patients with and without pulmonary embolism

	pulmonary embolism		
	yes (n = 13)	no (n = 264)	
Assay	mean	mean	p
APTT (sec)	57	69	0.140
Thrombin Time Ca^{++} (sec)	17	27	0.032
Thrombin Time Ci (sec)	8	10	0.369
Heparin conc (U/ml)	0.23	0.40	0.017

Antithrombin III during Heparin Treatment

It is a well known fact that antithrombin concentration tends to decrease during heparin treatment. Decrease in antithrombin concentration is shown in Table 8.

Table 8. Decrease in antithrombin concentration during heparin treatment (n = 237)

	Decrease in antithrombin conc (%) < 10	10–19	20–39	40–59
Number of pts.	74 (31 %)	79 (33 %)	81 (34 %)	3 (1 %)

Table 9 shows mean antithrombin concentration in 67 patients before, immediately after and approximately three months after heparin treatment. During this three months period the patients received warfarin therapy which tends to increase antithrombin concentration.

Table 9. Mean antithrombin concentration on three different occasions (n = 67)

	mean	SD
Before heparin	94.4	13.0
After heparin (one week)	74.7	9.7
After warfarin (3 months)	98.7	12.0

Conclusion

The low incidence in this material of major bleeding complications and pulmonary embolism suggests that the recommended dose regimen is well suited for heparin treatment of DVT.

Except for the thrombin time of citrated plasma, there is a weak, but definite correlation between biological parameters and the results of heparin assays. The results obtained with the chromogenic assay are more closely correlated to bleeding complications and to regress of the thrombotic process than those obtained with the coagulation assays.

The present results indicate that an adequate heparin concentration not only protects against pulmonary embolism, but even has a positive influence on the fate of the thrombus and clinical symptoms like pain and edema.

References

1. Teien, A. N., Lie, M., Abildgaard, U.: Assay of heparin in plasma using a chromogenic substrate for activated factor X. Thromb. Res. 8, 413 (1976).

2. Teien, A. N., Lie, M.: Evaluation of an amidolytic heparin assay method: Increased sensitivity by adding purified antithrombin III. Thromb. Res. 10, 399 (1977).

Discussion

Schöndorf referred to *Holm's* correlation of the heparin correlation of the heparin concentration to the incidence of deep vein thrombosis and wondered if he had also calculated the incidence of DVT in correlation to the decrease of the antithrombin III concentration.

Holm had not done that but considers it to be an important task. One should divide the material in those with low and those with high decrease and see if one group fares better than the other.

Schöndorf pointed out that this could eventually have therapeutical consequences, namely in substituting antithrombin III during heparin therapy.

Thaler asked if *Holm* had adjusted the dosage if heparinization was too high - as measured by APTT - or if he had followed a standard scheme of 400 units/kg/day.

Holm explained that in most clinics involved, they were not used to having assays, so they adjusted according to clinical criteria. If, for instance, there was bruising of the abdomen or any place else, they reduced the dosage. In some clinics there was a crude adjustment, usually according to APTT.

Duckert asked about the normal thrombin time.

Holm stated that it was up to 5-6 sec with this thrombin time method (30 U thrombin/ml).

Duckert felt that this is a high concentration of thrombin and therefore less sensitive to variations in concentration of heparin.

Holm agreed. The therapeutic range is probably not very steep in this assay. The concentration of thrombin should be less. This particular test was used because it is the one usually used in Norway.

Witt wanted to know if *Holm* had seen patients with low response to heparin and also patients with varying response during the heparin treatment.

Holm replied that special problems had not been taken into consideration in this study. They had not investigated individual patients. Such studies are planned, especially for that group of patients which had an increase of the thrombus during therapy. They will look for what was special with them aside from the fact that they received less heparin than the others.

Witt asked if the patients with high levels of antithrombin III had received cortisol.

Holm stated that drug administration was registered prior to and during treatment, but there were very few who received cortisol. He could not say if there is an influence on antithrombin III concentration, but this could be found out.

Witt pointed out that it is well known that patients receiving cortisol or patients with M. Cushing have elevated antithrombin III concentrations.

Verstraete asked if clinicians had been advised to give another dose to women than to males.

Holm answered that the general recommendation was to give a lower dose to older patients, especially to older women. A very strict recommendation had not been given.

Verstraete wished to know the basis of that recommendation concerning women.

Holm's recommendation was more or less empiric. His experience is that most often the major bleedings occur in women, especially in elderly women.

Verstraete wanted to know if the women seem to bleed more often or more severely on a given dose of heparin or if the basis of the recommendation had been that women need less heparin to get the same therapeutic effect.

Holm speculated that both mechanisms may be involved. The data indicate that the women who bled clearly received higher doses than recommended. One of the reasons may be that females in general have a smaller body volume.

Verstraete is afraid that it may be more complicated than that. Pharmacotherapeutic literature reports more and more evidence that drug handling is different for males and females. For the field of coagulation it became quite evident in the Canadian TIA study and in a number of other studies and amasingly it is not admitted for the human being. The differences are also evident, for instance, in rats and rabbits. This is also the opinion of the pharmacologists. In other fields of therapeutics, even in physiology, there are more receptors, for instance, in the smooth muscle cells of males than of females. This is just one example.

Verstraete said, 'so, in essence, what I am trying to say is that eventually I am forced to believe that females are not equal to men.'

Holm replied that from his study he cannot say that females are very differlent from males because they received higher doses than they should have, according to the general recommendation. 'But I agree with you that there are differences.'

Verstraete: 'The very interesting point is then, why? Is it because they have one x more or an x less?'

Holm: 'Or because they lost the y.'

Heparin-, Heparin Cofactor- and Platelet Factor 4 Plasma Levels Under Heparin Treatment

Norbert Bender, Jürgen Schlegel, Viola Hach, Carl Maximilian Kirchmaier, Hans Klaus Breddin
Department of Internal Medicine
University of Frankfurt a. M.
Division of Angiology
D-6000 Frankfurt

Introduction

Thrombin-time (1) and aPTT (2) are commonly used for monitoring heparin therapy. Although these assays are relatively insensitive to heparin (3, 4) and are influenced by various coagulation parameters as the presence of fibrin degradation products and the activity of clotting factors (5), they reflect the overall anticoagulant activity of heparin in the plasma. New amidolytic methods using chromgenic substrates, however, allow calculation of plasma heparin levels with the determination of the anti Xa-activity (6) and the rest-thrombin activity (7). It was the aim of our study to examine which of these three methods or which set of methods can be used in a routine laboratory to monitor heparin treatment.

Two other parameters, antithrombin III, the apoenzyme (8) of heparin and platelet factor 4, a platelet specific protein with high affinity to heparin (9, 10), which markedly influence the anticoagulative effect of heparin in vitro (11, 12) were determined simultaneously in patients.

Heparin · New Biochemical and Medical Aspects

Patients

We investigated blood samples from 39 patients under heparin treatment for different reasons. 25 patients received heparin subcutaneously two or three times daily. 14 patients were treated intravenously with an infusion pump over the whole period of heparin treatment. We did not interfere with the heparin dosage which was under the responsibility of the patients physicians. Before heparin treatment thrombine time, aPTT, heparin plasma level, heparin cofactor and platelet factor 4 were determined. These five parameters were controlled daily during the period of heparin therapy. Blood was collected at 8 a. m.; 10 ml of citrated blood were obtained for the determination of thrombin time, aPTT, plasma heparin level and heparin cofactor and 3 ml blood in a tube containing 0.1 ml of 10 % Na_2EDTA and 0.1 ml theophylline (5.4 mg/ml) for the determination of platelet factor 4. From five patients under subcutaneous heparin treatment, blood was taken 1, 4 and 11 hours after the morning injection of heparin.

Methods

aPTT was measured according to Proctor and Rapaport (13) using Pathrombin (Behring, Marburg, FRG). Normal range: 35 - 45 sec. The procedure for *thrombin time* determination based on the method originally described by Jürgens (13). We used diethyl-barbiturate-acetate buffer and thrombin (final concentration 10 U thrombin/ml) from Behring, Marburg, FRG. Normal range: 17 - 24 sec.

Heparin plasma levels were calculated using the Heparin Coatest from KABI, Stockholm, Sweden, according to the method of Teien and coworkers (6) for low dose heparin therapy.

Heparin cofactor was measured with the Boehringer Mannheim diagnostic kit AT III. The assay procedure was described by Witt (15).

Platelet factor 4 was determined with the radioimmuno assay kit from ABBOTT Diagnostic Products, North Chicago, USA as described by Handin et al. (16).

Results

In Fig. 1 the calculated plasma heparin levels are plotted against the heparin dosage indicated as IU Hep/kg body weight/24 hours.

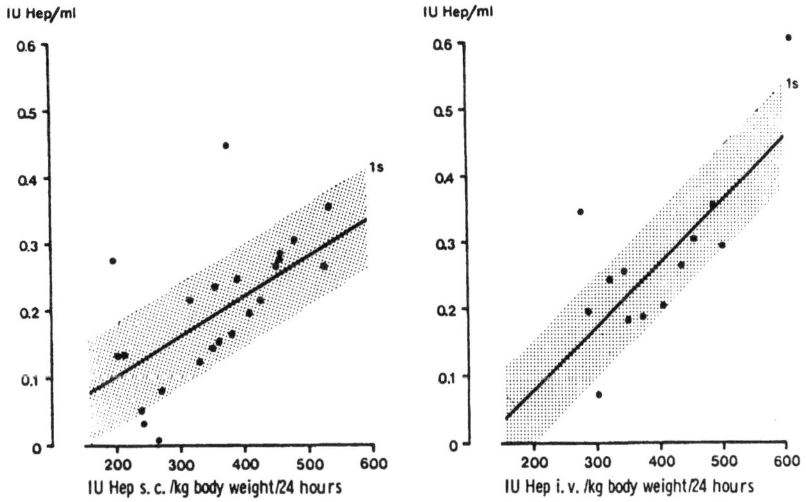

Fig. 1. Plasma heparin levels after heparin therapy, applicated subcutaneously and intravenously in different dosage

A rather good linear correlation is demonstrated between these two parameters over a dosage range of 200 IU Hep to 600 IU Hep/kg body weight/ 24 hours if heparin is applied subcutaneously or intravenously inspite of the heterogeneity of the patients. The different slope of the two regression curves may have been caused by the time of blood collection (blood was collected at 8 a. m. one hour after the subcutaneous heparin injections). Heparin plasma levels had not reached their maximum at that time. Compared with intravenous heparin application where resorption phenomena are negligible, heparin plasma levels determined one hour after subcutaneous heparin injections were lower.

A good correlation was also found between aPTT and heparin dosage as shown in Fig. 2. A prolongation of aPTT was found with heparin doses higher than 300 IU Hep/kg body weight/24 hours. The regression curve of the results from patients with subcutaneous heparin is steeper than that from the values obtained of the patients with intravenous heparin treatment.

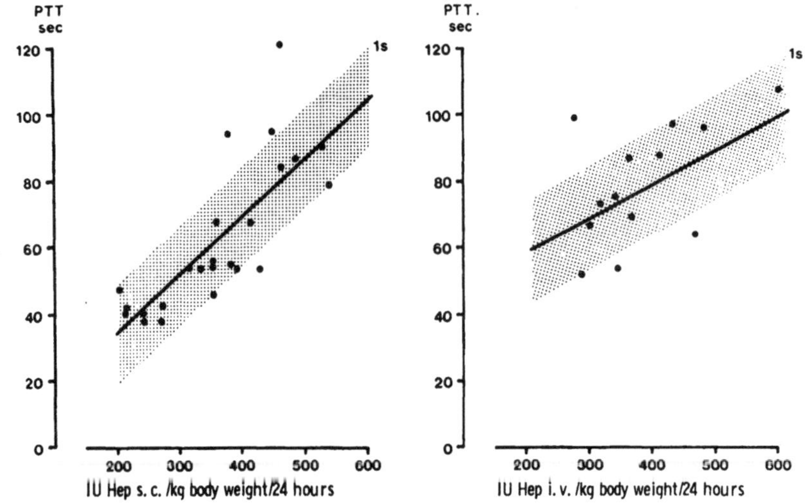

Fig. 2. PTT after heparin therapy, applicated subcutaneously and intravenously in different dosage

No linear regression was found if the thrombin time was plotted against the heparin dosage (Fig. 3). Up to heparin doses of 320 IU Hep/kg body weight/24 hours no prolongation of the thrombin time occurred. If higher heparin doses had been administered the prolongation of thrombin time was unpredictable.

Platelet factor 4 and heparin cofactor levels determined before heparin therapy seemed to have no effect on the values of thrombin time, aPTT and heparin plasma levels if they are in the normal range.

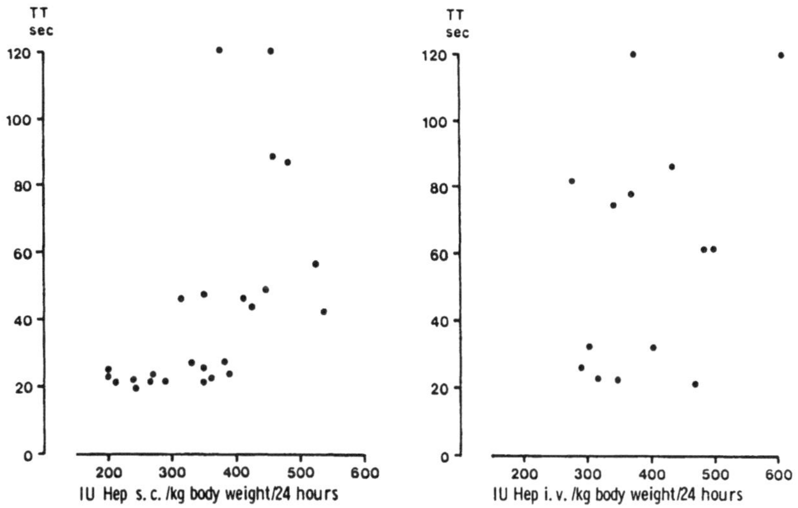

Fig. 3. Thrombin time after heparin therapy, applicated subcutaneously and intravenously in different dosage

If heparin was administered in a dosage between 300 and 400 IU Hep/kg body weight/24 hours, all three assays, thrombin time, aPTT and chromogenic substrate heparin level determination reacted very sensitively to changes in heparin doses. As shown in Fig. 4 and Fig. 5, even changes in a range of 10 % lead to marked changes in the assays.

In Fig. 6 and Fig. 7 platelet factor 4 and heparin cofactor levels are presented which were determined simultaneously with thrombin time, aPTT and heparin plasma levels of the two patients presented in Fig. 4 and Fig. 5. The results are controversial.

In a 66 year old patient (Fig. 6) high heparin levels seemed to elevate the heparin cofactor values and to reduce the platelet factor 4 values, whereas in the other patient heparin cofactor and platelet factor 4 were positively correlated with the heparin plasma level.

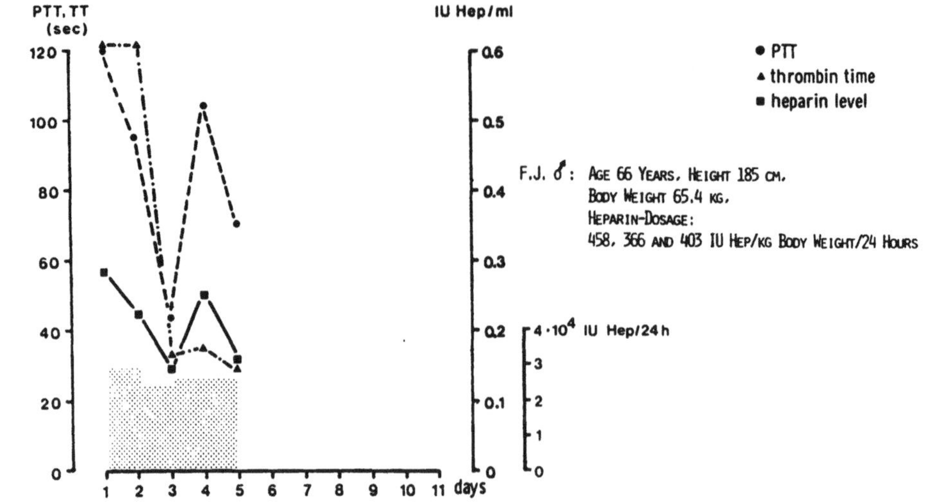

Fig. 4. PTT, thrombin time and plasma heparin levels after different heparin doses

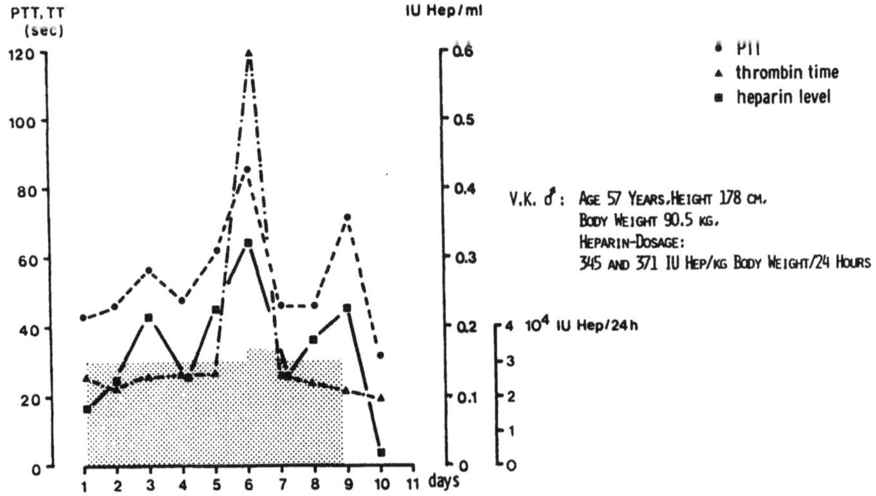

Fig. 5. PTT, thrombin time and plasma heparin levels after different heparin doses

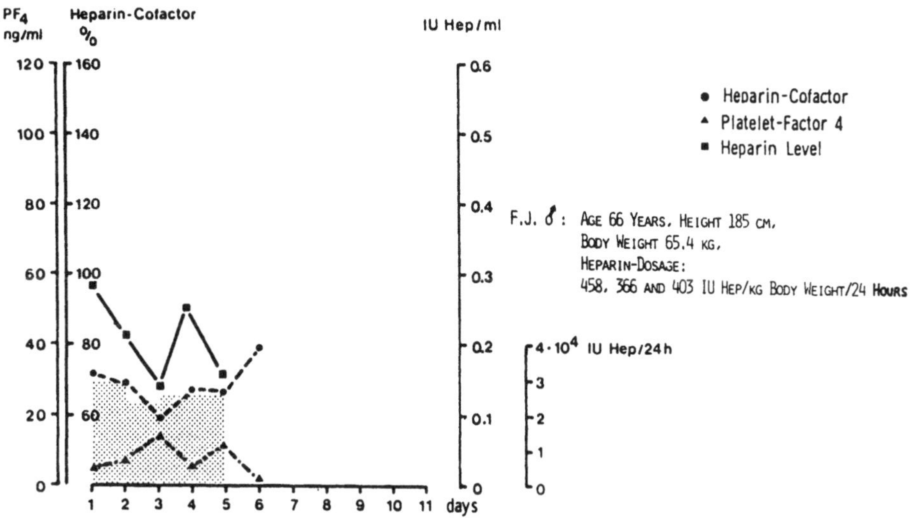

Fig. 6. Platelet factor 4, heparin cofactor and plasma heparin levels after different heparin doses

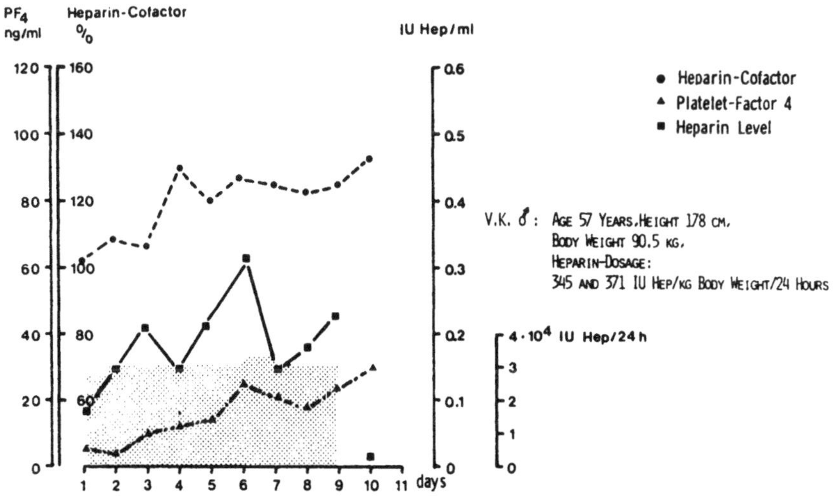

Fig. 7. Platelet factor 4, heparin cofactor and plasma heparin levels after different heparin doses

If the results are summarized no influence of heparin dosage on platelet factor 4 and heparin cofactor was found.

From five patients blood was collected three times daily, one, four and eleven hours after the morning heparin injection. Fig. 8 demonstrates that in a patient with a medium dosage of heparin the morning and evening values for the thrombin time and aPTT are in a normal range. Only at 11 a. m. was a prolongation in both assays. Heparin plasma levels were measurable at each time of blood collection. If higher doses of heparin were used (Fig. 9) a prolongation of thrombin time and aPTT at 8 a. m. and 6 p. m. was observed. At 11 a. m. the clotting time in both assays was lengthened up to more than two minutes indicating a certain bleeding risk at that time. Only the amidolytic method revealed a reliable value for anti-coagulation at that moment.

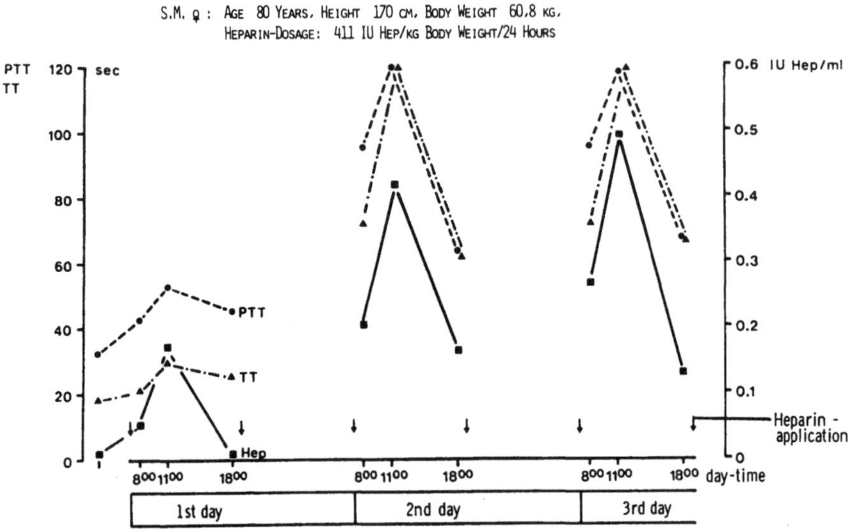

Fig. 8. Heparin levels, thrombin time and PTT during a three day period of subcutaneous heparin application

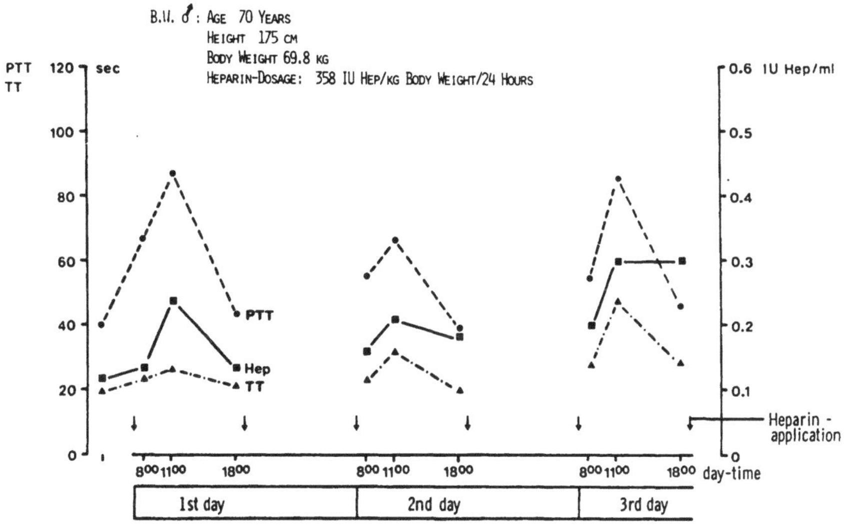

Fig. 9. Heparin levels, thrombin time and PTT during a three day period of subcutaneous heparin application

Fig. 9 shows that in some patients high heparin doses have a cumulative effect on the plasma heparin levels during the first days of therapy. Daily controls of anticoagulation with thrombin time, aPTT or the determination of heparin plasma levels seem to be neccessary especially within the first three days of heparin therapy to avoid both insufficient treatment and a bleeding risk.

Discussion

What assay should be used to monitor heparin therapy? Should an amidolytic method be offered in a routine laboratory in addition to the clotting methods (thrombin time or aPTT)? Which of the two clotting methods is the better assay for calculating the anticoagulant effect of heparin? Is it necessary to determine platelet factor 4 and heparin cofactor before starting heparin treatment to get more information about the heparin dosage?

During a period of three months we collected blood samples from patients who were to be treated with heparin. We calculated the heparin dosage in IU Hep/kg body weight/24 hours. We found a good correlation between heparin plasma levels determined with an amidolytic method and the heparin dosage and between the aPTT and the heparin dosage. The amidolytic method was more sensitive to heparin administration. Down to a dosage of about 200 IU Hep/kg body weight/24 hours (the upper range for low dose heparin) an elevated plasma heparin level is still detectable. The aPTT showed significant prolongation only at doses higher than 300 IU Hep/kg body weight/24 hours but is measurable (clotting time below two minutes) up to doses of about 600 IU Hep/kg/24 hours.

Thrombin time behaved differently. Comparable to the aPTT up to a dosage of 300 IU Hep/kg body weight/24 hours no prolongation occurred. But at higher heparin doses no correlation between heparin dosage and thrombin time was found.

If heparin is applicated in normal therapeutic doses, the amidolytic methods for determination of heparin plasma levels and the aPTT reflect with reliable values the anticoagulant state of a patient. Thrombin time, however, in the assay which is used in our laboratory reacted in an *all or nothing* manner and seemed to be independent of the heparin dosage the patient received. In a medium dosage range between 300 and 400 IU Hep/kg body weight/24 hours all three assays are sensitive and usable for the control of heparin therapy. Both clotting tests, however, are influenced by a variety of other coagulation parameters like fibrin degradation products and the content of other clotting factors (5). Before starting a heparin therapy therefore, base values of both assays are necessary to decide which of them should be used for monitoring the heparin therapy. So up to now we do not yet possess the ideal method for the control of heparin therapy and the question as to which one of the described assays should be used routinely, the amidolytic method with its calculated heparin plasma level or one or both of the two clotting assays which may better reflect an insufficient anticoagulation or a bleeding risk, still cannot be answered.

In a second part of the study we collected blood three times daily from patients who received subcutaneous heparin. The values of all three assays varied markedly over the whole range of values if blood was collected one, four and eleven hours after the last heparin injection, indicating the great change in the anticoagulant state of a patient during the day. Under medium heparin doses nearly no heparin effect could be measured at 8 a. m. and 6 p. m., whereas three to four hours after the subcutaneous injection a high anticoagulation was found in all patients. Since the risk of rethrombosis usually is more apparent than the risk of bleeding blood can be collected shortly before or shortly after heparin injection to monitor heparin treatment. An accumulation of heparin which eventually occurs under high heparin doses is also noticed. If a more constant anticoagulation is desired, heparin should, however, be administered intravenously as a continuous infusion.

Simultaneously to the thrombin time, aPTT and plasma heparin level we determined heparin cofactor and platelet factor 4 because they may influence the determination of heparin plasma levels (11, 12). In our material we could not find any influence of these two parameters on the plasma heparin levels. Before the first heparin application, heparin cofactor values of all patients varied within the normal range of 80 to 120 % and the highest platelet factor 4 level was 29 ng/ml. Within these normal ranges the influence of these two parameters on heparin treatment seemed to be negligible.

References

1. Godal, H. C.: Thromb. Diath. Haemorrh. 33, 77-80 (1974).

2. Teien, A., Abildgaard, U.: Thrombos. Haemostas. 35: 592-597 (1976).

3. Wenzel, E., Holzhüter, H., Bahre, G., Kleesiek, R., Saaredra, E., Nienhaus, K. H., Rommelspocher, G.: 9. Angiologisches Symposion Kitzbühel - Moderne Thromboseprophylaxe. Edited by Breddin, K., Gross, D.: F. K. Schattauer Verlag Stuttgart - New York, 80-92 (1976).

4. Vogel, G. E., Goodmann, F. L., Jelen, S., Tempel, G.: Med. Welt 28, 899-902 (1977).

5. Wenzel, E., Holzhüter, H., Muschietti, F., Angelkort, B., Ochs, H. G., Pusztai-Markos, S., Nowak, H., Stürner, H.: Dtsch. Med. Wschr. 99: 746-756 (1974).

6. Teien, A., Lie, M., Abildgaard, U.: Thromb. Res. 8: 413-416 (1976).

7. Bartl, K., Dorsch, E., Lill, H., Ziegenhorn, J.: Thrombos. Haemostas. 42: 1446-1451 (1979).

8. Rosenberg, R. D., Damus, P. S.: J. Biol. Chem. 248: 6490-6505 (1973).

9. Bolton, A. E., Ludlam, C. A., Pepper, D. S., Moore, S., Cash, J. D.: Thromb. Res. 8: 51-58 (1976).

10. Levine, S. P., Wohl, H.: J. Biol. Chem. 251: 324-328 (1976).

11. Teien, A. N., Lie, M.: Thromb. Res 10: 399-410 (1977).

12. Poplawski, A., Niewiarowski, S.: Thromb. Diath. Haemorrh. 13: 149-154 (1965).

13. Proctor, R. R., Rapaport, S. J.: Amer. J. Clin. Path. 36: 212-219 (1961).

14. Jürgens, J.: Dtsch. Arch. Klin. Med. 200: 67-85 (1952).

15. Witt, I., Hasler, K.: In: Prostaglandine und Plättchenfunktion, edited by Breddin, H. K.: F. K. Schattauer Verlag Stuttgart - New York, 227-243 (1978).

16. Handlin, R. I., McDonough, M., Lesch, M.: J. Lab. Clin. Med. 91: 340-349 (1978).

Discussion

Two related questions were discussed:

1. What is the most suitable time for measuring heparin activities in plasma after the administration?
2. How an even infusion had been achieved for intravenous administration.

Bender stated that they had used an infusion pump and that they had taken samples between eight and nine o'clock in the morning.

Holm related his experience with infusion pumps and said that they are not as reliable as the manufacturers say. He has found large variations. Even when the pumps were corrected in the night they were found to be two hours ahead or behind in the morning, indicating that the morning is the worst time to collect blood samples.

Concerning the best time for blood sampling after subcutaneous heparin administration, *Duckert* expressed the opinion that it is best to take the blood sample just before the next heparin administration.

Róka was very much surprised about the variation in the antithrombin III levels because his experience has been that after the administration of heparin to healthy persons the antithrombin III level does not change at all. He has only seen a drop in antithrombin III levels during open heart surgery with extracorporal circulation which returns slowly to normal after the operation. He felt that the fast decrease and the fast increase in Bender's cases is surprising and should be explained.

Bender had no explanation at the time

Marbet wondered about the good correlation between the different tests which is in contrast to his findings. He wanted to know if *Bender* sometimes saw discrepancies between the heparin determination and the APTT or the TT for instance.

Bender said that in the 5 patients who were controlled 3 times a day he did not see discrepancies, but in other patients he has seen them. In general in the very heterogenous group of patients the correlation was satisfactory.

Determination of Heparin, Partial Thromboplastin Time and Antithrombin III after Subcutaneous Heparin Administration

Theodor H. Schöndorf, Helena Paplham, Klaus Franz
Department of Medicine
Orthopedic Hospital
University Giessen

Introduction

The results of low dose heparin prophylaxis in hip surgery are controversial since the incidence of deep vein thrombosis ranges from 5 to 55 % (see review: Schöndorf (1)).

In the present trial coagulation studies were performed to obtain further information about the relationship between haemostaseological alterations and clinical findings such as deep venous thrombosis or bleeding complications under heparin prophylaxis.

The results were compared to previous investigations which studied changes of the blood coagulation system due to operations (Hedlund and Blombäck (2), Gitel et al. (3), Schöndorf and Lasch (4)), and administration of subcutaneous heparin (Tilsner et al. (5), Hedlund et al. (2), Kruse-Blinkenberg et al. (6), Brozović et al. (7), Zimmermann et al. (8) as well as the heparin sensitivity of various laboratory tests (Bounameaux et al. (9), Bruhn et al. (10), Zahavi and Smetana (11).

Patients

Group 1: 22 patients received 5000 U sodium heparin combined with 0.5 mg dihydroergotamine (DHE) preoperatively and in 8 hour intervals for 18 days after the operation. The mean body weight of the patients was 71 ± 12 kg.

Heparin · New Biochemical and Medical Aspects

Group 2: 22 patients received 5000 U sodium heparin preoperatively and in 8 hour intervals on the day of operation and on the first and second postoperative day. On the third day after the operation, the sodium heparin dosage was increased to 3 x 7500 U sodium heparin s.c./24 hours and administered until the 18th postoperative day. The patients' average body weight was 66 ± 11 kg.

In both groups heparin prophylaxis was given 10 and 2 hours before the operation.

Methods

1. Heparin activity (U/ml plasma) was determined by measuring the residual thrombin activity with Chromozym TH at 25 °C.

2. Heparin concentration (U/ml plasma) was determined by measuring the residual factor Xa activity with the chromogenic substrate S-2222.

3. For measuring the partial thromboplastin time (PTT, s), a caolin-cephalin activated reagent was used.

4. For the determination of the diluted thrombin time (TT, s), 2.5 units of thrombin were added to 0.2 ml citrated plasma.
Both clotting tests were performed immediately after withdrawal and centrifugation of the blood by a turbidimetric method (Fibrintimer II).

5. Antithrombin III (AT III) activity (U/ml) was measured by the substrate Chromozym TH at 37 °C.

6. Antithrombin III (AT III) concentration (mg/dl) and

7. Fibrinogen concentration (mg/dl) were measured antigenically by radial immunodiffusion (RID).
The amidolytic and immunological tests were performed from frozen plasma within one week after sampling.

Blood was withdrawn 2 and 8 hours after the subcutaneous injection of sodium heparin and heparin plus DHE respectively. It was collected in plastic syringes and mixed 1:10 with 0.1 mol/l sodium citrated buffer.

Statistics

The results were analyzed by the Student's t-test for paired or unpaired samples.

Results

1. Heparin activity (Chromozym TH) 8 hours after injection (Fig. 1)
The heparin activities determined 8 hours after injection of 5000 U sodium heparin plus DHE or sodium heparin alone revealed no statistical differences of the mean values between the two groups before the operation. On the morning of the third day after the operation, a further blood sample was collected from the patients of group 2 (heparin without DHE) before their heparin dosage was increased.

On the first and third day after the operation, the mean values of the plasma heparin were even lower in the heparin plus DHE-group than in the group which had received heparin alone, but the differences were not significant.

The widest range of the heparin levels were found in both groups on the first postoperative day. But the standard deviations were below 0.200 U heparin per ml plasma, which is considered to be the upper range for prophylaxis. The mean heparin activities of the heparin plus DHE-group had decreased on the third and seventh day after the operation; significant differences were not found.

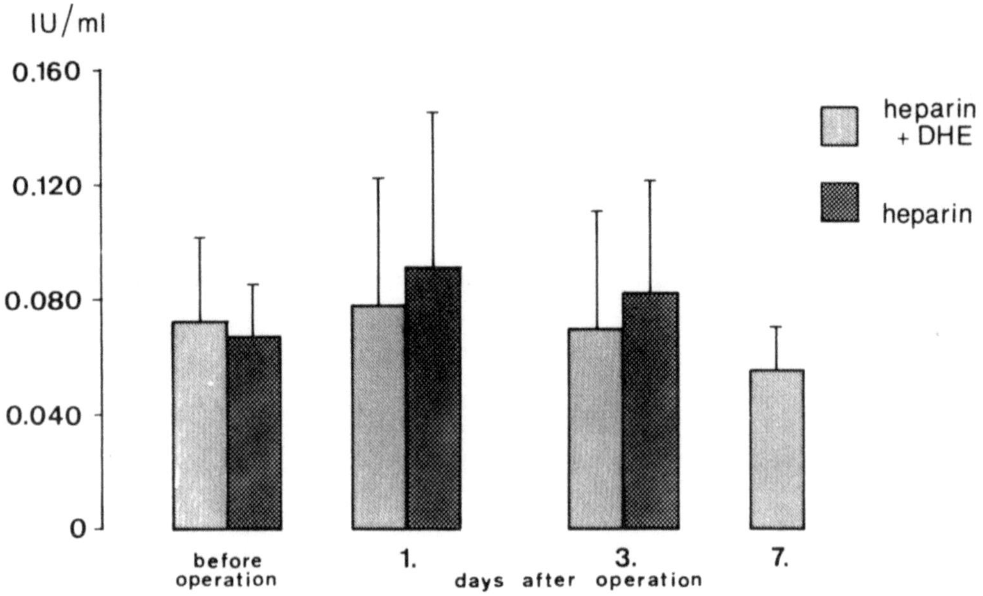

Fig. 1. Heparin activity (IU/ml plasma) (Chromozym TH) determined 8 hours after injection of 5000 U sodium heparin or combined with dihydroergotamine (DHE). Pre- and postoperative mean values ± 1 standard deviation.

2. Heparin activity (Chromzym TH) two hours after injection (Fig. 2)
Before operation and on the first day after operation, the mean values of the heparin determined two hours after the injection were higher in the group receiving heparin alone than in the group with the combination heparin plus DHE; the differences are not significant ($p > 0.5$).

On the third and seventh day after operation, a slight decrease of the mean heparin levels was found in the group with the combined prophylaxis (heparin plus DHE) when compared to the mean of the first postoperative day (Fig. 2).

The tendency of the mean values to decrease was similar to that found when heparin was determined 8 hours after the administration of 5000 U heparin plus DHE. The decreases were, however, statistically not significant. On the third postoperative day, 8 h blood samples of group 2 were collected in the morning (Fig. 2), thereafter the dosage of the heparin prophylaxis was increased. The mean values of the plasma heparin, determined two hours after the first injection of 7500 U heparin s.c. did not differ significantly from the mean value of the first postoperative day ($p > 0.5$) (Fig. 2). Mean value and standard deviation of the 2 h determination of the seventh day remained in the same range as on the third day after operation. Two hours after 7500 U heparin s.c., the mean values of the plasma heparin were significantly higher on the third ($p < 0.01$) and seventh ($p < 0.01$) postoperative day than the means of the group with the combination of 5000 U heparin plus DHE.

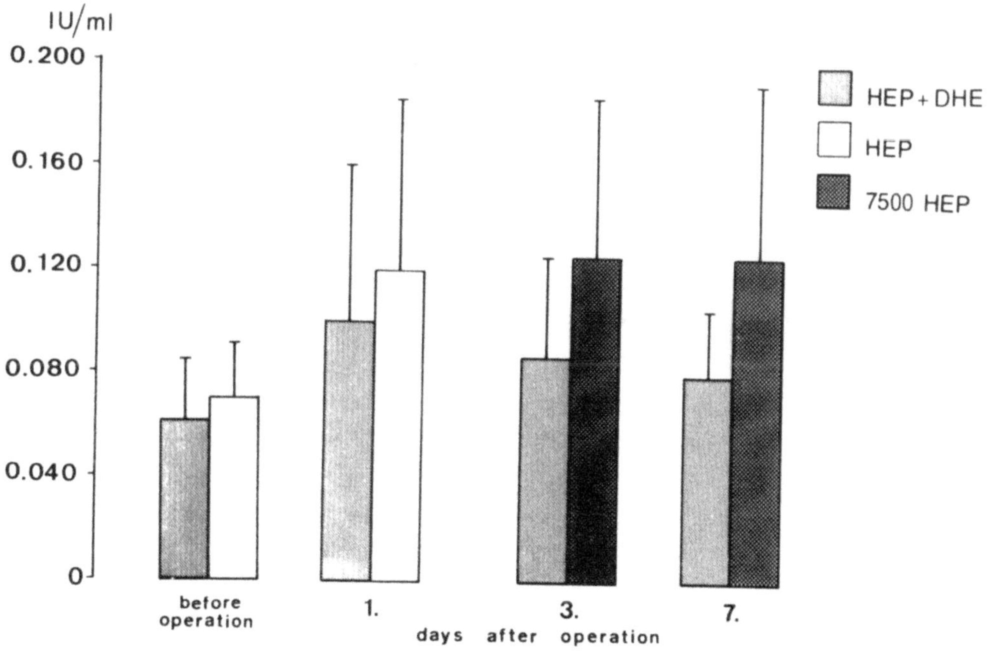

Fig. 2. Heparin activity (IU/ml plasma) 2 hours after injection of 5000 U sodium heparin without and with dihydroergotamine (DHE) and after increase to 7500 U heparin from the third postoperative day. Mean values ±1 standard deviation.

3. Antithrombin III activity and fibrinogen concentration (Fig. 3)
The parameters were determined because hyperfibrinogenaemia promotes stasis due to hyperviscosity and decreased AT III levels facilitate deep vein thrombosis. In addition, both coagulation parameters are reported to interfere with heparin administration (Zahavi et al. (11)). The fibrinogen concentration had significantly increased on the third ($p < 0.01$) postoperative day compared to the mean value before operation.

Concomitantly the AT III activity had significantly decreased on the first ($p < 0.001$) and third ($p < 0.001$) day after the hip operation in both groups (Fig. 3).

4. Range and coefficient of variation (Tab. 1)
After the subcutaneous injection of 5000 U sodium heparin, the coefficient of variation of the plasma heparin activity (Chromozym TH) determined before operation was 28 %. The PTT was more often prolonged than the thrombin time, which had the lowest coefficient of variation.

Heparin determinations by F Xa inhibition from the frozen plasma samples varied over such a wide range that they were of no practical use, particularly since no correlations to PTT, thrombin time and the heparin activity assayed by Chromozym TH were found (Tab. 1).

On the third day after operation and two hours after the injection of 7500 U sodium heparin, a plasma heparin activity (Chromozym TH) of 0.285 U/ml was detected in one female patient with a body weight of 59 kg. Thus the heparin activity ranged between a minimal value of 0.03 U/ml and a maximal value of 0.285 U/ml (Tab. 1).

The mean values of all the heparin sensitive tests, except the F Xa inhibition test, after the injection of 7500 U were significantly higher than the mean values before operation and after the administration of 5000 U heparin (p-values see Tab. 1). The coefficient of variation of the thrombin time had increased most. One might interpret this to mean that the heparin sensitivity threshold of the TT has been reached.

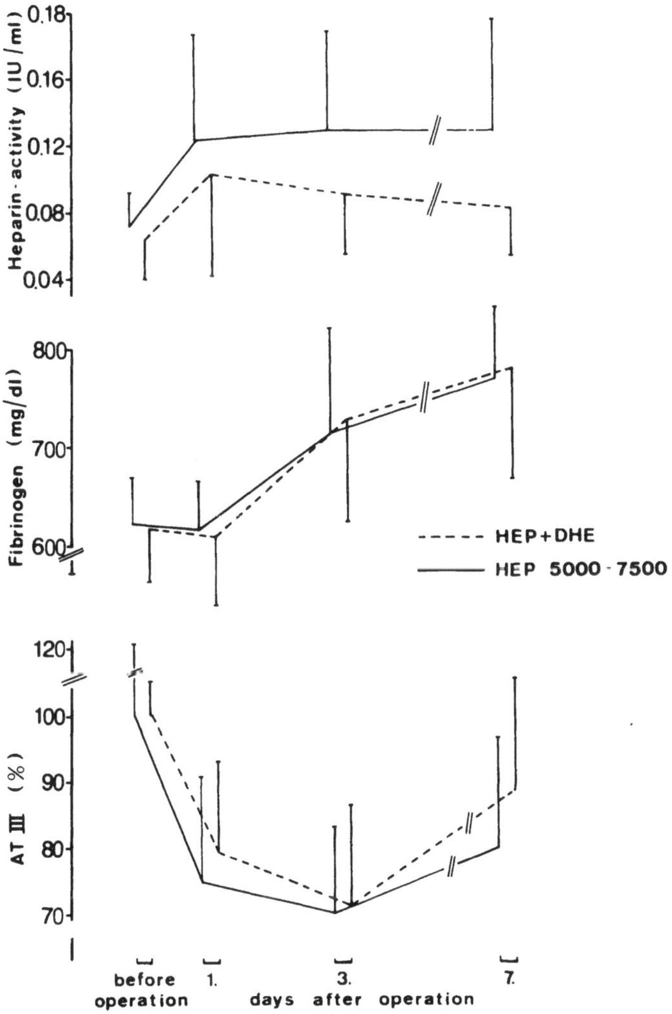

Fig. 3. Pre- and postoperative course of heparin activity (two hours after injection), of fibrinogen concentration and antithrombin III activity. Mean values ± 1 standatd deviation.

Table 1. Mean ($\bar{x}$), range (min. - max. value), and coefficient of variation (V C) of heparin activity, PTT, T T and F Xa inhibition. Comparison (p-values) 5000 U versus 7500 U sodium heparin s. c. 2 hours after injection. (n = 22)

		Heparin activity (IU/ml) (Chromozym TH)	P T T	T T	F Xa inhibition (IU/ml)
before OP (5000 U s.c.)	$\bar{x}$	0.067	32.6	17.8	0.166
	range	0.035-0.115	28-41	16-26	0-0.830
	V C %	28	12	2	141
3rd day after OP (7500 U s.c.)	$\bar{x}$	0.126	37.1	21.4	0.246
	range	0.030-0.285	25-58	14-53	0-0.890
	V C %	48	26	36	98
p-value		< 0.01	< 0.05	< 0.05	n.s.

Table 2. Correlation coefficients (r) and significance (p) between heparin activity, PTT, TT, AT III activity and concentration

		Heparin activity (Chromozym TH)	P T T	A T III (conc.)
P T T	r	0.641		0.390
	p	< 0.01		> 0.05
T T	r	0.739	0.680	0.260
	p	< 0.01	< 0.01	> 0.05
A T III	r	0.139	0.158	0.594
activity	p	> 0.05	> 0.05	< 0.01

(n = 22)

3rd postoperative day, 2 hours after 7500 U sodium heparin s.c.

5. Comparison of plasma heparin activity, partial thromboplastin time and thrombin time (Tab. 2)

The correlation coefficient between the tests was calculated by linear regression. The r-values obtained on the third day after operation and two hours after the first s.c. injection of 7500 U heparin were chosen for comparison of the different heparin sensitive tests as the highest heparin levels were found at that time. Elevated plasma heparin correlated best ($r = 0.739$) with prolongations of the thrombin time. Heparin acitivities and changes of the PTT as well as prolongations of the PTT and thrombin time also correlated significantly (Tab. 2).

Reduced AT III activities on the third postoperative day revealed no significant correlation to enhanced plasma heparin activity or prolonged PTT.

A good correlation was found between the AT III activity and the AT III concentration (Tab. 2).

Conclusions

1. After the subcutaneous injection of 5000 U heparin plus DHE, no higher heparin levels were found than after the administration of heparin alone in elderly patients operated upon for elective hip replacement.

2. The means of the plasma heparin levels revealed no significant differences between the determination two or eight hours after the injection of 5000 U heparin plus DHE. The plasma heparin decreased postoperatively compared to the value of the first day after the operation.

3. After the increase of the heparin dose to 7500 U heparin/8 h on the third postoperative day, the mean heparin activity of the first postoperative day was maintained and the + 1 standard deviation remained below 0.20 U/ml plasma.

Heparin levels depend on the individual response, but so far patients with a body weight under 60 kg had fairly consistently elevated heparin levels.

If the observed tendency can be confirmed, the heparin dosage should postoperatively not be increased in patients weighing less than 60 kg in order to avoid a bleeding tendency at the operation site.

4. After the s.c. injection of 5000 U heparin, the determination by Chromozym TH was more sensitive than the PTT or thrombin time in detecting heparin in the blood. The increase of the heparin dose to 7500 U/8 h on the third postoperative day, was registered by the clotting tests but less sensitively than by the amidolytic method with Chromozym TH.

5. Plasma heparin activity or changes of the PTT and elevated fibrinogen did not correlate to decreased AT III activity on the third postoperative day.

A conclusion cannot yet be drawn if changes of any of the laboratory tests are associated with increased bleeding episodes or thromboembolic complications.

References

1. Schöndorf, T. H., Hämostaseologie 1, 143-153 (1981)

2. Hedlund, P. O., Blombäck, M., Thrombos. Haemostas. 41, 337-345 (1979)

3. Gitel, S. N., Salvati, E. A., Wessler, S., Robinson, H. J., Worth, M. H., J. Bone and Joint Surg. 61-A, 653-656 (1979)

4. Schöndorf, T. H., Lasch, H. G. in: Lijnen, H. R., Collen, D., Verstraete, M. (eds.): Synthetic Substrates in clinical blood coagulation assays. The Hague, Boston, London, Devel. Haematol., Vol. 1, 51-57 (1980)

5. Tilsner, V., Müller, U., Reuter, H., Raedler, A., Thromb. Res. 17, 519-525 (1980)

6. Kruse-Blinkenberg, H. O., Bech-Jansen, P., Jensen, J., Schmidt, A., Gormsen, J., Haemostasis 6, 252-259 (1977)

7. Brozović, M., Stirling, Y., Abbosh, J., Brit. J. Haematol. 31, 461-466 (1975)

8. Zimmermann, R. E., Schwering, H., Wittrin, G., Hollenders, Th., Chirurg 52, 316-319 (1981)

9. Bounameaux, H., Marbet, G. A., Lämmle, B., Eichlisberger, R., Duckert, F., Am. J. Clin. Pathol. 74, 68-73 (1980)

10. Bruhn, H. D., Albert, J. P., Sachs, L., Timme, H., Dtsch. med. Wschr. 104, 1336-1339 (1979)

11. Zahavi, J., Smetana, S., Thrombos. Haemostas. 38, 107 (1977)

Discussion

Weber asked if *Schöndorf* had studied the time course of the different heparin preparations to see if they all have the maximum at the same time after administration.

Schöndorf said that he had found no differences between the one hour and two hour values. That means that the maximum is already reached after one hour. In previous studies with healthy volunteers, the activity was already lower after three hours.

Monitoring of Heparin During Extracorporal Circulation in Open Heart Surgery

Reiner Spaethe, Margot Naumann
Medical-scientific department
American Hospital Supply Deutschland GmbH
D-8000 München

Because of the high heparin dosages which have to be given to the patient, the control of heparin therapy during extracorporal circulation is very difficult. The heparin levels received can make it impossible to measure the final point of coagulation for thrombin time or APTT (1).

To perform heparin therapy with the minimal effective dosage, it is necessary to determine the minimum required level of plasma heparin (2, 3, 4).

After extracorporal circulation, a neutralization with protamine is usual necessary. A correct determination of the heparin level is only possible with synthetic substrates and is necessary in order to calculate the amount of protamine to be given and to control the effect of neutralization. It seemed to us to be desirable for the anesthesist, who carries out the heparinisation, to have the possibility of determining the heparin values immediately in the operating theatre. This possibility is given with the *Protopath proteolytic enzyme detection system*. With a fluorogenic synthetic substrate in a one-way cuvette and with the aid of a fluorometer, calibrated for this method, the determination of heparin is easily carried out (5).

The different methods will be discussed during this symposium (6). We had the possibility to measure the heparin and antithrombin level of 5 patients during an operation day at a cardio surgical clinic. We compared the results with coagulation tests. The therapy was effected in the usual manner of this hospital. An initial dosage of 300 IU/kg body weight (BW) was

Heparin · New Biochemical and Medical Aspects

given *in Bolus*. The continuous dosage was 150 IU/kg BW. The protamine total dosage conformed to the heparin dosage.

The operation of the first three patients mentioned above, lasted from less than one hour to a little more than one hour. Therefore, only one heparin dosage was injected. After the extracorporal circulation, the same unit of protamine was given. In all cases APTT (reference values: -45 sec.) was not measurable. The thrombin time (reference values: -21 sec.) only could be measured in two cases between 100 and 150 seconds, immediately after the injection. The thromboplastin time was rather long after heparin. During the administration of heparin antithrombin was diminished until three hours after the operation. Unfortunately, we could not closely observe the antithrombin in all cases. It surely would be intersting to measure such coursed for a longer period, because it can be assumed that after neutralization of heparin by protamine with very low antithrombin, there is a danger of thrombosis.

After establishing the extracorporal circulation the platelet values went down very quickly to half or less of the initial value. This reduction lasted even three hours after the operation, though with increasing tendency. The enzymatically measured heparin levels varied widely, though the heparin dosage was based on the body weight.

After administration of protamine, in all these cases, no heparin was measured, the APTT was more or less increased, the thrombin time could be measured in the normal range. If only the APTT had been available, in all these patients it could not have been clarified if a heparin effect still existed and therefore, during bleeding protamin would have been necessary again.

Case 1 (Fig. 1) shows such a typical course as discussed above. After injection of 12,000 IU heparin, the heparin level was 1.5 U/ml, before administration of protamine 0.7 U/ml. After protamine, up to three hours after the operation, no heparin could be measured; the APTT was slightly increased.

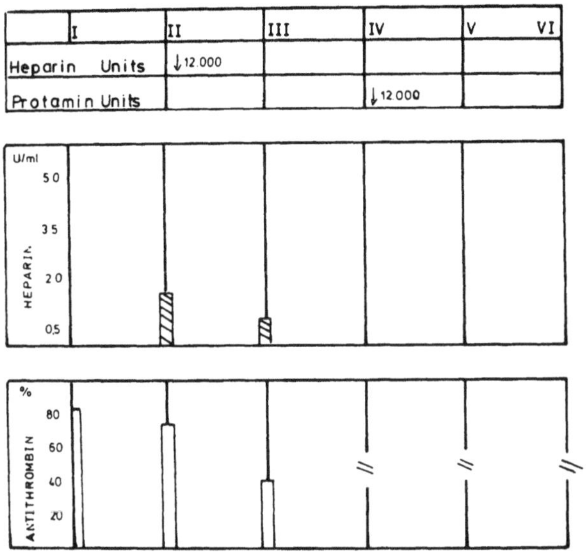

Patient J. Th.

Age 15 years

Weight 52 kg

Height 161 cm

Initial Dosage
Heparin 300 U/kg BW

Maintenance Dosage
Heparin 150 U/kg BW

Total Dosage Given
Heparin 12,000

Total Dosage Given
Protamine 12,000

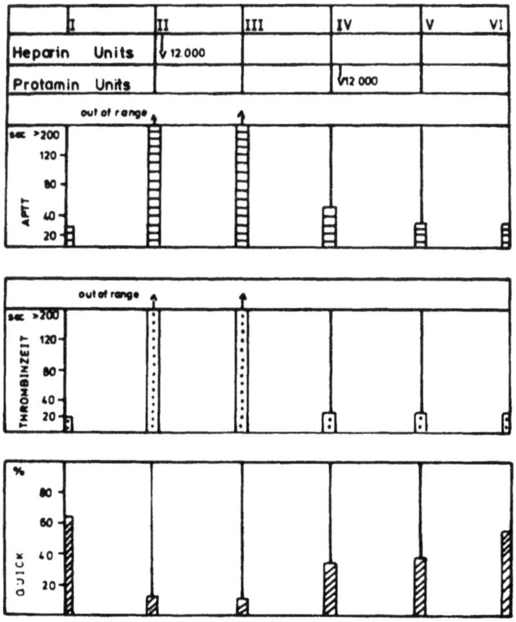

Fig. 1, 1 a

I. Preoperative

II. A few minutes after Heparin was given, beginning of the ECC*

III. End of ECC - before Protamine

IV. End of ECC - immediately after Protamine was given

V. One hour after ECC

VI. Three hours after ECC

*Extracorporal Circulation

≠ No measurement

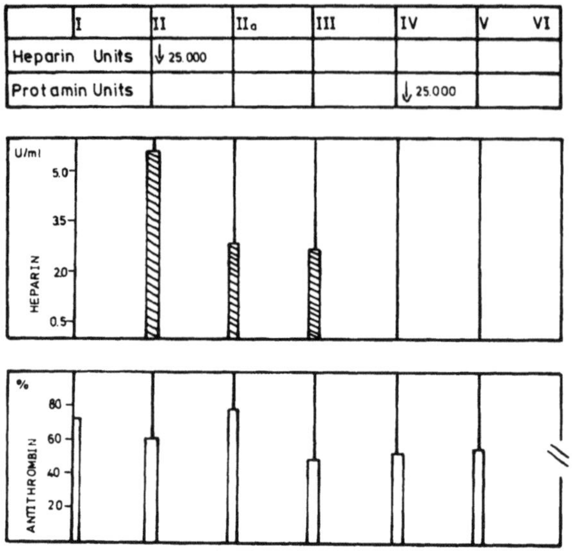

Patient E. H. G.

Age 41 years

Weight 94 kg

Height 185 cm

Initital Dosage
Heparin 300 U/kg BW

Maintenance Dosage
Heparin 150 U/kg BW

Total Dosage Given
Heparin 25,000

Total Dosage Given
Protamine 25,000

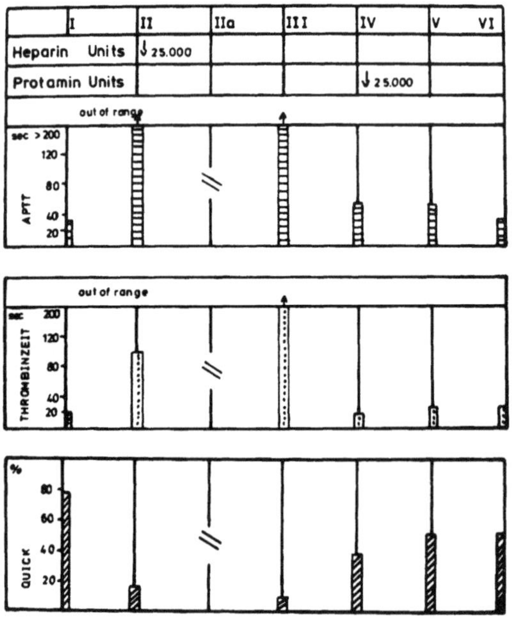

I. Preoperative

II. A few minutes after Heparin was given, beginning of the ECC*

IIA. One hour after start of ECC

III. End of ECC - before Protamine

IV. End of ECC- immediately after Protamine was given

V. One hour after ECC

VI. Three hours after ECC

*Extracorporal Circulation

⧣ No measurement

Fig. 2, 2 a

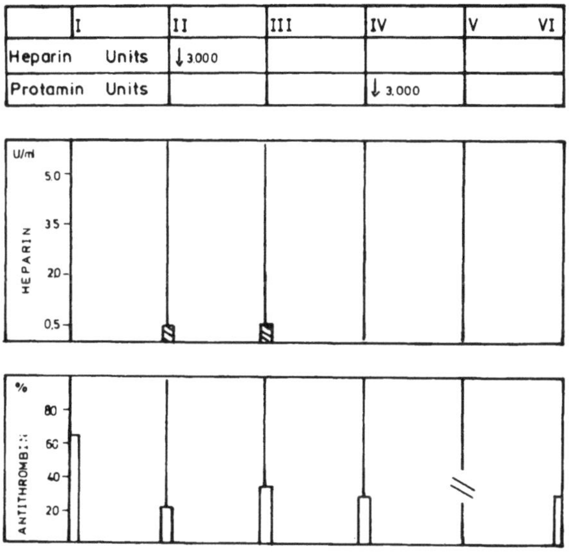

Patient B. N.

Age 6 months

Weight 6.2 kg

Height 65 cm

Initial Dosage
Heparin 300 U/kg BW

Maintenance Dosage
Heparin 150 U/kg BW

Total Dosage Given
Heparin 3,000

Total Dosage Given
Protamine 3,000

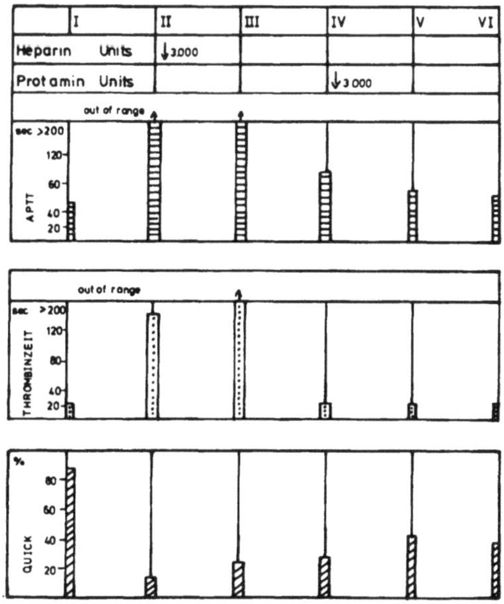

I. Preoperative

II. A few minutes after Heparin was given, beginning of the ECC*

III. End of ECC - before Protamine

IV. End of ECC - immediately after Protamine was given

V. One hour after ECC

VI. Three hours after ECC

*Extracorporal Circulation

╫ No measurement

Fig. 3, 3 a

In case 2 (Fig. 2) 25,000 IU heparin were injected which could be detected as 5.7 U/ml in the plasma. After one hour 2.2 U/ml were measured and before protamine 2.6 U/ml. After protamine no heparin could be determined any longer.

Case 3 (Fig. 3) is a six months old child, given 3,000 IU heparin. The extracorporal circulation was less than one hour. After heparin injection 0.45 U/ml were measured. Before protamine 0.48 U/ml were determined. After protamine the heparin level was zero, but the APTT with 91 seconds was still very long. Up to three hours this prolongation was still observable with 59 seconds APTT. Even during this period heparin could not be measured. All these heparin determinations were carried out by equalization of AT III in the test system, thus the lower AT III level of the patients did not have any influence on the measurement. Measuring the heparin zero value it was noticed that the remaining thrombin value, indicated was higher than 100 %.

Anido (7) could demonstrate that such a *minus heparin specimen* can be corrected to normal values by titration with heparin. In this way, a preceding administration of too much protamine was pointed out.

Fig. 4 shows the influence of protamine and heparin on APTT in a plasma sample. Not only protamine but also heparin have a prolonging influence on APTT. After further neutralization normal values can be obtained.

SPECIMEN CONCENTRATIONS

PROTAMIN	HEPARIN	APTT (NORMAL RANGE 21-29 SEC)
0,005 MG/ML	NONE	36,5 SEC
0,005 MG/ML	0,2 U/ML	35,2 SEC
0,005 MG/ML	0,4 U/ML	31,9 SEC
NONE	0,2 U/ML	58,9 SEC
NONE	0,4 U/ML	86,3 SEC

Fig. 4. (n. Anido)

Measuring a residual thrombin value of more than 100 % with the Protopath system it is shown that too much protamine was given. The prolonged APTT, demonstrated in case 3, can indicate not only various administrations of protamine but also residual heparin not neutralized. In such a case, enzymatically measuring a heparin level of zero, a titration with heparin can be carried out in vitro, which leads to a normalisation of the measured residual thrombin versus 100 % and to a normalisation of APTT. This finding can also be of importance for the patient, because in this way, a coagulation defect caused by protamine can be corrected in giving heparin.

In cases 4 and 5 heparin administration was necessary twice because of a longer operation time.

Case 4 (Fig. 5) shows heparin values of 1.0 U/ml one hour after starting the extracorporal circulation. After the second heparin dosage 1.7 U/ml heparin and before administration of protamine 2.2 U/ml were measured. After protamine administration 0.11 U/ml heparin were still detected. The slightly higher APTT value now reflects these findings. One hour after neutralization with protamine no heparin was measurable, after three hours 0.05 U/ml. Obviously heparin from other absorption sites was liberated.

In case 5 (Fig. 6) a heparin level of 1.0-1.5 U/ml was measured during the operation. The neutralization was satisfactory. There was no more heparin measured, but also no excessive protamine administration could be detected. The heparin rebound phenomenon was certainly more surprising in case 5 than in case 4. After three hours 0.1 U/ml heparin was evident, which could be seen also in a prolonged APTT and thrombin time.

The discussion of these cases clearly shows that the therapy with high heparin dosage could be improved by enzymatic measurements of the heparin level with synthetic substrates. The individual condition of the patients leads to variable reactions to the drug which cannot be demonstrated correctly by the coagulation test. The correct amount of protamine could only be estimated after an exact measurement of the heparin level.

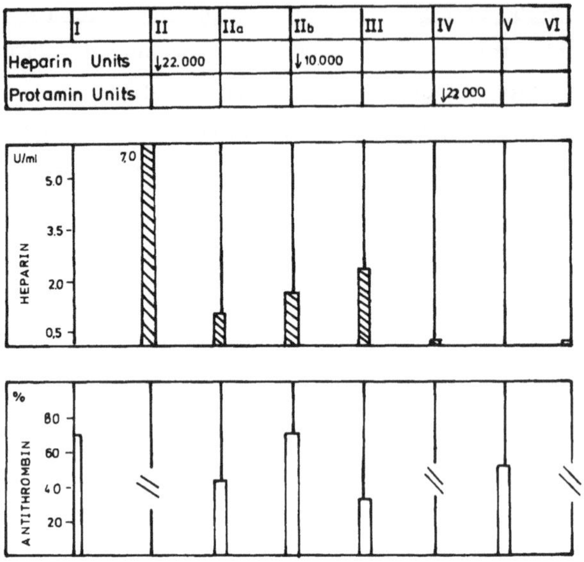

Blood transfusion

Patient R. S.

Age 43 years

Weight 75 kg

Height 170 cm

Initial Dosage
Heparin 300 U/kg BW

Maintenance Dosage
Heparin 150 U/kg BW

Total Dosage Given
Heparin 32,000

Total Dosage Given
Protamine 22,000

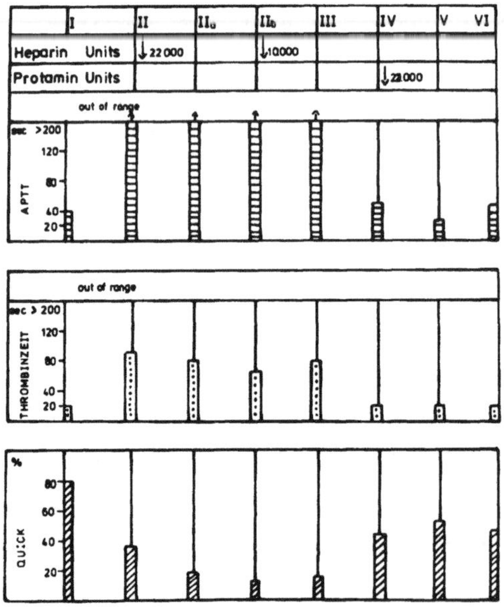

Blood transfusion

I. Preoperative

II. A few minutes after Heparin was given, beginning of the ECC*

IIA. One hour after start of ECC

IIB. After maintenance dosage Heparin

III. End of ECC- before Protamine

IV. End of ECC - immediately after Protamine was given

V. One hour after ECC

VI. Three hours after ECC

*Extracorporal Circulation

No measurement

Fig. 5, 5 a

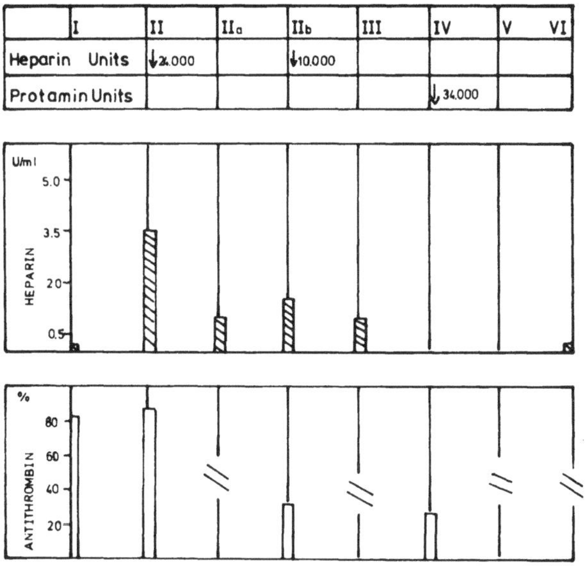

Patient K. B.

Age 41 years

Weight 80 kg

Height 174 cm

Initial Dosage
Heparin 300 U/kg BW

Maintenance Dosage
Heparin 150 U/kg BW

Total Dosage Given
Heparin 34,000

Total Dosage Given
Protamine 34,000

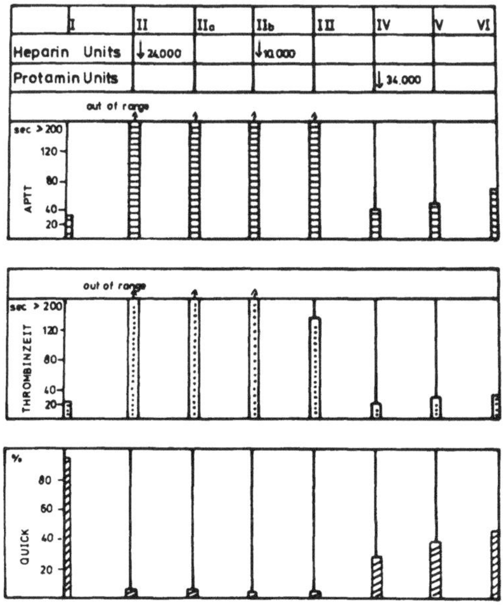

I. Preoperative

II. A few minutes after Heparin was given, beginning of the ECC*

IIB. After maintenance dosage Heparin

III. End of ECC - before Protamine

IV. End of ECC - immediately after Protamine was given

V. One hour after ECC

VI. Three hours after ECC

*Extracorporal Circulation

No measurement

Fig. 6, 6a

Because protamine disturbs coagulation, an exact dosage for very sick patients is necessary. Cobel-Geard et al. (8) could demonstrate that protamine not only disturbs the thrombin activity by affecting antithrombin but also has an inhibitory effect on thrombin itself. Therefore, the conversion of fibrinogen into fibrin id disturbed. This inhibition depends on the concentration and is also reversible.

Kitani et al. (9) showed that the protamine sulfate, added to the heparinized plasma, breaks the activated heparin-antithrombin-complex. The *liberated* antithrombin can again become an inhibitor of thrombin if heparin is given in excess to the now *neutralized* plasma. The same authors (10) found that in vivo-heparin-protamine-complexes are filtered in the lung. This finding surely can have clinical relevance.

Büller et al. (11) and Sturk et al. (12) demonstrated that AT III, plasminogen and α_2-antiplasmin decreased during major surgery (11) and during bypass operations (12). Coagulation factors II and X are decreased dependent on the operation. The authors found a decrease of 30 % in platelet count (corrected for hemodilution) and an increase of plasma β-thromboglobulin of 50 % after 15 min. bypass and 400 % after 60 min.

Our results show a similar behaviour. The changes in levels of coagulation factors, AT III and α_2-antiplasmin (12) may reflect an activation of coagulation and fibrinolysis during bypass. The lower levels of plasma factors and platelets during bypass are not only due to hemodilution.

The heparin therapy should be carried out with the minimal effective dosage to avoid bleedings and to enable neutralization of heparin by protamine in smallest amounts.

The measurement of the heparin level by means of synthetic substrates is the only possibility to watch the therapy exactly and to keep the side effects of the drug as low as possible.

References

1. Soloway, H. B.: Monitoring Heparin Therapy how and why. Diag. Med. Febr. 2 (1978).

2. Vogel, G. E.: Die Heparinisierung bei der Hämodialyse. Habilitationsschrift - Technische Universität München 1979.

3. Vogel, G. E., Kopp, K. F.: "Minimalintermittierende" Heparinisierung bei stark blutungsgefährdeten Hämodialysepatienten. Nieren und Hochdruckkrankheiten 6, 218 (1975).

4. Vogel, G. E., Buttermann, G., Komm, Ch., Kuhlencordt, M., Blümel, G., Oberdorfer, A.: Praktische Durchführung einer Heparinisierung im extracorporalen Kreislauf. In: Mikrozirkulation und Prostaglandinstoffwechsel. Verh. 25. Tg. der Dtsch. Arbeitsgemeinschaft f. Blutgerinnungsforschung, München 1981, Herausgeber: Blümel, G., Haas, S., F. K. Schattauer Verlag, Stuttgart.

5. Mitchell, G. A., Gargiulo, R. J., Huseby, R. M., Lawson, D. E., Pochron, S. P., Sehuanes, Z. A.: Assay for Plasma Heparin using a synthetic peptide substrate for thrombin: Introduction of the fluorophore amino-isophthalic acid, dimethylester. Thrombosis Research 13, 47 (1978).

6. Spaethe, R., Naumann, M., Strauß, J.: Measurement of Heparin with a fluorogenic synthetic substrate. In: I. Witt: Monitoring of heparin therapy. Walter de Gruyter Verlag, Berlin · New York (1982).

7. Anido, G.: Hematology Department Broward General Medical Center, Fort Lauderdale, Florida, USA. Personal information.

8. Cobel-Geard, R. J., Penner, J. A., Hassouna, H. J.: Introduction of protamine sulfat with thrombin. Department of Medicine, Michigan State University. In press.

9. Kitani, T., Nagarajan, S. C., Shamberge, J. N.: Effect of protamine on heparin-antithrombin III complexes. In vitro studies. Thrombosis Research 17, 367 (1980).

10. Kitani, T., Nagarajan, S. C., Shamberge, J. N.: Effect of protamine on heparin-antithrombin III complexes, in vivo studies. Thrombosis Research 17, 375 (1980).

11. Büller, H. R., Henny, Ch. P., Ritzen, M., Kahlé, L. H., Ten Cate, J. W.: Intraoperative antithrombin III, plasminogen and α_2-antiplasmin behaviour. Thrombos. Haemost. 46 (1), 300 (1981).

12. Sturk, A., Hoogendijk, E. M. G., Schaap, M. C. L., Sebel, P. S., Bovill, J. G., Beiboer, J. L., TenCate, Z. W.: Platelet and coagulation behaviour during open heart surgery. Thrombos. Haemostas. 46 (1), 318 (1981).

Discussion

Aronson asked concerning the meaning of the heparin-protamine complexes in the lung.

Spaethe said that work on this problem was published in 1980 by Kitani in Thrombosis Research (T. Kitani et al. Thromb. Res. 17, 367 and 375, 1980). He had performed studies using radioactive labelled protamine and found protamine-heparin complexes in the lung. Because it is possible that these complexes may have side effects in the lung it is advisable to give only the amount of protamine which is necessary for neutralization but not more.

Another interesting observation described in this paper is that protamine can break the antithrombin III-heparin complex. In addition, it is possible that protamine has an effect on coagulation by itself. Surgeons often observed bleedings after operations, although the heparin was neutralized by protamine.

Duckert was unable to understand why so many people have difficulties with the extracorporal circulation. The standard procedure used in his hospital since 1967 is as follows: the patient is heparinized and the machine also receives heparin. In operations lasting longer than two hours, the same dose of heparin is given again, and after the operation the heparin is neutralized by protamine chloride.

Two hours later the effectiveness of neutralization is monitored. For nearly 15 years there have been no problems with bleeding or other complications.

Thaler asked if platelet functions are disturbed. This may be a reason for bleeding. Some centers give platelet concentrates.

Spaethe and *Duckert* were of the opinion that the platelet count can drop during the operation and remain low for more than two hours but then raise again. So there is a rebound rather than a dysfunction of platelets.

Róka pointed out that the clearance of heparin differed greatly in the patients reported by Spaethe. He wanted to know if there was a correlation to the decrease in platelet count.

Spaethe agreed that this may be a possibility. No data on the correlation are available.

Spaethe replied to *Witt's* question if the reported values were corrected for haematocrit that the preoperative values were corrected to 50 % haematocrit and the values during operation to 38-40 %.

Róka wondered why the quick values had remained low, even when the APTT had returned to normal.

Spaethe had no explanation, but he pointed out that factor II and V were also in the range of 60 % after operation. The quick values were even lower.

Witt asked for the fibirnogen concentration since it might explain the low quick values.

Fibrinogen had not been measured.

Róka reported that he had made the same observations and found no alterations in fibrinogen levels but also did not know how to explain it.

Heene pointed out that these changes during extracorporal circulation are well known since about 20 years ago. The decrease in coagulation factors is caused by coagulation processes in the machine and also by the dilution effect.

Spaethe does not believe in the dilution effect because the haematocrit does not decrease much.

Heene urged that there is a complex situation involving disseminated intravascular coagulation, dilution, contact activation and alteration of the circulation in the liver.

Chromogenic and Fluorogenic Assays - A Challenge for Conventional Monitoring of Heparin Therapy?

German A. Marbet, François Duckert
Coagulation Laboratory
Kantonsspital Basel
CH-4031 Basel

Introduction

Several chromogenic and fluorogenic assays for the measurement of heparin concentrations have been developed in the last years. These are functional tests based on the acceleration of antithrombin III by heparin present in the plasma sample. Heparin treatment has traditionally been monitored by clotting tests such as activated partial thromboplastin time (APTT) and thrombin time (TT). Several arguments favour these conventional tests: They reflect the heparin induced impairment of the coagulation process, they require only simple equipment, can easily be performed as an emergency test and are very cheap. On the other hand, there are some problems:
differences between test systems, different heparin sensitivities of APTT reagents, limited precision and reproducibility. In a previous paper (1) our group has compared TT and APTT with an assay measuring the total concentration of functional heparin (2, 3). Although highly significant correlations were found between the three methods there were some disquieting discrepancies. We have, therefore, separately analysed our own results obtained during a multicentre study for the evaluation of new assays measuring the concentration of heparin bound to the patient's own antithrombin III, the so-called *active heparin*. In a small number of plasma samples heparin concentrations have been measured with a fluorogenic assay. Our analysis will focus on the relationship between clotting tests and heparin concentrations.

Heparin · New Biochemical and Medical Aspects

Materials and Methods

Blood sampling. Blood collection by venipuncture in Vacutainer tubes containing sodium citrate (3.8 %), blood to citrate ratio 9 : 1. Separation of platelet poor plasma by centrifugation at 3,000 x g for 5 min. Coagulation tests were performed immediately after centrifugation. Aliquots were frozen and stored at -20 °C for heparin concentration assays.

Clotting tests. Activated partial thromboplastin times were measured with PTT-Reagenz Boehringer Mannheim (method H) and ACTIN Dade (method I) according to the prescriptions of the manufacturers. Normal values for method H are 30-40 sec (given by the manufacturer) and 25-35 for method I (our laboratory).

Thrombin times using bovine thrombin solutions (F. Hoffmann-La Roche & Co., Ltd., Basle, Switzerland) with 3.33 and 33.3 NIU/ml (method K). With the lower concentration 0.1 ml thrombin solution added to 0.2 ml plasma at 37 °C gives thrombin clotting times (TT) of 14-18 sec with normal plasma. If TT exceeds 2 min in heparinized plasma a second assay is done with 0.1 ml of the 33.3 NIU/ml thrombin solution. The result is reported as e. g. > 2 min/8 sec, the first figure denoting the TT with the lower and the second the TT with the higher thrombin concentration.

TT using the Thrombin-Reagenz Boehringer Mannheim (method G) dissolved in 1 ml aqua bidest. TT with normal plasma 10-12 sec according to the manufacturer.

Heparin concentrations. The concentrations of *active heparin* are measured using the chromogenic thrombin substrate Tos-Gly-Pro-Arg-pNA according to the prescriptions of Beohringer Mannheim given to the participants of a multicentre study evaluating these methods in comparison with COATEST HEPARIN Kabi. Method A is the kinetic and method B the endpoint version of the same assay (4). In principle only heparin bound to the endogenous antithrombin III is measured.

COATEST HEPARIN Kabi (method C) is performed according to the prescriptions of the manufacturer (2, 3). It aims at measuring the *total* plasma heparin concentration in the presence of an excess of purified antithrombin III. The enzyme is bovine factor Xa and its substrate is Bz-Ile-Glu-Gly-Arg-pNA (S 2222).

PROTOPATH HEPARIN Dade (method D) measures plasma heparin concentrations in antithrombin III excess, human thrombin as the enzyme and the fluorogenic substrate D-phenylalanine-proline-arginine-5-amidoisophthalic acid dimethyl ester. The test is done with the PROTOPATH Fluorometer (Dade) according to the instructions of the manufacturer (5).

All heparin concentrations are expressed as USP-U/ml.

Patients. In-patients of the university clinics of the Kantonsspital Basle, treated with sodium heparinate (Liquemin Roche) for venous thromboembolism, arterial occlusions, myocardial infarction or for thrombosis prevention. Heparin administration either by continuous intravenous infusion or subcutaneously 2-3 times a day. A first group of 30 patients with daily doses of 15,000 to 45,000 USP-U was the plasma source for the assays included in the Boehringer Mannheim multicentre study comparing methods A, B, C, G and H. Only one plasma sample was obtained from 11 patients, two samples on subsequent days from 13 patients, 3 from 4 patients, 4 from 1 patient and 5 from 1 patient. The samples of the 19 patients with two and more blood collections were used for the mututal comparison of the within-patient changes of the different test values from day to day, totally 28 changes. 20 plasma samples of a second patient group including 6 with low dose heparin were involved in our comparison of methods C, D and I.

Statistical analysis. Assumption: The structural relationship between APTT (methods H and I) as well as thrombin time (method G) and heparin concentration (methods A, B, C, D) can be adequately approximated by a simple exponential function (6)

$$y = y_o e^{kx} \qquad (1)$$

where y = clotting time, x = heparin concentration, k = constant defining the steepness of the curve and y_o = basal value of y at x = 0. This relationship non only holds for in vitro experiments but also for test results ex vivo. After transformation of y into natural logarithms the data can easily be subjected to a linear regression analysis.

$$\ln = \ln y_o + kx \qquad (2)$$

Between the within-patient changes of x (Δx) and y a simple relationship follows from:

$$\ln y_1 = \ln y_o + kx_1$$
$$\ln y_2 = \ln y_o + kx_2$$
$$\ln y_1 - \ln y_2 = \Delta \ln y = kx_1 - kx_2 = k \cdot \Delta x$$
$$\Delta \ln y = \ln (y_1/y_2) = k \cdot \Delta x \qquad (3)$$

This is a straight line through 0 with slope k.

Simple relations between clotting results evolve:

$$\ln y^Q = \ln y_o^Q + k_Q x \text{ and } \ln y^R = \ln y_o^R + k_R \cdot x$$

where Y and R denote different clotting assays.

$$x = 1/k_Q \cdot \ln (y^Q/y_o^Q)$$
$$\ln y^R = \ln y_o^R + (k_R/k_Q) \cdot \ln (y^Q/y_o^Q)$$
$$\ln y^R = \underbrace{\ln y_o^R - (k_R/k_Q) \ln y_o^Q}_{a} + \underbrace{(k_R/k_Q)}_{b} \ln y^Q \qquad (4)$$

which is linear between $\ln y^R$ and $\ln y^Q$ with intercept a and slope b. A similar linear relationship for $\Delta \ln y^Q$ can be derived as follows:

$$\ln y_1^R = a + b \ln y_1^Q \text{ and } \ln y_2^R = a + b \ln y_2^Q$$
$$\Delta \ln y^R = \ln(y_1^R/y_2^R) = b \cdot (\ln y_1^Q - \ln y_2^Q) =$$
$$b \cdot \ln(y_1^Q/y_2^Q) = b \cdot \Delta \ln y^Q$$
$$\Delta \ln y^R = b \Delta \ln y^Q \qquad (5)$$

This is a straight line through 0 with slope $b = k_R/k_Q$.

Based on these derivations the data, after logarithmic transformations of clotting times, are subjected to linear regression analysis (7).

The following symbols will be used: a = intercept on ordinate, b = slope of regression line (regression coefficient), s_a = standard deviation of intercept a, s_b = standard deviation of slope b, r = correlation coefficient, $s^2_{y \cdot x}$ = residual mean square, $s_{y \cdot x} = \sqrt{s^2_{y \cdot x}}$ = standard error of estimate y, s_y^2 = total variance of y, $s^2_{y \cdot x}/s_y^2$ = fraction of total variance of y *not* explained by linear regression, $\bar{y}$ = arithmetic mean of the dependent variable y of linear regression, $\bar{x}$ = arithmetic mean sample, s = sample standard deviation, $s_{y \cdot x}/\bar{y}$ = ratio approximating the coefficient of variation of method y at $\bar{y}$, if $s_{y \cdot x}$ is only due to errors of method y, assuming absolute precision for method x.

Results and Comments

In Table 1 the thrombin time results of method K (Basle) in 56 patients have been classified as appropriate, strong and excessive according to our clinical experience based on several thousand patients getting heparin for venous and arterial thromboembolism, haemodialysis, charcoal perfusions and open heart surgery (13).

The concentrations of *active* (methods A and B) and of *total* (method C) heparin concordantly increase from *appropriate* to *excessive* as demonstrated by the statistically significant differences of the mean values ($p = < 0.05$, sometimes $p < 0.001$). On the other hand the ranges show a large overlap between the groups with clearly different anticoagulation intensity as measured by method K.

The results obtained in the patients on sequential controls might even look quite frightening to the clinical user of laboratory tests. As Tables 2 and 3 demonstrate there are several contradictory judgements by the different methods, one indicating increase and the other decrease of heparin concentration or heparin action respectively.

Table 1. Heparin concentrations (methods A, B, C) in 56 plasma samples and their anticoagulant effect assessed by thrombin time (method K)

Anticoagulation judged by thrombin time (K) as	A	B	C
appropriate, N = 37	0.240 ± 0.142	0.257 ± 0.120	0.200 ± 0.153
(>2'→2'/10")	(0.065 - 0.620)	(0.090 - 0.735)	(0.000 - 0.680)
strong, N = 12	0.337 ± 0.103	0.383 ± 0.145	0.416 ± 0.196
(>2'/11"->2'/25")	(0.165 - 0.480)	(0.145 - 0.665)	(0.070 - 0.720)
excessive, N = 7	0.637 ± 0.125	0.625 ± 0.139	0.651 ± 0.201
(>2'/>25")	(0.395 - 0.780)	(0.405 - 0.850)	(0.350 - 0.920)

Table 2. Contradictory results by different methods about the fluctuations of heparin concentrations (methods A, B, C) and of heparin anticoagulation (methods G, H, K). Discrepancy means increase by one method and decrease by the other. Comparison of 28 pairs of subsequent within patient observations

	heparin concentrations			coagulation tests		
Methods	A/B	A/C	B/C	G/H	G/K	H/K
Number of discrepancies	1	4	3	6	7	13

Table 3. Contradictory results between changes of heparin concentrations (A, B, C) and variations of clotting tests (G, H, K). Discrepancy means increase by one method and decrease by the other. Comparison of 28 pairs of subsequent within patient observations

Methods	A/G	A/H	A/K	B/G	B/H	B/K	C/G	C/H	C/K
Number of discrepancies	4	9	7	4	8	8	7	5	11

Table 4. Heparin concentrations (USP-U/ml) by three chromogenic substrate assays (A, B, C) and heparin effects on coagulation expressed by natural logarithms of thrombin time (G) and APTT (H). Distribution characteristics.

methods	N	$\bar{x}$	s	range
A	58	0.300	0.185	0.040 - 0.715
B	58	0.319	0.178	0.080 - 0.735
C	58	0.287	0.230	0.000 - 0.920
ln G	49	3.344 (28 sec)	0.846	2.303 - 5.165 (10 sec) (175 sec)
ln H	49	3.956 (52 sec)	0.299	3.434 - 4.644 (31 sec) (104 sec)

What method can reliably be used for the management of heparin therapy? The clinical experience of thirty years is probablv in favour of the clotting assays although their predictive value concerning rethrombosis or bleeding is at least not straightforward (8, 9. 10). Table 2 shows as much contradiction between the different clotting assays themselves as between clotting assays and heparin concentrations. As some of these discrepancies might quantitatively not be more than slight fluctuations we have used the linear regression model for a quantitative analysis of the deviations between methods. The assumption of an exponential relationship between heparin concentration and clotting times approximate the dose response relationship as known from studies in vitro (7) and ex vivo (6).

In the same patient with assays at various heparin concentrations this relationship is expected to be optimally realized with a fairly low ratio of $s_{y \cdot x}^2/s_y^2$ (see "statistical analysis") and a correlation coefficient near 1.0. r-values below 1.0 would be due to imprecisions of the method and to the fact that the *true* structural relationship would be a more complicated, actually unknown mathematical expression. For the individual case the k-value of $y = y_0e^{kx}$ not only reflects the heparin sensitivity of the test system but also the heparin tolerance of the patient. If the regression analysis is applied to our data from different patients the correlation coefficients, the $s_{y \cdot x}^2/s_y^2$-ratios and the variation of k-values will depend on differences of individual characteristics (clotting variables, heparin tolerance, antithrombin III, platelet factor 4 etc.) in addition to the precision of the methods.

Table 4 contains means, standard deviations and range of heparin concentrations and natural logarithms of clotting times of our first patient group. Clotting times exceeding 180 sec have been excluded from the statistical analysis.

The correlation coefficient (Table 5) between methods of similar type (clotting or chromogenic assay) are all highly significant ($p < 0.001$).

Table 5. Linear regression characteristics of the comparison of 3 heparin assays (A, B, C) by chromogenic substrates and of clotting assays (H, G) for heparin effects.

y/x	N	a	s_a	b	s_b	r	$s_{y \cdot x}$	$\frac{s_{y \cdot x}^2}{s_y^2}$	$\frac{s_{y \cdot x}}{\bar{y}}$
B/A	58	0.072	0.023	0.826	0.066	0.860	0.092	0.265	0.287
C/A	58	-0.015	0.034	1.009	0.096	0.813	0.135	0.344	0.470
C/B	58	-0.085	0.027	1.166	0.074	0.902	0.100	0.189	0.348
lnH/lnG	49	3.108	0.124	0.254	0.036	0.717	0.211	0.496	0.053

The comparisons in pair of heparin concentration do not deviate largely from the line of identity. The correlation coefficient between "total heparin" (method C) and "active heparin" (method A) is lowest but between method C and B("active heparin", endpoint assay) it is highest. Therefore, no clearcut difference between "active heparin" and "total heparin" can be demonstrated. If the standard error of estimate $s_{y \cdot x}$ were solely due to imprecisions of the measurement of y, the ratio $s_{y \cdot x}/\bar{y}$ would provide an approximation of the coefficient of variation for y-values near $\bar{y}$ (see "statistical analysis"). As the regression of y on x assumes absolute precision for x-values, which is not true for our data, the true coefficient of variation for y-values near $\bar{y}$ would certainly be smaller. Assuming coefficients of variation of 10 % for the precision of heparin assays and natural logarithms of coagulation times, $s_{y \cdot x}/\bar{y}$ ratios above 0.20 will probably indicate the presence of additional reasons for the deviation from the regression line.

The values for $s_{y \cdot x}$ and $s_{y \cdot s}/\bar{y}$ are fairly large (Table 5). They might only be explained by lack of precision if coefficients of variation of 20 % and more are assumed. All chromogenic assays had been performed in one series and the largest within series coefficient of variation of our laboratory in the multicentre study had been 13 %. Therefore, additional influences from individual plasma characteristics must be considered.

For the natural logarithms of clotting times (APTT versus TT) the $s_{y \cdot x}/\bar{y}$ ratio can be well explained by the precision of these methods (coefficients of variation of less than 10 % for logarithms corresponding to 10 % and more (7) for original clotting times).

The correlation coefficients between the log-transformed clotting times and the heparin concentrations are highly significant (Table 6) and confirm the previous assumptions. Thormbin times are related to heparin concentrations by a relatively steep exponential curve with k-values between 3-6 (corresponding to slope b in Table 6). The curves relating APTT to heparin concentration are less steep (k-values around 1.5, see slope b in Table 6).

Table 6. Linear regression characteristics of the comparison of heparin concentrations by methods A, B, C with the natural logarithms of thrombin time (G) and APTT (H)

y/x	N	a	s_a	b	s_b	r	$s_{y \cdot x}$	$\frac{s_{y \cdot x}^2}{s_y^2}$	$\frac{s_{y \cdot x}}{\bar{y}}$
lnG/A	49	2.372	0.209	4.005	0.764	0.608	0.679	0.644	0.203
lnG/B	49	1.823	0.170	5.715	0.583	0.819	0.490	0.336	0.147
lnG/C	49	2.505	0.131	3.809	0.471	0.763	0.555	0.427	0.166
lnH/A	58	3.576	0.065	1.668	0.184	0.770	0.258	0.414	0.063
lnH/B	58	3.545	0.074	1.653	0.203	0.736	0.273	0.467	0.067
lnH/C	57	3.675	0.054	1.408	0.151	0.782	0.250	0.395	0.062

Looking at the $s_{y \cdot x}/\bar{y}$ ratios of APTT vs heparin concentrations additional influences distorting the exponential relationship beside imprecisions of the measurement cannot be detected.

For the thrombin time the $s_{y \cdot x}/\bar{y}$ ratio is clearly higher but can probably still be explained by the combined lack of adequate precision of methods G and A, B, C respectively.

Table 7 and 8 give the preliminary results of our first experience with a fluorogenic heparin assay. Despite a large scatter of values around the line of identity between the fluorogenic and the chromogenic method for "total heparin" the correlation coefficient is statistically significant at $p < 0.001$. But the $s_{y \cdot x}/\bar{y}$ ratio is fairly high either pointing to unacceptably low precisions of the measurement or to different influences of the individual plasma samples on the two assay systems. The natural logarithms of APTT method I are exponentially related to both heparin concentration methods with k-value of about 2 (slope b), the corresponding correlation coefficients being statistically significant at less than $p = 0.01$. The $x_{y \cdot x}/\bar{y}$ ratio is fairly low.

The analysis of within patient changes according to equations (3) to (5) is given by Tables 9 to 11. The changes of heparin concentrations by the different methods correlate with high statistical significance and the regression line does not differ from the line of identity (Table 10). The measures of dispersions $s_{y \cdot x}$ and $s_{y \cdot x}^2/s_y^2$ are large. As vairation coefficients of differences tend to increase without limit the influence of precision can no longer be considered.

The relation between $\Delta \ln H$ and $\Delta \ln G$ approximates equation (5) quite well with a slope corresponding to the ratio of the k-values of APTT divided by those of thrombin time (see b values in Table 6).

Equation (3) describing the relation between changes of logarithms of clotting times and those of heparin concentrations is realized fairly well (Table 11). The intercept a barely deviates from 0, the slopes b tend to be somewhat lower than in Table 6, but considering the large values of s_b in both tables the concordance with the previous calculations is acceptable.

Table 7. Heparin concentrations by chromogenic substrate assay C and fluorogenic substrate assay D and heparin effects on coagulation expressed by the natural logarithm of APTT method I. Distribution characteristics.

methods	N	$\bar{x}$	s	range
C	20	0.148	0.134	0.000 - 0.740
D	20	0.199	0.149	0.000 - 0.650
lnI	19	3.732 (42 sec)	0.440	3.091 (22 sec) - 4.787 (120 sec)

Table 8. Linear regression characteristics of the comparison of heparin assays C and D and the natural logarithms of APTT method I

y/x	N	a	s_a	b	s_b	r	$s_{y \cdot x}$	$\frac{s_{y \cdot x}^2}{s_y^2}$	$\frac{s_{y \cdot x}}{\bar{y}}$
D/C	20	0.057	0.026	0.956	0.134	0.860	0.078	0.276	0.394
lnI/C	19	3.430	0.095	1.821	0.393	0.747	0.301	0.467	0.081
lnI/D	18	3.301	0.149	2.214	0.728	0.605	0.333	0.673	0.090

Table 9. Within patient-changes of heparin concentrations (methods A, B, C) and of natural logarithms of thrombin times (method G) and APTT (method H). Distribution characteristics.

methods	N	$\bar{x}$	s	range		
ΔA	28	-0.004	0.194	-0.530	-	+0.405
ΔB	28	-0.050	0.255	-0.445	-	+0.340
ΔC	28	-0.027	0.291	-0.730	-	+0.690
$\Delta \ln G$	20	-0.027	0.872	-2.079	-	+1.869
$\Delta \ln H$	28	-0.161	0.425	-0.979	-	+0.768

Table 10. Fluctuations within patients of heparin concentrations (methods A, B, C) and of clotting test values (methods G and H). Linear regression analysis for ΔA, ΔB, ΔC and for $\Delta \ln G$ and $\Delta \ln H$.

y/x	N	a	s_a	b	s_b	r	$s_{y \cdot x}$	$\frac{s_{y \cdot s}^2}{s_y^2}$
$\Delta B / \Delta A$	28	-0.045	0.029	1.059	0.151	0.808	0.153	0.360
$\Delta C / \Delta A$	28	-0.022	0.033	1.204	0.174	0.804	0.176	0.366
$\Delta C / \Delta B$	28	+0.015	0.039	0.840	0.152	0.735	0.201	0.477
$\Delta \ln H / \Delta \ln G$	28	-0.101	0.047	0.289	0.039	0.827	0.243	0.328

Table 11. Within-patient fluctuations of heparin concentrations (methods A, B, C) compared to the corresponding changes of thrombin time (method G) and APTT (method A). Linear regression analysis of $\Delta \ln G$ and $\Delta \ln H$ on A, B, C respectively.

y/x	N	a	s_a	b	s_b	r	$s_{y \cdot x}$	$\frac{s_{y \cdot x}^2}{s_y^2}$
$\Delta \ln G/\Delta A$	20	-0.022	0.134	4.600	0.972	0.745	0.598	0.470
$\Delta \ln G/\Delta B$	20	+0.051	0.168	2.169	0.756	0.560	0.742	0.724
$\Delta \ln G/\Delta C$	20	-0.027	0.146	3.243	0.813	0.685	0.652	0.560
$\Delta \ln H/\Delta A$	20	-0.154	0.061	1.454	0.319	0.666	0.323	0.578
$\Delta \ln H/\Delta B$	28	-0.102	0.059	1.170	0.233	0.702	0.308	0.527
$\Delta \ln H/\Delta C$	28	-0.141	0.071	0.737	0.247	0.505	0.374	0.774

Conclusions

Our data confirm the existence of the expected structural relationship between ex vivo clotting assays sensitive for heparin action and ex vivo heparin concentrations. This relationship can be approximated by the simple exponential function $y = y_o e^{kx}$ which is very suitable for statistical calculations. The large deviations from the regression line as expressed by $s_{y \cdot x}$ and $s_{y \cdot x}^2 / s_y^2$ are probably explained by shortcomings of precision. As demonstrated by the multicentre study (22 centres) coefficients of variation for the heparin assay (method A) in the range of 1.7 - 26.8 % (within series) and of 2.6 - 28.9 % (day to day) can be seen. A reduction of these values to 5 % might be obtained by modifications of the methods and by getting quite familiar with the assay. For APTT and thrombin time coefficients of variation below 10 % are difficult to realize (11). Further studies should be done with repeated plasma sampling in the same patients if possible at varying heparin concentrations. The precision of clotting tests and heparin assays should be checked repeatedly and kept at an optimum. Differences between assays for "total" or "active" heparin and between chromogenic and fluorogenic substrate assays might then be better visible than in the present analysis. Finally a suitable approach to the problems of the individual heparin tolerance might be found.

At present the future of heparin concentration assays is open. They cost much more than the familiar clotting tests. This will probably change by their more frequent use, especially if performed on autoanalyzers. But now priority must be given to trials which demonstrate their clinical relevance concerning bleeding and rethrombosis. The trial of Dr. Holm and coll. (12) is a promising start in this direction.

References

1. Bounameaux, H., Marbet, G. A., Lämmle, B., Eichlisberger, R., Duckert, F.: Am. J. Clin. Pathol. 74, 68-73 (1980).

2. Teien, A. N., Lie, M., Abildgaard, U.: Thromb Res. 8, 413-416 (1976).

3. Teien, A. N., Lie, M.:Thromb. Res. 10, 399-410 (1977).

4. Bartl, K., Dorsch, E., Lill, H., Ziegenhorn, J.: Thromb. Haemostas. (Stuttg.) 42, 1446-1451 (1979).

5. Mitchell, G. A., Gargiulo, R. J., Huseby, R. M., Lawson, D. E., Pochron, W. P., Sehuanes, J. A.: Thromb. Res. 13, 47-52 (1978).

6. Simon, T. L., Hyers, T. M., Gaston, J. P., Harker, L. A.: Brit. J. Haematol. 39, 111-120 (1978).

7. Poller, L., Thomson, J. M., Yee, K. F.: Brit. J. Haematol. 44, 161-165 (980).

8. Basu, D., Gallus, A., Hirsh, J., Cade, J.: N. Engl. J. Med. 287, 324-327 (1980).

9. Salzman, E. W., Deykin, D., Shapiro, R. M., Rosenberg, R.: N. Engl. J. Med. 292, 1046-1050 (1975).

10. Mant, M. J., O'Brien, B. D., Thang, K. L., Hammong, G. W., Birtwhistle, R. V., Grace, M. G.: Lancet 2, 1133-1135 (1977).

11. Denson, K. W. E., Bonnar, J.: Thrombos. Diathes. haemorrh. 30, 471-479 (1979).

12. Holm, H. A., Abildgaard, U., Laerum, F., Wolland, T.: Synthetic Substrates in Clinical Blood Coagulation Assays. Martinus Nijhoff Publishers, The Hague, Boston, London 1980.

13. Nyman, D., Duckert, F.: Thrombos. Diathes. haemorrh. (Stuttg.) 33, 221-225 (1975).

V. Concluding Discussion

The first topic proposed for the concluding discussion was the question if treatment with heparin will be carried out with different types of heparin, for instance, low or high molecular weight, in the future.

Róka pointed out that especially for subcutaneous administration higher plasma levels can be reached in a shorter time with low molecular weight heparin. In spite of this plasma heparin is maintained at levels as high and for about the same length of time as with unfractionated heparin.

The question is if low molecular weight heparin is an improvement in subcutaneous heparin therapy. In connection with this question one has to consider if the methods for monitoring heparin therapy have to be adapted. For instance, do the calibration curves have to be changed.

Bhargava commented that hitherto all pharmacopeia methods have depended on the anticoagulatory effect of heparin. There are certain problems connected with the standardisation of low molecular weight heparin by the current mandatory pharmacopeia methods which have to be solved before it can be put on the market.

The low molecular weight preparation has very low values of USP units. This could have clinical consequences for handling the dosage. Different methods are needed for the standardisation of low molecular weight heparin.

A further question is if the anti-Xa methods reveal the antithrombotic action of heparin. It has been proven in rabbits. The number of human patients hitherto investigated seems to be too small.

Heene commented that if unfractionated heparin is injected subcutaneously the body performs an in vivo chromatography to get the same product which is expensive to produce in vitro. He expressed the opinion that it is worthwhile to look at the biological activity of this fraction and its metabolic pathway from the subcutaneous tissue to the blood. What happens along this route seems to have a positive effect on the heparin.

Róka raised two important points which had been presented in the lectures of *Rosenberg* and *Kakkar*. *Rosenberg* had said that the best way to evaluate heparin therapy would be to look at the inhibition of clotting reactions in the body. One possibly would be to measure peptide A.

Kakkar had shown the measurement of peptide A in his study. The fibrinopeptide A levels were exactly the same for the low molecular weight heparin as for the unfractionated heparin. From this point of view there also seems to be little difference in these two preparations.

Concerning the proposal of *Witt* to discuss if the different heparin types differ in bleeding complications no experience was available.

Róka recommended that the procedure used in *Holm's* study should be applied to larger multicenter trials. *Holm's* study has shown that it is important to stick to a certain scheme of therapy, that means: the use of the same heparin, the same dosage, the same route of administration and the same clinical criteria. If this is achieved in a multicenter trial each laboratory could use its method of preference for measuring the heparin level or the influence of heparin on the blood coagulation system. In this way one could obtain a reliable comparison of the different methods and their correlations with the clinical outcome of the patients. This would help to find the best method for predicting overresponders and non-responders.

At present different therapeutic strategies are followed which makes it difficult to compare the monitoring methods.

In contrast *Dawes* proposed applying the various methods to the same samples. This would be less expensive than investigating enormous numbers of patients with the same therapy and assaying the heparin by different methods. One could perform this on few patients and compare the methods on the same samples.

Duckert agreed with *Dawes* that one should perform as many tests as possible but felt that the number of patients should not be reduced. It is the frequency of the occurrence of bleeding and rethrombosis which determines the numbers of patients needed for statistical significance. This cannot be achieved by increasing the number of tests.

Holm pointed out that it is cumbersome to carry out such a clinical study. The established dose regimen used, which is not very different from that used in other countries, was so good that there were actually very few complications. This confirmed the hypothesis that there should be some correlation between the tests and the clinical result of the treatment.

On the other hand one should have better methods for the evaluation of the fate of a thrombus: may be by applying radioactive methods for exact quantitation of the thrombus before and after treatment with heparin.

Witt pointed out that it would also be necessary to collect all data of a patient, especially concerning other drugs.

Holm replied that such data had been collected but not yet evaluated.

Róka expressed the opinion that it is still necessary to compare clotting methods and colorimetric methods as well as colorimetric methods with each other. One should find out which clotting method gives the best results and also which colorimetric method gives the same information or new information.

Spaethe asked if anyone present could specify the therapeutic range for heparin.

The opinion was expressed that a separate therapeutic range should be found for each method of heparin determination, similar to the way in which *Holm* has done for the Kabi-Coatest.

Heene explained that when one gives the standard dosage of 1500 USP as a bolus followed by 400 USP/kg body weight, as was used in Holm's study also, in 70 % of the patients a prolongation of APTT and TT is achieved.

The discussion stressed that it is not possible to give a standard amount of heparin to each patient. The dosage depends on the individual patient. Therefore exact monitoring of plasma heparin levels is necessary.

Holm stated that the primary aim of treating the patients is preventing pulmonary embolism. In his study the incidence of pulmonary embolism was rather low. The patients with pulmonary embolism were consistently low in their mean heparin activity in both the clotting tests and the Kabi-Coatest. With the Kabi-Coatest the mean heparin value was 0.23 USP/ml. That means that one should normally have a little higher lower limit, at least 0.3 USP/ml. Then there is a low risk of bleeding. Especially during the first 3 - 4 days of heparin treatment, the risk of pulmonary embolism is very low under this regimen. Major bleedings usually occur later. Therefore one should not be afraid to give more heparin during the first three days.

Bender asked if an upper limit exists where bleeding starts.

Holm replied that the sensitivity and specificity of the tests have to be further evaluated. The experience up to now has shown that regarding bleeding complications the sensitivity is good; all patients with bleedings had long clotting times and high heparin concentrations. The specificity seems, however, not to be so good, some patients with long clotting times and high heparin concentrations did not have bleedings.

Subject Index

Afibrinogenemia
- platelet aggregation 208, 209, 210

α_2-Antiplasmin 338

Antithrombin III 95, 96, 99, 100, 104, 105, 112, 113, 117, 120, 140, 141, 149, 150, 153, 154, 155, 163, 169, 175, 181, 195, 197, 264, 275, 278, 295, 296, 302, 316, 320, 321, 323, 324, 329, 330, 331, 332, 333, 334, 336, 337, 338, 343, 344, 345, 351
- abnormal 212, 214
- binding to heparin 5f., 51
- concentration during surgery 186, 187
- heparin activated 139, 140, 141
- influence of heparin 296
- interaction with factor IXa 15
- interaction with factor Xa 15, 21, 23
- interaction with plasmin 15
- interaction with thrombin 8f.

Antithrombin
- progressive 139, 140, 141

Aspirin 210, 217, 219
- platelet aggregation 210

Atherogenesis 261f.

Bleeding
- after heparin administration 193, 194, 198, 239f., 292, 296

Bleeding time 178, 182, 189, 191

Catecholamines 243

Chondroitinase 135

Chondroitin 4-sulphate 131, 132

Chondroitin 6-sulphate 131, 132

Chondroitin sulphate lyase 265

Chromogenic substrates 95, 96, 97, 119, 151, 289, 292

Chromozym TH 95, 96, 97, 315, 317, 318, 320, 322, 323, 325, 344

Deep vein thrombosis 175f., 289f., 315, 320

Dermatan sulphate 132

Dextran sulphate 132, 133, 134

Dihydroergotamine 315, 317, 318, 319, 321, 324

Endoglucuronidase 35

Endoglycosidase 265, 268, 269

Endothelium 154, 196, 217, 221, 261f., 277
- cell surface 53
- binding of heparin 52, 53
- binding of platelet factor 4 53, 54
- electronegative charge 51, 52, 129

Eosinophil basic protein 70

Factor IXa 176, 197
- inactivation by antithrombin III 15

Factor Xa 176, 195, 197
- inactivation by antithrombin III 15, 21, 23

Factor XIa 176, 197

Factor XIIa 176, 197

Factor VIII 208

Fatty acids 243

Fibrinogen 320, 321, 325

^{125}-Fibrinogen
- uptake test 197

Fibrinopeptide A 181, 186, 188, 189

Fluorescence spectroscopy 6, 7

Fluorogenic substrates 105, 106, 109, 329f.

Glucocorticoids 243

D-Glucuronic acid 16f., 36f., 177

D-Glucosamine
- N-acetylated 16f., 36f., 177
- N-sulphated 16f., 36f., 177
- O-sulphated 36f.

Glycosaminoglycans 263, 266
- platelet aggregation 210
- platelet release reaction 213

Growth factor
- platelet derived 261, 268

Growth hormone 243

Heparan sulphates 46, 51, 131, 132, 135, 217, 221
Heparin
- action 3f.
- administration 275
- allergic reactions 246, 247
- anti-thrombin activity 151, 152, 154, 155
- anti-Xa activity 149f., 163, 164, 165, 166, 168, 169, 175, 177, 182, 183, 184, 185, 195, 196, 211, 277, 279
- anticoagulant activity 49
- antithrombotic activity 49, 197, 277
- binding site for antithrombin III 16f., 37, 40, 46
- binding to antithrombin III 5f.
- binding to thrombin 7f., 51
- binding with platelet factor 4 49, 50, 54
- biological activities 47
- biosynthesis 35f.
- bleeding complications 193, 194, 197, 277, 292, 296
- cardiac arrythmias 243
- catabolism 55f.
- clearance 55f., 77, 78, 79
- desulphation 55, 56, 70, 72, 75, 80
- determination 89f.
- - activated partial thromboplastin time (APTT) assay 90, 93, 104, 149f., 162f., 175, 177, 181f., 195, 211, 227f., 289, 292f., 302f., 315, 320, 322f., 329f., 343, 344, 350, 353f., 360, 361,
- - anti-factor Xa-assay 91, 93, 117f., 149f., 162f., 175, 177, 182f., 195, 196, 229f., 301, 316, 320, 322
- - anti-thrombin assay 92, 93 95f., 139
- - calcium thrombin time 292, 293 294, 295
- - chromogenic assays 91, 92, 93, 95, 96, 103, 117, 139, 162, 181, 227, 235, 236, 289, 292f., 301, 305, 310, 316, 317, 318, 320, 329f., 343, 344, 350f.
- - clotting assays 89, 90, 91, 93, 152, 197, 344, 348f., 361
- - competitive binding assay 129f.
- - fluorogenic assays 103f., 343, 355, 356
- - fluorogenic substrate 345
- - influence of antithrombin III 95, 96, 99, 100, 104, 105, 112, 113, 117, 120, 139
- - low dose activity 139
- - photometric assays 91, 92, 93 95, 96, 103, 117, 139
- - protamine neutralization test 227
- - thrombin time 90, 93, 104, 149, 152, 163, 167, 227, 231, 235, 292f., 301f., 316, 320, 322, 324, 325, 329f., 343, 344, 347, 348, 350, 353, 354, 355, 358, 360, 361
- - titration assays 91, 93
- - whole blood clotting time 227, 231, 232, 233, 235
- different species 5f., 46, 210, 227, 229, 230
- drug interactions 250f.
- effect on clotting time 197
- effect on biological systems 240
- endogenous 46, 51, 52, 57, 279
- endothelium 50, 51, 53, 79
- extracorporal circulation 329f.
- function 3f.
- half life 55, 79, 278
- high activity 5f., 297, 228
- high affinity 229, 230, 231, 236
- high molecular weight 162, 163, 169, 196
- history 89
- inhalation 275
- international standard 181
- internalisation 71, 72, 73, 80
- intravenous administration 176, 177, 182, 183, 195, 196, 227, 231, 233, 276, 291, 302, 303, 304, 311
- levels during surgery 186, 187, 191, 192, 321f.
- levels in plasma 293, 294, 295, 301f., 317f., 331f., 348f.
- low dose 176f.
- low molecular weight 5f., 149f., 162, 163, 167, 168, 169, 175f., 211, 213
- - affinity to antithrombin 150, 153, 154, 155
- neutralization 71, 72, 73f., 80
- osteoporosis 244
- pharmacokinetics 77, 79
- physiological 46, 51, 52, 57
- platelet count 216, 217, 248, 249

- platelet factor 4 49, 50, 53, 54
- proteoglykan 46
- proteoglykan biosynthesis 35, 37
- radioactive labeled 55
- rebound 69, 73f., 78, 79, 80
- recycling 10
- relatively inactive 5f.
- reticuloendothelial system 50, 55, 79
- semisynthetic 279
- side effects 239f.
- structure 35f., 45
- subcutaneous administration 176, 177, 178, 182, 184, 185, 191, 195, 196, 275, 302, 303, 304, 305, 308, 309, 311, 315, 317, 320, 322, 323
- substances bound 48
- sulphated 135
- thrombocytopenia 207, 215
- thyroseine in serum 251
- transaminases in serum 245
- ultra low dose 276
- unfractionated 149f., 162, 163, 175f., 211, 213, 228, 261, 262
- - affinity to antithrombin 150, 153, 154, 155
- uptake 69, 70, 71, 72, 73
- urinary 56
- vitamin D metabolites 245

^{125}J-heparin 129, 130, 133
Heparin-antithrombin complex 5f., 278
Heparin Cofactor 301, 302, 304, 305, 307, 308, 309
Heparin-thrombin complex 5f.
Heparinoids 52
Heparitinase 20, 56, 265, 268
Heparitins 46, 51, 52, 53, 57
Histones 70f.
Hyaluronidase 265

L-Iduronic acid 16f., 36f.

Keratan sulphate 132

Lipases 154
Lipoproteins
- binding to heparin 51, 53
Lipoprotein lipase 154, 181, 186, 188, 189, 196, 243, 279
- binding to heparin 51, 53, 54
Low density lipoproteins 195
Lysosomes 268

Macrophages 261, 268, 275
Mast cells 70f., 268

Pentosan sulphate 132
Phlebography 290, 291, 293, 294
Plasma prekallikrein 181, 186, 188, 196, 197
Plasmin 77
- inactivation by antithrombin III 15
Plasminogen 338
Platelet
- count 330, 338
- release reactions 212, 213, 215, 216
Platelet aggregation
- ADP induced 208
- adrenalin induced 208, 209
- collagen induced 208, 209, 210
- ristocetin induced 208
Platelet factor 4 49, 51, 53, 54, 112, 118, 119, 141, 151, 181, 189, 190, 196, 214,f., 268, 269, 301f.
Platelet functions 181, 189, 190, 196, 207, 215, 216, 249, 250, 263
- influence of heparin 207, 215, 216
Polycythemia vera 214
Poly-DL-lysine 70, 71, 72, 75
Poly-L-ornithine 70, 72, 75
Polysaccharids
- sulphated 130f.
Prekallikrein 181, 186, 188, 196, 197
Pronase 131, 133, 135, 136
Prostaglandins 196, 248
Protamine 70f., 129, 130, 131, 133, 329f.
- fractionation 75
- substitutes 75
Protaminolysis 74, 76, 77
Pulmonary embolism 176, 193, 198, 295, 296

Quick time
- influence of heparin 331, 332, 333, 336, 337

S-2222 151, 164, 165, 166, 181, 289, 292, 316, 345
S-2238 164, 181
Serotonin 208, 209, 210, 212, 213, 214, 217, 218, 220, 250

Smooth muscle cells 261f.
Sulphated polysaccharids 130f.

Thrombelastography
- influence of heparin 227, 228, 229, 236
Thrombin 96, 97, 107, 108, 112, 139, 140, 197
- binding to heparin 7f.
- inactivation 10, 21
- inhibition by heparin 197
- interaction with antithrombin III 8f.
Thrombin inhibitors 279
Thrombocytopenia 207, 214, 215, 218, 248, 249, 250
Thrombocytosis 218
β-Thromboglobulin 181, 189, 190, 197, 214, 215, 216, 218, 219, 220, 338
Thromboxan 181, 189, 190, 196

Uroheparin 56

Vessel wall 262, 263, 264, 268

White-clot-syndrome 248f.

Bei Fragen zur Produktsicherheit wenden Sie sich bitte an:
If you have any questions regarding product safety,
please contact:

Walter de Gruyter GmbH
Genthiner Straße 13
10785 Berlin
productsafety@degruyterbrill.com